PREGNANCY AND SKIN

PREGNANCY AND SKIN

Editors

Sanjeev Gupta MD DNB MNAMS
Professor and Head
Department of Dermatology
Maharishi Markandeshwar Institute of Medical Sciences and Research, MMDU
Mullana, Ambala, Haryana, India

Rohit Batra MD
Consultant Dermatologist
Sir Ganga Ram Hospital
Director, Dermaworld
Skin and Hair Clinics
New Delhi, India

Mudita Gupta MD
Associate Professor
Department of Dermatology
Indira Gandhi Medical College and Hospital
Shimla, Himachal Pradesh, India

Forewords

Dedee F Murrell
Jenny Murase

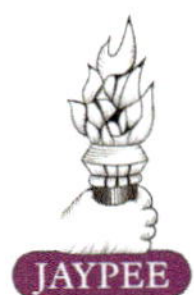

JAYPEE BROTHERS MEDICAL PUBLISHERS
The Health Sciences Publisher
New Delhi | London

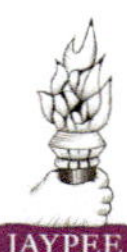

JAYPEE Jaypee Brothers Medical Publishers (P) Ltd

Headquarters
EMCA House
23/23-B, Ansari Road, Daryaganj
New Delhi 110 002, India
Landline: +91-11-23272143, +91-11-23272703
+91-11-23282021, +91-11-23245672
E-mail: jaypee@jaypeebrothers.com

Corporate Office
4838/24, Ansari Road, Daryaganj
New Delhi 110 002, India
Phone: +91-11-43574357
Fax: +91-11-43574314
E-mail: jaypee@jaypeebrothers.com

Overseas Office
J.P. Medical Ltd.
83, Victoria Street, London
SW1H 0HW (UK)
Phone: +44-20 3170 8910
E-mail: info@jpmedpub.com

EU GPSR Authorised Representative
Logos Europe, 9 rue Nicolas Poussin
17000, La Rochelle, France
Phone: +33 (0) 6 67 93 73 78
E-mail: Contact@logoseurope.eu

Website: www.jaypeebrothers.com
Website: www.jaypeedigital.com

Inquiries for bulk sales may be solicited at: jaypee@jaypeebrothers.com

Pregnancy and Skin / ***Sanjeev Gupta, Rohit Batra, Mudita Gupta***

First Edition: 2025
Reprint: **2026**

ISBN: 978-93-6616-500-4

Printed in India

Dedicated to

Our teachers

For nurturing our academic aspirations

Our parents

For their belongings, affection and unconditional love

Our family

Dr Sunita Gupta, Namya, and Gauri (Sanjeev Gupta)
Dr Neha Batra, Aarna (Rohit Batra)
Dr Jagdish Gupta, Dr Archit and Dr Archita (Mudita Gupta)
For their understanding, forbearance, unconditional support and love

Our patients

For providing us an opportunity to serve them and learn from them.

Contributors

Aakansha Sharma MD
Senior Resident
Department of Dermatology and Venereology
Shri Lal Bahadur Shastri Government Medical College
Mandi, Himachal Pradesh, India

Aditi Dabhra MD
Resident
Department of Dermatology
Maharishi Markandeshwar Institute of Medical Sciences and Research, MMDU
Mullana, Ambala, Haryana, India

Aishwarya Dua MD DNB
Consultant Dermatologist
Department of Dermatology
Dermaworld Skin and Hair Clinics
New Delhi, India

Ankur Talwar MD
Professor and Head
Department of Dermatology
Hind Institute of Medical Sciences
Lucknow, Uttar Pradesh, India

Anushka Lohariwala MBBS MD
Resident
Department of Dermatology
Maharishi Markandeshwar Institute of Medical Sciences and Research, MMDU
Mullana, Ambala, Haryana, India

Biju Vasudevan MD
Professor and Head
Department of Dermatology
Command Hospital, Chandimandir
Panchkula, Haryana, India

Chaithra Shenoy MD
Senior Consultant and Lead Aesthetic Dermatologist
Department of Dermatology
CUTIS Academy of Cutaneous Sciences
Bengaluru, Karnataka, India

Chander Grover MD DNB
Director and Professor
Department of Dermatology and STD
University College of Medical Sciences and GTB Hospital
New Delhi, India

Debdeep Mitra MD DNB
Professor
Department of Dermatology
Command Hospital Air Force
Bengaluru, Karnataka, India

Deepika Pandhi MD
Director and Professor
Department of Dermatology and STD
University College of Medical Sciences and GTB Hospital
New Delhi, India

Devyani Sapra MD
Assistant Professor
Department of Dermatology
Base Hospital Delhi Cantt and Army College of Medical Sciences
New Delhi, India

Diksha Goyal MD
Senior Resident
Department of Dermatology
All India Institute of Medical Sciences
Rishikesh, Uttarakhand, India

Divya Seshadri MD MRCP(UK)
Assistant Professor
Department of Dermatology
Sri Madhusudan Sai Institute of Medical Sciences and Research
Chikkaballapur, Karnataka, India

Gagandeep Kaur MD
Senior Resident
Department of Dermatology
Dayanand Medical College and Hospital
Ludhiana, Punjab, India

Hima Gopinath MD
Associate Professor
Department of Dermatology
All India Institute of Medical Sciences
Mangalagiri, Andhra Pradesh, India

Himani Chawla MD
Senior Resident
Department of Dermatology
All India Institute of Medical Sciences
Bathinda, Punjab, India

Kshama Talwar MD
Associate Professor
Department of Dermatology
Hind Institute of Medical Sciences
Lucknow, Uttar Pradesh, India

Kuldeep Verma MD DNB
Assistant Professor
Department of Skin and Venereal Disease
Government Medical College
Orai, Uttar Pradesh, India

Madura C MD
Medical Director
Consultant Dermatologist
Dematosurgeon and Hair Transplant Surgeon
Department of Dermatology
CUTIS Academy of Cutaneous Sciences
Bengaluru, Karnataka, India

Meghna Khatri MD
Senior Resident
Department of Dermatology
Maharishi Markandeshwar Institute of Medical Sciences and Research, MMDU
Mullana, Ambala, Haryana, India

Mudita Gupta MD
Associate Professor
Department of Dermatology
Indira Gandhi Medical College and Hospital
Shimla, Himachal Pradesh, India

Namya Gupta MBBS(Student)
Kalpana Chawla Government Medical College
Karnal, Haryana, India

Neha Rani MD
Senior Resident
Department of Dermatology
Maharishi Markandeshwar Institute of Medical Sciences and Research, MMDU
Mullana, Ambala, Haryana, India

Nidhi Jindal MD
Consultant Dermatologist
Department of Dermatology
Tata Medical Centre
Kolkata, West Bengal, India

Nikita Gupta MBBS MD
Resident
Department of Dermatology
Maharishi Markandeshwar Institute of Medical Sciences and Research, MMDU
Mullana, Ambala, Haryana, India

Parul Verma MD
Additional Professor
Department of Dermatology, Venereology and Leprosy
King George's Medical University
Lucknow, Uttar Pradesh, India

Payal Chauhan MD DNB MNAMS
Associate Professor
Department of Dermatology,
Venereology and Leprosy
All India Institute of Medical Science
Jammu, Jammu and Kashmir, India

Pratika Goyal MD
Senior Resident
Department of Dermatology
Christian Medical College and Hospital
Ludhiana, Punjab, India

Preeti Garg BDS MDS
Associate Professor
Department of Oral Medicine and
Radiology
Maharishi Markandeshwar College of
Dental Sciences and Research, MMDU
Mullana, Ambala, Haryana, India

Reena Kumari Sharma MD
Assistant Professor
Department of Dermatology,
Venereology and Leprosy
Dr Rajendra Prasad Government
Medical College
Kangra, Himachal Pradesh, India

Resham Vasani MD DNB
Consultant Dermatologist
Department of Dermatology
Bhojani Clinic, Matunga
BJ Wadia Children's Hospital and
Nowrosjee Wadia Maternity Hospital
Mumbai, Maharashtra, India

Ritu Rani MD DNB
Senior Resident
Department of Dermatology,
Venereology and Leprosy
Dr Rajendra Prasad Government
Medical College
Kangra, Himachal Pradesh, India

Rohit Batra MD
Consultant Dermatologist
Sir Ganga Ram Hospital
Director, Dermaworld
Skin and Hair Clinics
New Delhi, India

Sandhya Chauhan MD
Assistant Professor
Department of Dermatology,
Venereology and Leprosy
Indira Gandhi Medical College and
Hospital
Shimla, Himachal Pradesh, India

Sanjeev Gupta MD DNB MNAMS
Professor and Head
Department of Dermatology
Maharishi Markandeshwar Institute of
Medical Sciences and Research, MMDU
Mullana, Ambala, Haryana, India

Santanu Banerjee MD DNB
Professor
Department of Dermatology,
Venereology and Leprosy
Armed Force Medical College
Maharashtra University of Health
Sciences
Pune, Maharashtra, India

Senkadhir Vendhan MD
Specialist
Department of Dermatology
Dr Babasaheb Ambedkar Memorial
Hospital (Central Railway)
Mumbai, Maharashtra, India

Shivani Bansal MD DNB MNAMS
Assistant Professor
Department of Dermatology
All India Institute of Medical Sciences
Bathinda, Punjab, India

Shivani Gauba Wadhwa MD
Specialist Dermatologist
Department of Dermatology
Fakeeh University Hospital
Dubai, UAE

Sivasankari M MD
Graded Specialist
Department of Dermatology
Military Hospital
Jodhpur, Rajasthan, India

Sucheta Pathania MD
Consultant Dermatologist
Department of Dermatology
Medical College Mandi
Ner Chowk, Himachal Pradesh, India

Sunil Kumar Gupta MD
Professor and Head
Department of Dermatology and Venereology
All India Institute of Medical Sciences
Gorakhpur, Uttar Pradesh, India

Sunita Gupta MD
Professor and Head
Department of Medicine
Maharishi Markandeshwar Institute of Medical Sciences and Research, MMDU
Mullana, Ambala, Haryana, India

Swati Suman MD
Senior Resident
Department of Dermatology and Venereology
All India Institute of Medical Sciences
Gorakhpur, Uttar Pradesh, India

Varsha R Koti MD DNB
Fellow Dermatosurgery
Department of Dermatology
CUTIS Academy of Cutaneous Sciences
Bengaluru, Karnataka, India

Vikram K Mahajan MD
Professor
Department of Dermatology, Venereology and Leprosy
Dr Radhakrishnan Government Medical College
Hamirpur, Himachal Pradesh, India

Vishal Pal MD
Senior Resident
Department of Dermatology and STD
University College of Medical Sciences and GTB Hospital
New Delhi, India

Vishal Sharma MD DNB
Professor and Head
Department of Dermatology
Maharishi Markandeshwar University
Solan, Himachal Pradesh, India

About the Editors

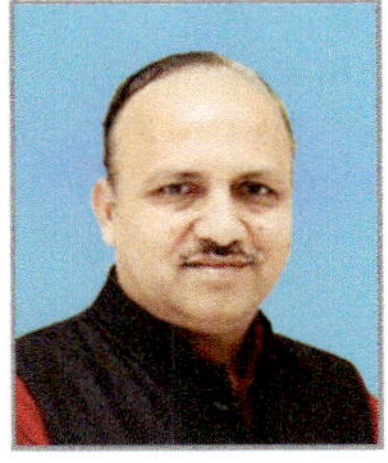

Sanjeev Gupta MD DNB MNAMS is working as Professor and Head, Department of Dermatology, Maharishi Markandeshwar Institute of Medical Sciences and Research, MMDU, Mullana, Ambala, Haryana, India. He is a member of most of national and international academic societies. He has around 170 publications, 8 books and 17 book chapters to his credit. He has invented many dermatosurgical techniques and instruments to simplify the procedures and reduce the cost. Twenty-six of such inventions have been published one of the most prestigious journal of dermatology—Journal of the American Academy of Dermatology USA. He was awarded with "Making a Difference" award by the American Academy of Dermatology, USA. He is the first Indian to be honoured with this prestigious award. He has served his professional association [Indian Association of Dermatologists, Venereologists, and Leprologists (IADVL)] as Executive Committee Member at the state level as Treasurer, Secretary, Vice President, and President and also at the National level as Joint Secretary and Vice President IADVL. He was honoured with the LN Sinha Award by IADVL in 2013 and the ACSI Innovation Award 2021 by the Association of Cutaneous Surgeons of India (ACSI). He is the recipient of the Dr BM Ambady Oration awarded at DERMACON 2025 Jaipur.

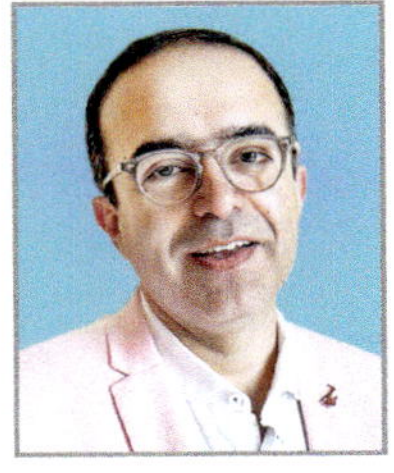

Rohit Batra MD is a renowned Dermatologist associated with Sir Ganga Ram Hospital, New Delhi, and is head and founder of Dermaworld Skin and Hair Clinics, New Delhi, India. His areas of interest are clinical dermatology, pediatric dermatology, aesthetic dermatology, trichology and multidisciplinary care of dermatological disorders. He has numerous presentations at various national and international conferences. He has been the architect of two of the most famous Dermatology Conclaves—Dermatology and Allied Specialities Summit (DAAS) and Acne India Summit. A prominent organizational guru and a mentor for many, he has held various roles and posts in the IADVL including the President of the IADVL – Delhi State Branch.

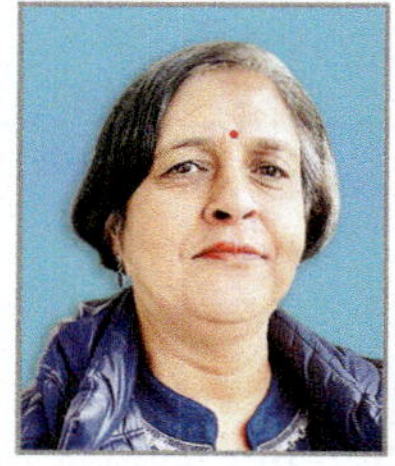

Mudita Gupta MD is currently working as Associate Professor, Dermatology Department, Indira Gandhi Medical College and Hospital, Shimla, Himachal Pradesh, India. In addition to clinical practice, she is a prolific researcher in the field of dermatology, with innumerable publications in various prestigious journals. She has given many presentations at various national conferences and authored chapters in dermatology textbooks. Her research mainly focuses on sexually transmitted diseases, immunobullous disorder, and pediatric dermatology and has contributed to advancements in both diagnostic techniques and treatment strategies.

Foreword

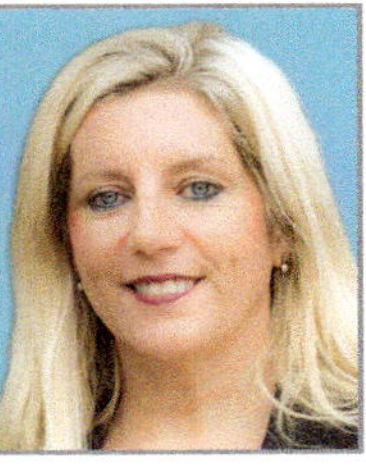

The understanding of skin disorders in pregnancy was a "black box" when I was training as a dermatology resident in the USA in the 1990s. This book, edited by leading dermatology educators from excellent institutions, Drs Sanjeev Gupta, Rohit Batra, and Mudita Gupta, is a pleasure to read. It is coauthored by some three dozen experts and rising stars in dermatology from all over India. With a population of a billion, high fertility rate, and a relatively young population, dermatologists in India are particularly experienced in pregnancy dermatoses.

The book contains simple explanations of complex topics, such as how the immune system is downregulated during pregnancy in order for the fetus not to be attacked since at least 50% of its DNA is foreign to the mother. It was interesting to learn that the Th2 pathways are induced, while Th1 pathways are reduced, explaining why we see more atopic eruptions of pregnancy in those who are predisposed and the development of pemphigoid of pregnancy in some patients, and why psoriasis, a Th1-mediated disease, typically improves during pregnancy. The imbalance between these two arms of the immune system as well as vascular pathways are what exacerbates systemic lupus erythematosus (SLE) during pregnancy.

The chapter on novel biomarkers in SLE was particularly interesting as to why it is important to keep women with SLE on certain safer immunosuppressants/ modulators at conception and during pregnancy, such as hydroxychloroquine. The early recognition of lupus erythematosus in girls and young women is important because there is such a high rate of maternal mortality in those with pulmonary arterial hypertension and it is advised for them to avoid pregnancy altogether. This made me wonder if some of these diagnoses warranted grounds for approval of surrogate deliveries of IVF-generated embryos in couples where the future mother has SLE, just as occurs if she has a congenitally defective uterus. Mothers with scleroderma are also at a high risk of maternal complications.

The chapters on blistering diseases in pregnancy were of particular interest to me, given my professional interest in these disorders. Each medication that may be needed is clearly covered in useful tables with the doses, including IVIG. As delivery approaches, the reduction in estrogen and proinflammatory state of increasing Th1 and Th17 cytokines increases the chance of urticarial eruptions, illustrated with easy-to-remember diagrams.

This book has excellent sections on infections during pregnancy, particularly those that are sexually transmitted, including syphilis, gonorrhea, HPV, chlamydia, and herpes. Since leprosy and fungal infections are still prevalent in India, these chapters are very comprehensive. This book also covered the management of intrahepatic cholestasis very well, including the doses of ursodeoxycholic acid and, if needed, rifampicin.

In addition, this book covers general skin, nail, and hair care during pregnancy, all the medicines' ratings during pregnancy and lactation, and what is appropriate for surgery during pregnancy.

In conclusion, if you see many pregnant women in your practice, whether you are a dermatologist or not, this book is a must-have.

Dedee F Murrell MA BMBCh FAAD MD FRCP FACD DSc
Professor and Chair
Department of Dermatology
St George Hospital, University of NSW
Sydney, Australia

Foreword

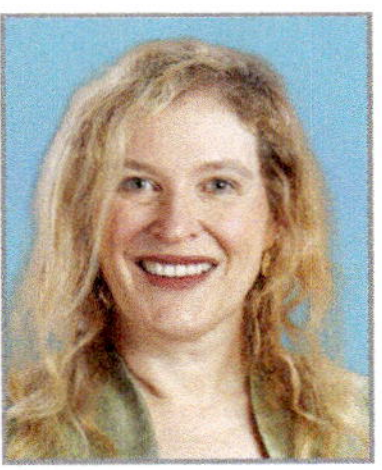

As our field of dermatology continues to evolve, it is increasingly important to recognize how the care of special populations, such as pregnant women, differs from that of the general dermatologic patient. Pregnancy represents a unique and vulnerable state, requiring special considerations when diagnosing and treating dermatologic conditions. During this time of profound physical transformation, the skin, hair, and nails undergo noticeable changes. Additionally, the hormonal and immunological shifts associated with pregnancy can significantly influence dermatologic conditions, potentially giving rise to new concerns or exacerbating pre-existing disease.

The content of this book encompasses a broad spectrum of concerns—addressing common skin conditions like acne, rosacea, psoriasis, and melasma, as well as more rare and complex disorders like immunobullous diseases and connective tissue disorders. From the physiological skin changes that naturally occur in pregnancy to autoimmune conditions such as systemic lupus erythematosus, scleroderma, and vasculitis, each chapter provides expert knowledge on the impact of pregnancy on both maternal and fetal health. It also explores the significant role of lifestyle factors in maintaining skin health, emphasizing the importance of a proper skincare routine during pregnancy.

Special attention is given to infections that can complicate pregnancy, including sexually transmitted diseases like syphilis, herpes, gonorrhea, and HIV, as well as other infections such as leprosy, fungal infections, and varicella. Each topic is discussed with the depth and care necessary to equip healthcare professionals and expectant mothers with the information needed for safe and effective management.

As pregnancy can also bring about changes in the hair and nails, the book covers conditions such as hair disorders and nail disorders that may arise during this period. It also explores the impact of genodermatoses, providing insight into how genetic skin conditions interact with pregnancy. Additionally, the book addresses key topics like orodental care, dermatologic surgery, aesthetic treatments, and the safe use of dermatological drugs, both topical and systemic, during pregnancy and lactation. This holistic approach ensures that healthcare providers can make well-informed decisions in guiding their patients through the various aspects of skin health and treatment during pregnancy.

Written by leading experts in our field, this book offers a well-rounded and accessible guide for clinicians caring for the dermatologic expectant mother. By combining scientific rigor with practical advice, it empowers healthcare professionals to offer tailored care for pregnant women, ensuring optimal outcomes for both mother and child.

As we move toward more specialized and evidence-based approaches in maternal health, this book stands as an indispensable resource, offering the latest knowledge on how to safely navigate the complexities of pregnancy-related dermatological concerns. I commend Editors Sanjeev Gupta, Rohit Batra, and Mudita Gupta for developing this text which provides such a comprehensive and in-depth exploration of the intricate relationship between pregnancy and skin health, offering an extensive range of topics that provide valuable insights into managing common and complex dermatological conditions.

Jenny Murase MD
Associate Clinical Professor
University of California, San Francisco
Department of Dermatology
Director of Medical Consultative Dermatology and Patch Testing
Palo Alto Foundation Medical Group
Co-Editor in Chief Emeritus
International Journal of Women's Dermatology

Preface

"Beneath the glow, the skin may bear,
Marks of change and signs of care.
From itch to flare, or spots that stay,
Each tells of life in its own way."

Pregnancy is a remarkable journey, a time of profound transformation that touches every aspect of life. Among the many changes that occur during these months, the skin—our largest and most visible organ—undergoes unique and often surprising transformations. It stretches, adapts, and responds to the myriad hormonal, physical, and environmental shifts that accompany pregnancy. These changes, while natural, can bring both wonder and challenges.

This book has been designed as a comprehensive resource to bridge the fields of dermatology and obstetrics. It delves into the spectrum of dermatological conditions seen in pregnancy, from physiological changes to pregnancy-specific dermatoses. We aim to simplify the understanding of pathogenesis, clinical manifestations, and treatment strategies for dermatological conditions linked to pregnancy, offering evidence-based methods for their diagnosis and care. The text also addresses the overlap between systemic diseases with dermatological manifestations and pregnancy, equipping practitioners with the tools to navigate complex cases.

In addition to disease management, this book highlights the critical issue of safety. Expectant mothers often have heightened concerns about the medications, skincare, and cosmetic products they use. This text offers a detailed evaluation of commonly prescribed drugs, topical treatments, and everyday products, including cosmetics, sunscreens, moisturizers, and cleansers. Clinicians will find clear guidance on the safety profiles of various treatments, empowering them to make informed decisions that prioritize both maternal and fetal well-being.

By combining clinical insights, practical strategies, and the latest research, this book aims to serve as a valuable companion for healthcare providers involved in the care of pregnant patients. Whether you are a dermatologist addressing skin concerns, a gynecologist guiding holistic prenatal care, or a clinician seeking clarity on treatment safety, this text provides the knowledge needed to navigate the unique intersection of pregnancy and skin health.

We hope this book enhances your practice and helps you support your patients with confidence, empathy, and expertise during one of the most transformative times in their lives.

We extend our heartfelt gratitude to all the contributors who made this monumental task possible within the given timeframe. Collaborating with an outstanding team of editorial board members and authors has been both an enriching and a rewarding experience. We also wish to express our sincere appreciation to our patients and postgraduate students (especially Dr Aditi Dabhra), whose insights and encouragement inspired us to undertake and complete this challenging endeavor. We also thank our family who supported, motivated and tolerated for stealing their precious family time.

The work would not have been possible without the support of Shri Jitendar P Vij (Group Chairman), Mr Ankit Vij (Managing Director), and Somoshri Banerji (Development Editor).

Happy reading!
Jai Maa Bharti!

Sanjeev Gupta
Rohit Batra
Mudita Gupta

Contents

CHAPTER 1

Immuno-Hormonal Changes in Pregnancy

Mudita Gupta, Sanjeev Gupta

"Everything grows rounder and wider and weirder, and I sit here in the middle of it all and wonder who in the world you will turn out to be."

—Carie Fisher

INTRODUCTION

Pregnancy is the remarkable journey where a fertilized egg develops into a fetus within the mother's womb, typically lasting around 9 months. To nurture this semiforeign fetus, the mother's body undergoes a carefully orchestrated series of adjustments. These adaptations go beyond anatomical changes, like the growing uterus and breasts. They encompass metabolic shifts (for nutrient supply), immunological tuning (to prevent fetal rejection while safeguarding the mother from infections), and hormonal changes (play a maestro role, coordinating these physiological changes throughout pregnancy). All these physiological changes work in harmony to optimize the health of both the mother and the developing fetus.

HORMONAL CHANGES

Hormones play a critical role in maintaining pregnancy and supporting fetal development. The interplay of various hormones ensures the proper physiological changes needed for a successful pregnancy. Endocrine environment of pregnancy is complex and involves various hormones. Human chorionic gonadotropin (hCG), progesterone, estrogen, prolactin, relaxin, oxytocin, and human placental lactogen (hPL) are the principal hormones of pregnancy.

Human Chorionic Gonadotropin

Human chorionic gonadotropin is a crucial hormone in pregnancy. Initially produced by the blastocyst, hCG can be detected in the mother's blood and urine as early as 11 days after conception. Following implantation, hCG levels double approximately every 2–3 days, peaking by the end of the first trimester (25.7×10^3 to 288×10^3 mIU/mL). In the second trimester, these levels begin to decline and then plateau (1.2×10^3 to 55×10^3 mIU/mL), further decreasing in the third trimester to levels lower than those at the beginning of the first trimester (1.1×10^3 to 56×10^3 mIU/mL) **(Fig. 1)**.

Human chorionic gonadotropin has following major actions:
- hCG supports pregnancy by maintaining the corpus luteum for progesterone production, stimulating fetal gonadal development, modulating the maternal immune response to protect the fetus, and promoting the development of placental blood supply.
- Additionally, hCG is linked to increased hormonal activity, contributing to breast tissue growth, morning sickness, stimulation of thyroid function, and production of inhibin and relaxin by the corpus luteum.

- Pregnancy heralds a cascade of hormonal transformations crucial for maternal health and fetal development
- hCG, progesterone, estrogen, hPL, prolactin, and relaxin are the six hormones which help in maintenance of pregnancy, maternal adaptations, and fetal growth
- hCG is the first hormone to appear and opens the door to rest of the hormonal changes in pregnancy
- hCG is responsible for supporting early pregnancy
- Morning sickness seen in early pregnancy is due to hCG

Progesterone

Progesterone is initially secreted by corpus luteum but after 10 weeks this function is taken over by placenta. Throughout gestation, progesterone levels exhibit a steady rise. In the first trimester, they elevate from approximately

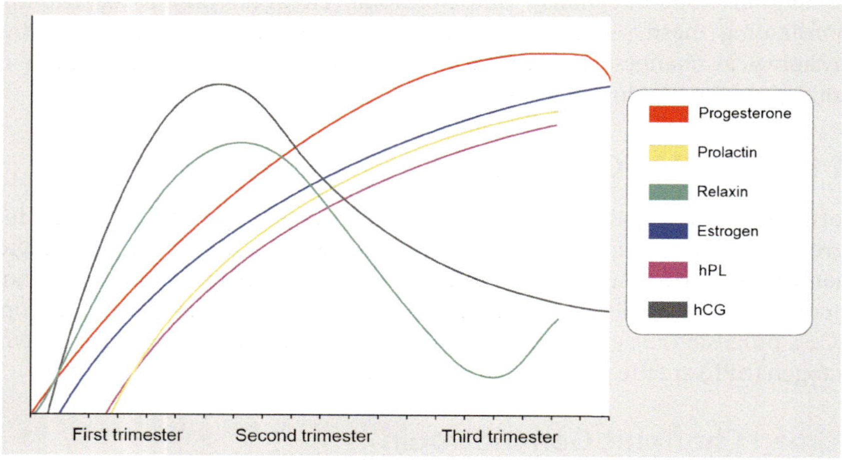

FIG. 1: Trends of various hormones in pregnancy.

(hCG: human chorionic gonadotropin; hPL: human placental lactogen)

10–30 ng/mL to 30–50 ng/mL. This upward trend continues into the second trimester, reaching levels between 25 and 90 ng/mL, and culminates in the third trimester with a peak range of 100–200 ng/mL. Progesterone level falls immediately before delivery.

Progesterone plays a pivotal role in pregnancy by maintaining the uterine lining, mitigating uterine contractions to prevent premature labor, fostering placental development, modulating the maternal immune response to safeguard the fetus, and facilitating breast tissue growth in readiness for lactation. Progesterone is responsible for various physiological dermatological changes in pregnancy, e.g., hyperpigentation, acne, and vascular changes (e.g., pregnancy glow, spider vein, and varicose vein). It also prolongs anaphase of hair.

- Progesterone secretion by placenta starts at 10 weeks and levels rise exponentially till immediately before term
- Progesterone is crucial for maintaining the uterine lining, preventing premature labor, and supporting breast tissue growth for lactation
- Progesterone is responsible for various dermatological physiological changes

Estrogen

Estrogen production in pregnancy originates initially from the maternal ovaries, adrenal glands, and peripheral conversion. In the early stages of the first trimester, estrogen levels hover around 0.3 ng/mL until reaching a gestational age of 6–10 weeks, after which they steadily escalate until term (2–30 ng/mL).

- Estrogen levels keep on increasing till term
- Estrogen exists in three different forms-of which estradiol is the most potent
- Estrogen promotes uterine and placental growth, regulates other hormones, and supports cardiovascular and breast tissue development

Three distinct types of estrogen operate during pregnancy: (1) Estradiol (E2), (2) estrone (E1), and (3) estriol (E3). Among these, estradiol stands out as the most potent. Estrone exists in relatively minor quantities and can also derive from androstenedione in adipose tissue. Estriol emerges as the predominant estrogen during pregnancy, synthesized by the placenta from 16-hydroxydehydroepiandrosterone sulfate (16-OH DHEAS).

Throughout pregnancy, estrogen assumes a myriad of roles, including the promotion of uterine and placental growth, regulation of other hormonal processes, initiation of breast tissue development for lactation, and facilitation of cardiovascular adaptations to meet the augmented demands imposed by fetal growth.

Prolactin

Increased estradiol leads to increase of prolactin which is ten times nonpregnant state. Prolactin levels rise progressively throughout pregnancy, starting in the first trimester and peaking in the third trimester, preparing the body for lactation. Prolactin's primary functions include stimulating mammary gland development and milk production, regulating immune tolerance to the fetus, influencing maternal behavior, and adjusting metabolic processes to support breastfeeding. Prolactin rises from a nonpregnant level of 25 μg/mL to up to 400 μg/L.

- *Prolactin* prepares the body for lactation by stimulating mammary gland development and milk production, and it also regulates immune tolerance to the fetus
- *hPL* and other hormones such as *relaxin* and *oxytocin* modulate maternal metabolism, support cardiovascular adaptations, and prepare the body for labor and breastfeeding
- In addition to anatomical, metabolic, hematological alterations, these hormones modify maternal immunological response

Human Placental Lactogen

Human placental lactogen is also known as human chorionic somatomammotropin (hCS). hPL production starts at fifth week of gestation and continuously rises thereafter. This hormone is responsible for increasing insulin-like growth factor-1 and modulates maternal metabolism to ensure a steady supply of glucose and amino acids to the fetus. It increases lipolysis leading to more availability of free fatty acids for mother hormone responsible for insulin resistance in the mother, increasing blood glucose levels for fetal use. It also has growth hormone-like and prolactin-like action.

Relaxin

Relaxin is a hormone crucial for human pregnancy, with levels peaking in the first trimester and follows hCG pattern, stabilizing at elevated levels throughout gestation. It facilitates cervical ripening, reduces uterine contractility to prevent premature labor, and promotes the growth and remodeling of reproductive tissues. Additionally, relaxin aids cardiovascular adaptations by increasing cardiac output and renal function, and it helps loosen joints and ligaments in the pelvis for childbirth. Its role in angiogenesis supports increased blood flow, essential for both maternal and fetal health.

Androgens

There is a progressive increase of testosterone with pregnancy. This increased androgen is produced by maternal ovary, both maternal and fetal adrenal glands. Pregnant female is protected from signs of hyperandrogenism because of increased production of sex hormone-binding globulin (SHBG) by liver during pregnancy leading to no change in free testosterone in first and second trimester **(Fig. 2)**. But there may be increased testosterone in third trimester. Testosterone in the presence of aromatase produced by placenta gets converted into estrogen thus preventing hyperandrogenism during pregnancy.

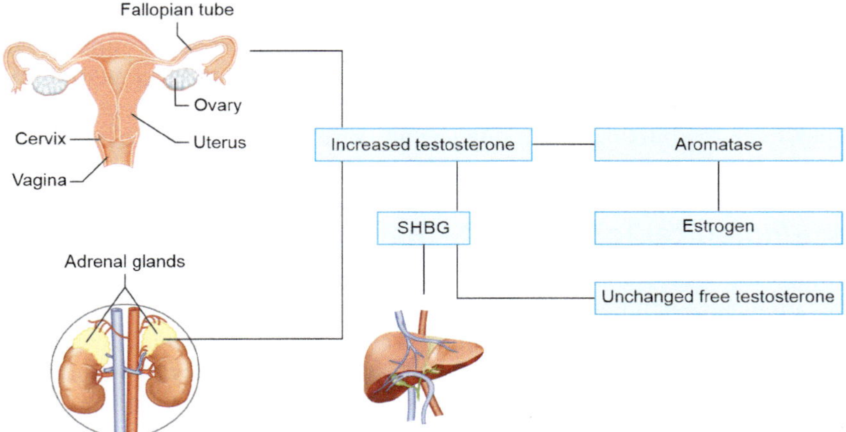

FIG. 2: Testosterone production and prevention of hyperandrogenism.
(SHBG: sex hormone-binding globulin)

Oxytocin

Increased production of oxytocin by posterior pituitary in third trimester helps in induction of labor.

Other Hormones

During pregnancy, there is a hypercortisolism (three times nonpregnant state) due to increase in production of cortisol, adrenocorticotropic hormone (ACTH), corticosteroid-binding globulin (CGB), and deoxycorticosterone. Progesterone has antiglucocorticoid action which balances this hyper cortisone activity.

Reduced vascular resistance and blood pressure lead to increase aldosterone production.

Stimulating effect of hCG in first trimester lead to decrease in thyroid-stimulating hormone. In second trimester, estrogen leads to increases production of thyroid-binding globulin which leads to increased levels of thyroxine (T4) and triiodothyronine (T3). But overall pregnancy is a euthyroid state. Parathyroid hormone secretion also increases leading to increased predisposition of hypocalcemia in conditions like pustular psoriasis of pregnancy. There is also a significant increase in insulin-like growth factor binding protein-1 (IGFBP-1), peaking at second trimester with a slight rise again near term.

PHYSIOLOGICAL IMMUNE SYSTEM CHANGES

Why the mother does not reject a fetus which is semi-allogeneic? Is pregnant female immunocompromised? Recent research reveals that maternal-fetal interface is not immunologically inert but possesses a series of active immune processes to sustain balance of the maternal-fetal tolerance and antipathogen defense. An alteration of this intricate balance may lead to either preterm births, abortion, preeclampsia or TORCH (toxoplasma, rubella, cytomegalovirus, herpes/hepatitis/human immunodeficiency, varicella, parvovirus b19, syphilis) or some other infections.

Immunological Tolerance Mechanisms

Mother's immune system as well as trophoblast immunomodulation participates in generating tolerance. There is alteration of both innate and adaptive immunity. Maternal immune tolerance varies with the gestation with early pregnancy requiring acceptance of fetus and later pregnancy precipitation of labor. Thus the immune response in pregnancy is complex and unique.

Maintaining immunological tolerance during pregnancy necessitates adjustments in the maternal immune system. These adaptations aim to sustain the pregnancy without compromising the mother's ability to combat infections. However, these changes also entail an increased susceptibility to certain infections. Furthermore, immune alterations can impact the course of inflammatory, autoimmune diseases, or coagulopathies, potentially leading to either improvement or worsening of these conditions.

- Hormonal changes lead to immunological changes for fetal tolerance
- Alteration in maternal immune system may lead to coagulopathies, alteration in autoimmune, inflammatory, and infective diseases

INNATE IMMUNITY

Complement

While there is an increase in cleaved complement proteins (C3a, C4a, C5a, C4d, C3a, C3, C9, and C5b9), complement inhibitors also see a rise **(Fig. 3)**. Notably, the elevation of C3 and C5 is minimal in the first trimester but becomes significant in subsequent trimesters. Complement proteins play crucial roles in placentation, maintaining vascular integrity, and regulating adaptive immunity. However, an imbalance in these proteins may lead to complications such as preeclampsia.

Pregnancy induces a hypercoagulable state, with fibrinogen and factor VII levels increased fourfold compared to the nonpregnant state. Additionally, elevated acute-phase reactants, complement, and coagulation proteins synergistically heighten the risk of deep vein thrombosis.

Granulocytes

Neutrophilic alterations lead to change in the number, function, or activity of neutrophils. They start increasing by 13 weeks of gestation, keep on increasing till second and remain more than nonpregnant till delivery **(Fig. 2)**. Some studies show that there is impaired neutrophil chemotaxis and phagocytosis.

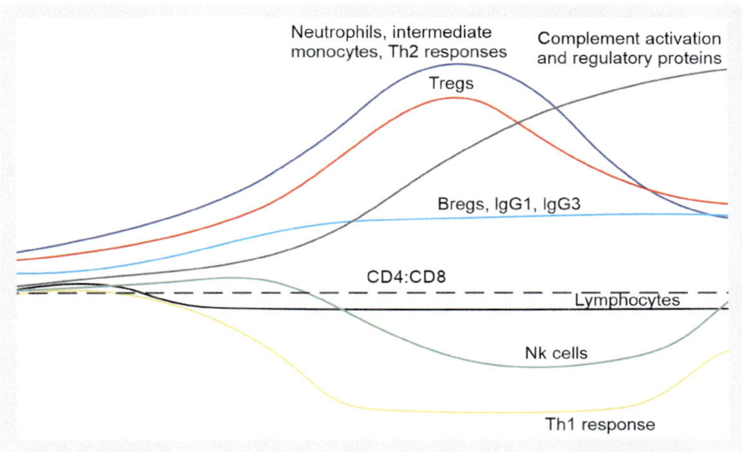

FIG. 3: Variation of immune cells in different trimesters.

While neutrophils are essential for host defense against infections, excessive neutrophil activation and inflammation can be detrimental.

Monocytes

Monocytes, while remaining fairly constant in terms of number, experience significant changes in their activation profile in pregnancy. Monocytes can be classified into different subpopulations based on the expression of cell surface markers. The three main subsets are classical ($CD14^{++}CD16^{-}$), intermediate ($CD14^{++}CD16^{+}$), and nonclassical ($CD14^{+}CD16^{++}$) monocytes. While classical monocytes have mainly phagocytic action, nonclassical have inflammatory activity. It is the intermediate monocytes which are increased in pregnancy **(Fig. 2)**. Intermediate monocytes are responsible for antigen presentation and inflammation.

Major adaptation is a shift in cytokine production toward an anti-inflammatory profile, with increased levels of cytokines like interleukin-10 (IL-10), which help prevent an immune attack on the fetus **(Fig. 4)**. Additionally, the phagocytic activity of monocytes is enhanced, allowing them to more effectively clear apoptotic cells and pathogens, thus reducing the risk of infections that could jeopardize the pregnancy. Furthermore, monocytes modulate their antigen presentation capabilities, promoting immune tolerance to fetal antigens and facilitating a harmonious maternal-fetal relationship.

Natural Killer Cells

During the first trimester of pregnancy, there is heightened natural killer (NK) cell activity. Mature NK cells increase in the peripheral blood, while immature NK cells become more prevalent in the decidua. Decidual NK cells play a crucial role in maintaining immune tolerance at the maternal-fetal interface, promoting

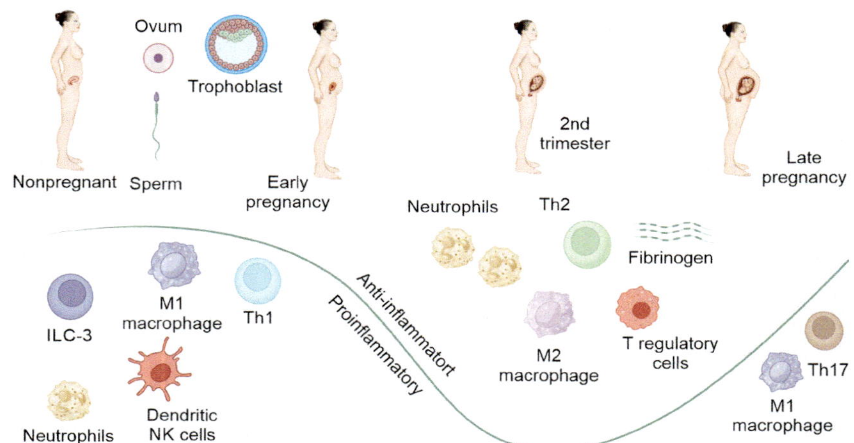

FIG. 4: Cellular changes during different trimesters of pregnancy shifting TH1 to TH2 immunity. (ILC-3: innate lymphoid cell type 3; NK: natural killer; Th1: type 1 T helper; Th2: type 2 T helper; Th17: type 17 T helper)

trophoblast invasion, and remodeling spiral arteries. Mature NK cells are more cytotoxic, facilitating antibody-dependent cellular cytotoxicity, whereas immature NK cells enhance the production of interferon-γ (IFN-γ), tumor necrosis factor-β (TNF-β), IL-10, IL-13, and granulocyte-macrophage colony-stimulating factor (GM-CSF), which contributes to antipathogen defense.

As pregnancy progresses into the second trimester, NK cell activity gradually decreases **(Fig. 2)**. This reduction is influenced by the increased expression of trophoblastic human leukocyte antigen (HLA)-G, HLA-E, and HLA-C, which further dampen NK cell activity. By downregulating NK cell activity, the maternal immune system fosters a state of immune tolerance toward the fetus and shifts toward a more anti-inflammatory state. During this period, the number of NK cells decreases, and their phenotype changes to a less cytotoxic type. The production of anti-inflammatory cytokines, especially IL-10 and transforming growth factor-β (TGF-β), increases. NK cells also interact with regulatory T cells (Tregs) and dendritic cells to maintain immune balance.

Alteration in innate immunity comprises of:
- Increase in cleaved components of complement and complement inhibitory proteins
- Hypercoagulable state
- Increased number and function of neutrophils
- Conversion of M1 predominant macrophages to M2 type
- Decrease in NK cell to a conversion to a less cytotoxic type
- Modulation of toll-like receptor (TLR) signaling to prevent excessive inflammation and fetal harm

ADAPTIVE IMMUNITY

T Cells

There is a decrease in absolute lymphocyte count during pregnancy, especially affecting T helper (Th) 17 cells and cytotoxic T cells **(Figs. 2 and 3)**.

B Cells

B cells decrease in pregnancy due to suppression of B cell lymphopoiesis and deletion of autoreactive B cells. This decrease persists till 1 month postpartum. B cell in pregnancy can be protective or harmful. Protective B cell produces asymmetric antibodies that bind to paternal antigens but do not destroy them. Harmful autoantibodies, e.g., antiphospholipid antibodies may terminate pregnancy.

Immunoglobulins

Immunoglobulin G1 (IgG1) and IgG3 levels are higher in pregnancy compared to nonpregnant women. IgG1 can cross placenta, providing protection against infections for both the mother and the fetus. However, there is an overall decrease in total Ig during pregnancy. Depression of cell-mediated immunity, loss of protein in urine, hemodilution, transfer of IgG from mother to fetus across the placenta, or pregnancy-associated hormones, especially steroid hormones (decreasing protein synthesis) may be various reasons for decreased total Ig.

T Regulatory Cells

The second trimester is characterized by a significant peak in Treg levels followed by a decline **(Fig. 2)**. Tregs are increased in maternal circulation as well as decidua. They produce anti-inflammatory cytokines such as IL-10 and TGF-β, which help to suppress immune activation and inflammation. They express molecules such as cytotoxic T-lymphocyte-associated protein 4 (CTLA-4) and programmed cell death protein 1 (PD-1), which interact with their ligands on effector T cells and dendritic cells to suppress immune responses.

B Regulatory Cells

A type of B regulatory cell (Breg) increase during pregnancy ($CD19^{+}CD24^{hi}CD27^{+}$) while IL-10 producing ones decrease in third trimester.

Th1 to Th2 Shift

There is conversion of Th1 dominance to Th2 cell type. Th2 cells secrete anti-inflammatory cytokines including IL-4, IL-5, IL-10, and IL-13 are produced more during pregnancy. These cytokines promote B cell activation, antibody production, and suppression of inflammatory responses. Th1 cytokines such as

IFN-γ, IL-2, and TNF-α are downregulated to reduce proinflammatory responses that could harm the fetus. While Th2 responses are effective against extracellular pathogens, they are less effective against intracellular pathogens (e.g., viruses and some bacteria). Pregnant women may be more susceptible to infections by intracellular pathogens due to the Th1 suppression. Listeria monocytogenes, Toxoplasma gondii, and leprosy, malaria are more severe and there is increased mortality rates due to influenza and varicella.

Impact on adaptive immunity:
- Expansion of Tregs and Bregs
- Alterations in antibody production
- Shift toward a Th2-type cytokine profile
- Expression of immune checkpoint molecules (e.g., PD-1, CTLA-4) to dampen immune activation

Other Immune Modulators

Indoleamine 2,3-dioxygenase (IDO), an enzyme responsible for the breakdown of tryptophan, is produced by both trophoblast cells and macrophages. This enzyme is crucial in inhibiting the activation of decidual α/β T cells. Additionally, the expression of IDO may be regulated by cytotoxic T lymphocyte antigen 4 (CTLA4), a protein expressed by Tregs. Overall pregnancy shows accelerated anti-inflammatory response with suppression of proinflammatory changes **(Table 1)**.

Trophoblast immunomodulation:
- Expression of immune-inhibitory molecules (e.g., HLA-G, PD-L1)
- Production of factors like IDO, which suppresses T cell activation

Impact of gestational age: Maternal immune adaptations vary throughout pregnancy, with distinct changes occurring during different trimesters:
- Early pregnancy—immune tolerance mechanisms to establish fetal-maternal tolerance
- Later stages of pregnancy involve a resurgence of immune activity to prepare for labor and delivery

TABLE 1: Other immune modulators in pregnancy.

Increased anti-inflammatory response	Decreased proinflammatory response
IL-4, 5, 10	IL-12,2
• TGF-beta • PIBF	• TNF-alpha • NK cells • Classical monocytes
• Intermediate monocytes • T regulatory cells • Th2	Th17Th1

(IL: interleukin; NK: natural killer; PIBF: progesterone-induced blocking factor; TGF-beta: transforming growth factor-beta; Th: T helper; TNF-alpha: tumor necrosis factor-alpha)

IMMUNO-HORMONAL INTERACTION

Hormonal fluctuations have a significant impact on the differentiation of Th cells. While lower levels of estradiol favor Th1 response the surge in this hormone during pregnancy promotes Th2 differentiation. Estrogen receptors (ERs) are present on lymphocytes, macrophages, and dendritic cells. Estrogen receptor α are present more on lymphocytes and Erβ on B cells. Estrogen also causes expansion of Treg and suppression of surface markers and secretion of granzyme and Fas ligand (FasL) on NK cell.

- Hormone receptors are present on immune cells
- Effect of estrogen on immunity is determined by its concentration
- Progesterone induces an anti-inflammatory response
- Progesterone increases the risk of genitourinary infections and that of acquiring HIV infection

Progesterone receptors are found on epithelial cells and various other immune cells such as mast cells, eosinophils, macrophages, dendritic cells, and lymphocytes. Progesterone can also bind to glucocorticoid receptor. Progesterone in pregnancy inhibit Th1 cytokine production and favor those of Th2. It also dampens TLR-induced cytokine production, innate immune responses, and the production of nitrite, nitric oxide, and TNF-α, resulting in an overall anti-inflammatory response in maternal circulation. However, progesterone also alters genital mucosal immune responses, potentially increasing the risk of acquiring HIV infection during pregnancy. Furthermore, progesterone and progesterone-induced blocking factor (PIBF) directly stimulate the production of IL-10, further contributing to immune modulation during pregnancy.

SUGGESTED READINGS

1. Abu-Raya B, Michalski C, Sadarangani M, Lavoie PM. Maternal Immunological Adaptation during Normal Pregnancy. Front Immunol. 2020;11:575197.
2. Robinson DP, Klein SL. Pregnancy and pregnancy-associated hormones alter immune responses and disease pathogenesis. Horm Behav. 2012;62:263-71.
3. De la Morena MT. Immunologic Changes During Pregnancy. In Stiehm's Immune Deficiencies; Elsevier Inc.: Amsterdam, The Netherladns; 2014. pp. 815-22.

CHAPTER 2

Physiological Skin Changes in Pregnancy

Mudita Gupta, Sanjeev Gupta

INTRODUCTION

During pregnancy, a woman's body undergoes significant hormonal and physiological transformations to support fetal development and prepare for childbirth. These changes impact almost every organ system, including the skin. Key hormonal changes involve increase in levels of estrogen, progesterone, human chorionic gonadotropin (hCG), and melanocyte-stimulating hormone (MSH). Additionally, there are alterations in blood flow, immune function, and metabolic processes. These changes can result in a variety of dermatological manifestations.

- Pregnancy is a state of transformation.
- Certain changes in skin are quite commonly seen and are named as physiological.
- Knowledge of these physiological changes is essential for the patient and the health provider.
- Broadly these physiological changes involve pigmentation, vascular system, connective tissue, hair, nail, and appendageal structures.

"Physiological dermatological changes" are called so because they are alterations that occur as part of the body's response to pregnancy. Certain cutaneous alterations are so common that they are not considered abnormal and are accepted as physiological. These changes are driven by hormonal shifts and other internal mechanisms that are inherent to the pregnancy process.

Understanding dermatological changes during pregnancy is crucial for both healthcare providers and pregnant individuals. For healthcare providers, this knowledge is essential for accurately diagnosing and differentiating between normal physiological changes and pathological conditions, providing appropriate treatment options, and offering preventive care advice. Educating pregnant individuals about these changes can reduce anxiety by setting realistic expectations and promoting proactive skin care practices. This understanding improves communication between patients and healthcare providers, leading to better management of skin-related issues and overall enhanced care during pregnancy.

CLASSIFICATION OF PHYSIOLOGICAL CHANGES

Physiological changes in pregnancy

- *Pigmentary changes*:
  - Chloasma (75%)
  - Linea nigra (32–92%)
  - Secondary areola
  - Darkening of nevi, freckles, recent scars, and dermal melanocytosis
  - Group B pigmentary lines
  - Melanonychia
  - Diffuse hyperpigmentation
- *Vascular changes*:
  - Spider nevi (11–66%)
  - Palmar erythema (33%)
  - Granuloma gravidarum (4–5%)
  - Varicosities (40%)
  - Hemangioma and purpura (5%)
  - Worsening of preexisting vascular tumors
  - Vasomotor instability disorders
  - Physiological edema (50%)
  - Gingival hyperemia (80–100%)
  - Nasal congestion (40%)
  - Unilateral nevoid telangiectasia
- *Structural changes*:
  - Striae
  - Skin tags
- *Hair changes*:
  - Telogen effluvium
  - Hirsutism
  - Frontoparietal hair loss
- Nail changes
- *Appendiceal changes*:
  - Increased eccrine gland activity
  - Decreased apocrine activity
  - Sebaceous gland activity increased/decrease

Pigmentary Changes

Hyperpigmentation affects approximately 90% of pregnant women, with these changes being more prevalent among those with Fitzpatrick skin type III–V. More commonly localized areas can show hyperpigmentation; this could be because of regional differences showing increased density of melanocytes. One of the most recognizable forms of hyperpigmentation during pregnancy is melasma, also known as chloasma/melasma gravidarum or the "mask of pregnancy", which appears as dark patches on the face particularly on the malar area, upper lip, and chin **(Fig. 1)**. This condition is observed in about 75% of pregnant women. Additionally, darkening of existing ephelides, nevi, and recent scars is common. Another typical manifestation is the linea nigra, a dark linear macule running from the xiphoid process to the pubic region, seen in 32–92% pregnant females **(Fig. 2)**. It corresponds to the pigmented linea alba and is often accompanied by a slight rightward displacement of the umbilicus, known as the "ligamentum teres sign". This line may persist postpartum until the abdominal muscles regain their tone.

Hyperpigmentation can affect areas that are normally more pigmented, such as the areolae (secondary areola) **(Fig. 3)**, genitalia, perineum, axillae, and inner thighs, becoming even darker. Longitudinal melanonychia may also appear and preexisting dermal melanocytosis darkens.

Pigmentary demarcation lines (PDLs) also known as Futcher's line or Voigt's line mark abrupt transitions between more deeply pigmented and lighter areas of the skin. In 1913, Matsumoto first described these lines. PDL appear because of neural control of melanin synthesis. As these neural territories do not show overlap leading to appearance of PDL. There are eight different PDLs; group B are more common in pregnancy, though type A have also been reported. Group B lines are present on lower limbs **(Fig. 4)**. Neurogenic compression and inflammation of sacral nerve root 1 and 2 by the enlarging gravid uterus has been speculated to be the cause of appearance of group B PDL in pregnancy. In a study, it was observed that occipitoposterior presentation further increases compression and hence appearance of these PDL.

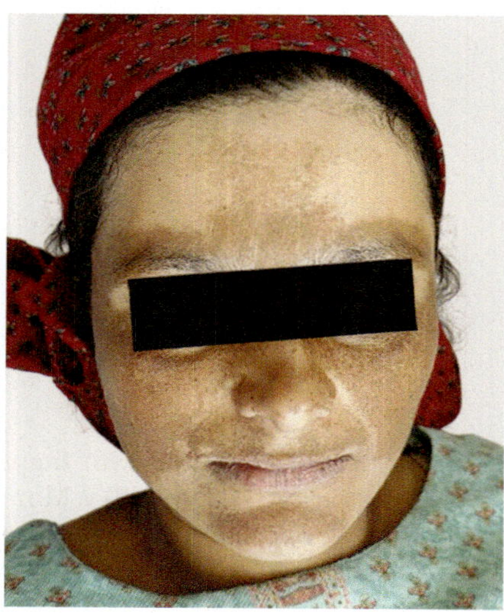

FIG. 1: Melasma.

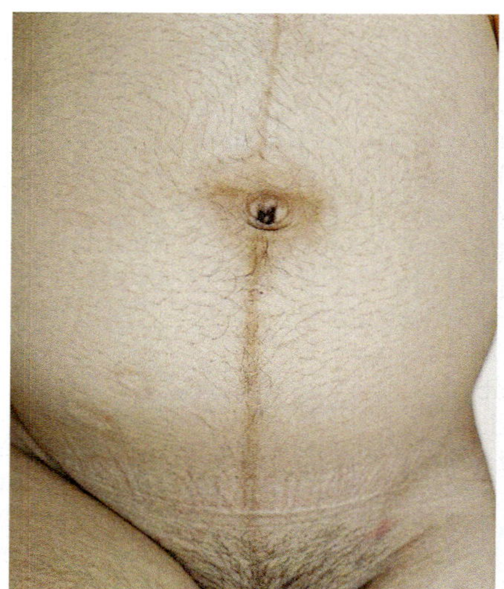

FIG. 2: Linea nigra.

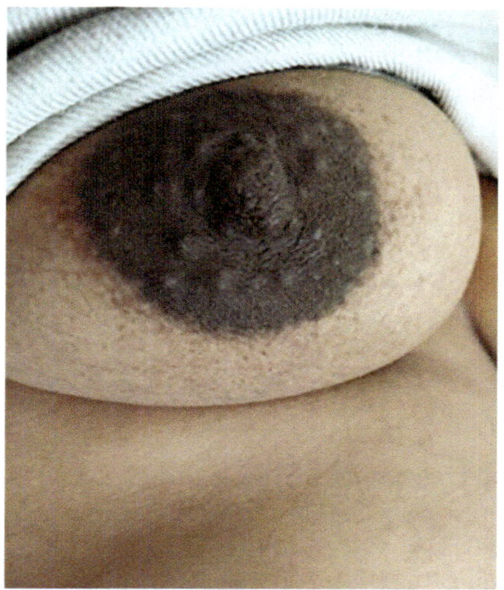

FIG. 3: Seconary areolae and montogomery's tubercle.

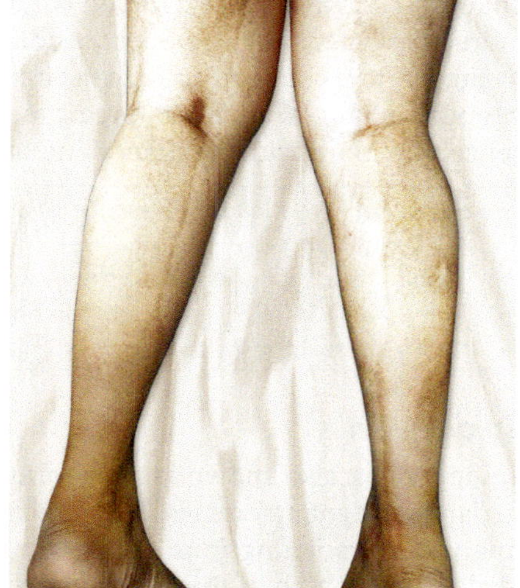

FIG. 4: Group B pigmentary demarcation lines.

- Hyperpigmentation is a common physiological change seen in pregnancy.
- Localized areas of hyperpigmentation in areas rich in melanocytes specifically darken during pregnancy.
- Chloasma, linea nigra, secondary areolae, darkening of previous nevi, ephelides, scars, dermal melanocytosis, PDLs, etc., are the various physiological PDLs.
- Surge in hormones, enzymes, and sphingolipids secreted by placenta are the main reason behind hyperpigmentation.

If pigmentation is generalized then other causes should be sought before labeling it as physiological.

The exact cause of pregnancy-related hyperpigmentation is not entirely understood. Increased estrogen and progesterone during pregnancy lead to increased melanogenesis. The details of this will be discussed later in this book. Increased MSH from the pituitary gland is no longer thought to be contributory. Along with melanogenic enzymes such as tyrosinase and tyrosinase-related proteins 1 and 2, are upregulated by bioactive sphingolipids secreted by the placenta. Not only this sensitivity of melanocytes to estrogen and progesterone receptors also increase during pregnancy.

Although hyperpigmentation often lightens after childbirth, it may persist in about 30% of cases. There are high chances of recurrence of these hyperpigmentary disorders in subsequent pregnancies. Treatment of melasma will be discussed later in this book.

Vascular Changes

Vascular changes during pregnancy are primarily attributed to estrogen surge, particularly blood vessel dilation and increased skin vascularity. Hemodynamic changes, such as increased blood volume and venous pressure from the growing uterus have a synergistic effect. Additionally, altered liver function, often seen in pregnancy, can lead to higher circulating estrogen levels, further promoting vascular changes. Genetic predisposition and individual variations in skin sensitivity, along with pregnancy-induced immune system changes, also play role.

- Hormonal surge leads to vascular dilatation, angiogenesis, increased blood volume, and venous pressure.
- Gravid uterus increase venous pressure and capillary permeability in lower limbs.
- Increased VEGF, bFGF, and angiopoietin are also increased during pregnancy.
- Also response of vessels to various stimulants is altered leading to vasomotor instability.

Spider Nevi

Spider nevus, also known as nevus araneus develops in 66% fair skinned and 11% in darker pregnant females. They are bright red, blanchable, small arterioles with fine vessels radiating from the center **(Fig. 5)**. Pressure on the central arteriole leads to blanching of the surrounding vessels. They typically appear during the second to fifth month and gradually increase in size throughout pregnancy. These lesions are usually seen on skin areas drained by the superior vena cava, particularly around the eyes. Most spider nevi regress postpartum within 3 months. However, for those that persist, treatment options include ablation by electrocautery or laser therapy.

Palmar Erythema

Palmar erythema presents as mottled redness of the thenar and hypothenar eminences only or the other type with involvement of whole of palms. This condition characterized by redness and warmth of the palms with no pain or

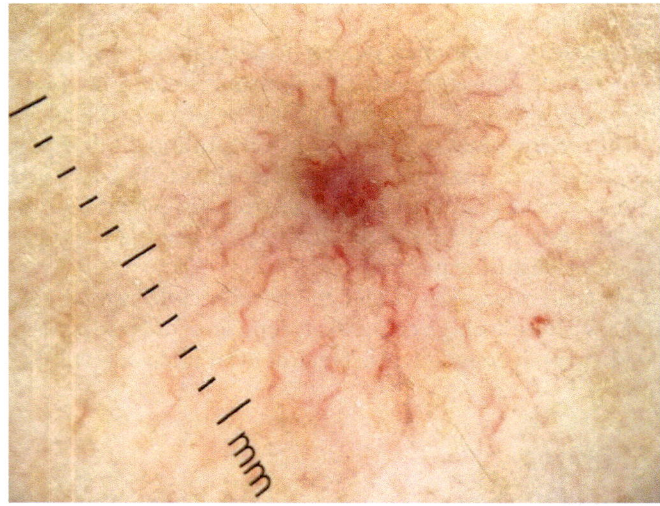

FIG. 5: Spider nevi.

itching. It is observed in approximately 66% of white and 33% of black women during pregnancy. Palmar erythema in pregnancy needs to be differentiated from palmar erythema due to liver failure and in systemic lupus erythematosus.

- *Spider nevus*: Appears in ~66% of fair-skinned and 11% of darker pregnant women, often regressing postpartum; persistent cases can be treated with electrocautery or laser.
- *Palmar erythema*: Affects ~66% of white and 33% of black pregnant women, presenting as painless redness of the palms and requiring differentiation from liver disease and lupus.

Pyogenic Granuloma

Pyogenic granuloma during pregnancy, also known as granuloma gravidarum or epulis gravidarum, is thought to result from a combination of hormonal influences and local irritation or trauma **(Figs. 6A and B)**. It is seen in 4–5% of pregnancies. The term pyogenic granuloma is a misnomer; actually nodular granulation tissue is formed. Increased estrogen in pregnancy leads to upregulation of basic fibroblast growth factor (bFGF), vascular endothelial growth factor (VEGF), and angiopoietin-2 (Ang-2) promoting angiogenesis. Progesterone has immunosuppressant action resulting in inability for acute inflammatory response instead a chronic tissue reaction occurs. Clinically it presents as a red, flesh colored tumor which bleeds when traumatized. It can be surgically excised/ scooped out, and cauterized.

Varicosities

Distension of the superficial venous vasculature in the legs (varicose veins) **(Fig. 7)**, vagina, vestibule (Jacquemier-Chadwick sign), and rectum (hemorrhoids) is common during pregnancy, affecting about 40% of pregnant women. Lack of valves in perineal veins increases the risk of varices in perineal area. Increased

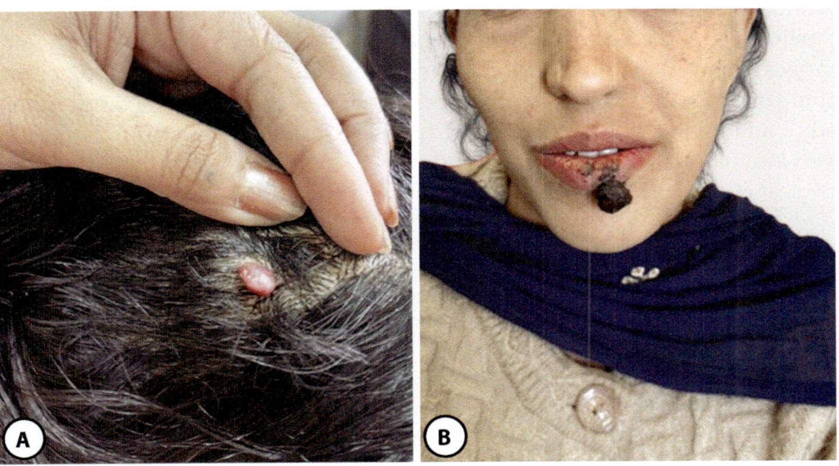

FIGS. 6A AND B: Pyogenic granuloma of scalp and on lips.

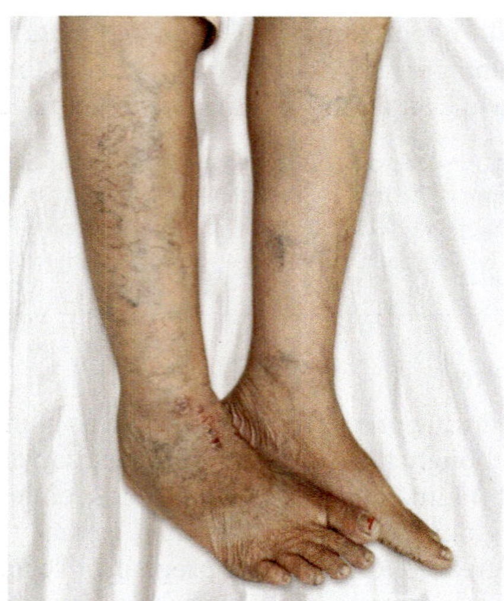

FIG. 7: Varicosities on lower legs.

vascularity of the cervix causes a bluish discoloration known as Goodell's sign. For varicose veins during pregnancy measures such as elevating the legs, using the Trendelenburg position, and wearing compression stockings can reduce varicosity. It is advisable to avoid prolonged sitting and standing. Varicose veins often regress postpartum, but persistent cases may require sclerotherapy.

Vasomotor Instability Disorders

During pregnancy, various vasomotor instability disorders can occur due to hormonal and physiological changes. Cutis marmorata, characterized by an intermittent reticulated cyanotic appearance of the legs when exposed to cold, is common. Pregnant women may also experience episodes of facial flushing or pallor, hot and cold sensations, and a noticeable facial glow, all attributed to changes in blood flow and hormonal fluctuations. Additionally, dermatographism, itching on the palms are often observed. These benign conditions result from the body's adaptation to pregnancy and typically resolve postpartum as hormone levels and blood flow return to normal.

- *Pyogenic granuloma*: Occurs in 4–5% of pregnancies due to hormonal influences and trauma, presenting as a red or flesh-colored tumor that bleeds easily; it can be excised and cauterized if needed.
- *Varicosities*: Affect ~40% of pregnant women, commonly seen in the legs, perineal area, and rectum; measures like leg elevation and compression stockings can help, with most cases regressing postpartum.
- *Vasomotor instability*: Includes cutis marmorata, facial flushing, and hot or cold sensations, caused by hormonal and circulatory changes; these benign conditions typically resolve after delivery.

Physiological Edema of Pregnancy

Physiological edema of pregnancy is a common condition characterized by the accumulation of fluid in the tissues, leading to swelling, particularly in the extremities and face. This nonpitting edema affects about 50% of pregnant women, especially during the third-trimester. The primary causes include increased capillary permeability, water and sodium retention, and elevated hydrostatic pressure. The growing uterus exerts pressure on the inferior vena cava, which contributes to the elevated hydrostatic pressure and subsequent fluid accumulation. Although generally benign, physiological edema can cause discomfort. It typically resolves postpartum when the body's fluid balance returns to normal.

Hemangiomas

Hemangiomas are benign vascular lesions that occur spontaneously in about 5% of pregnancies, usually during the second- or third-trimester. Other preexisting vascular like subcutaneous hemangioendotheliomas, glomangiomas worsen during pregnancy. They typically appear on the hands and neck. These lesions are characterized by an abnormal proliferation of blood vessels and tend to regress after childbirth.

Purpura

Purpuras are red spots which appear due to extravasation of red blood cells. In pregnancy, purpura can develop due to elevated hydrostatic pressure and increased capillary fragility, particularly in the lower limbs. This is often a result of the pressure exerted by the growing uterus on the blood vessels, leading to increased pressure in the capillaries and small blood vessels, causing them to rupture easily.

Hyperemia of Gingiva

Hyperemia of the gingiva is seen almost universally in pregnancy. Peaking during second to fourth month of pregnancy this hyperemia clinically manifests as erythematous, glossy smooth, and swollen interdental papilla, especially of central lower teeth. There is a predisposition to dental caries because of altered salivary pH and increased oral microflora. Gingival hyperemia is characterized by increased blood flow to the gums due to effect of hormones on blood vessels. Gum tissues also become more sensitive and reactive to plaque and bacteria. Additionally, changes in the immune system during pregnancy can alter the body's response to bacterial plaque, leading to gum inflammation. Increased plaque accumulation due to less effective oral hygiene practices, often resulting from morning sickness or altered habits, further contribute to gum irritation. Managing pregnancy gingivitis involves maintaining good oral hygiene through regular brushing and flossing, seeking professional dental care for regular checkups and cleanings and avoiding foods and drinks that can irritate the gums.

Nasal Congestion

Increased nasal congestion is seen in 30% pregnancies. Mucosal edema and relaxation of smooth muscles lead to this change.

Unilateral Nevoid Telangiectasia

Unilateral nevoid telangiectasia appears as fine delicate telangiectasias mainly located on the upper body in the C3, C4, and trigeminal region. This is under the effect of estrogen surge. These lesions are blanchable.

- *Purpura*: Red spots in the lower limbs caused by increased capillary fragility and elevated hydrostatic pressure due to the growing uterus; results from capillary rupture.
- *Hyperemia of gingiva*: Common in pregnancy, peaking in the second to fourth month, presenting as swollen, erythematous gums with increased sensitivity to plaque and bacteria; managed through good oral hygiene and professional care.
- *Nasal congestion*: Affects ~30% of pregnancies due to mucosal edema and smooth muscle relaxation caused by hormonal changes.
- *Unilateral nevoid telangiectasia*: Estrogen-induced blanchable telangiectasias appearing on the upper body, especially in the C3, C4, and trigeminal regions.

Structural Changes

Stria Gravidarum

Striae gravidarum are linear atrophic marks, wrinkled, erythematous, and purplish bands frequently appearing on the abdomen, thighs, buttocks, and breasts of pregnant women. To start with these striae are pink and shiny, whereas later they become white and atrophic. They are seen in up to 90% cases. The pathogenesis of striae formation is not fully understood. As explained later in this book striae result because of interplay between various factors such as overdistension, genetic factor, ethnicity, demographic factors, hormonal, obstetric causes and prepregnant weight, and nutrition, etc. These hormones cause thinning of elastin fibers and fibrillin microfibrils in the dermis, resulting in a shift in fiber orientation from perpendicular to parallel relative to the dermal-epidermal junction.

Currently, there is no effective treatment for striae. Various therapies which have been tried and are detailed later in this book.

Molluscum Fibrosum Gravidarum

Molluscum fibrosum gravidarum are firm tan to brown sessile/pedunculated fleshy growths 1–5 mm in size most commonly located on neck, axilla, and other flexures such as groin and inframammary area. They were first described by Brickner in 1906. The occurrence of molluscum fibrosum gravidarum is believed to be influenced by hormonal changes during pregnancy, particularly increased levels of estrogen and progesterone. Risk factors include a family history of skin tags, obesity, and the presence of diabetes, which can increase the likelihood of their appearance. Clinically and histopathologically they resemble acrochordon but unlike latter they are associated with pregnancy appearing in fourth to sixth month and regressing postpartum. But occasionally they may persist. They can be surgically excised or cauterized or destroyed by cryotherapy.

- *Striae gravidarum*: Present in up to 90% of pregnancies, these atrophic, purplish marks on the abdomen, thighs, breasts, and buttocks result from hormonal, genetic, and mechanical factors affecting dermal elastin fibers; no effective treatment exists.
- *Molluscum fibrosum gravidarum*: Hormone-related skin tags appearing in the neck, axilla, and flexures during the fourth to sixth months of pregnancy, often regressing postpartum but treatable by excision or cryotherapy if persistent.

Other Soft Tissue Tumors

There may be exacerbation of preexisting lesions such as keloid, dermatofibroma, neurofibroma, and leiomyoma. Increased collagen and fibroblast activity are responsible for this predisposition.

- Connective tissue alterations are common in pregnancy.
- Increased fibroblast growth factor, activity of fibroblasts, insulin-like growth factor, etc., lead to alteration in amount of collagen fibers and their arrangement.
- Elastic fiber disorganization is also seen.
- Overdistension of skin is also an important contributory factor.

Hair Changes during Pregnancy

During pregnancy, women often experience notable changes in hair growth, texture, and shedding. These changes are primarily driven by the hormonal fluctuations that occur during this period. Increased estrogen prolongs anagen and reduces conversion of anagen hair into telogen leading to thick and voluminous hair. Progesterone increases sebaceous secretions leading to improved texture of hair. Increased blood circulation can enhance nutrient delivery to hair follicles, supporting healthier hair growth. Iron deficiency and other vitamin and mineral deficit can lead to hair thinning and loss. After childbirth, the abrupt drop in estrogen levels triggers a large number of hair follicles to enter the telogen phase simultaneously (telogen effluvium), typically peaking around 3–6 months postpartum returning to normal pattern within 6–12 months **(Figs. 8A and B)**. Reassuring and counseling the pregnant patients about reversibility of hair changes is of utmost importance. Ensuring adequate intake of essential nutrients, including vitamins and minerals such as iron, zinc, and biotin is required. Hyperandrogenism can lead to hirsutism. In rare cases, some women may experience alopecia areata (patchy hair loss) during pregnancy, potentially triggered by an autoimmune response to hormonal changes. Details of hair changes in pregnancy will be dealt with in later chapters in this book.

Nail Changes

During pregnancy, women often experience various changes in their nails due to hormonal fluctuations, increased blood circulation, and metabolic changes. These changes can affect the growth rate, texture, and overall health of the nails.

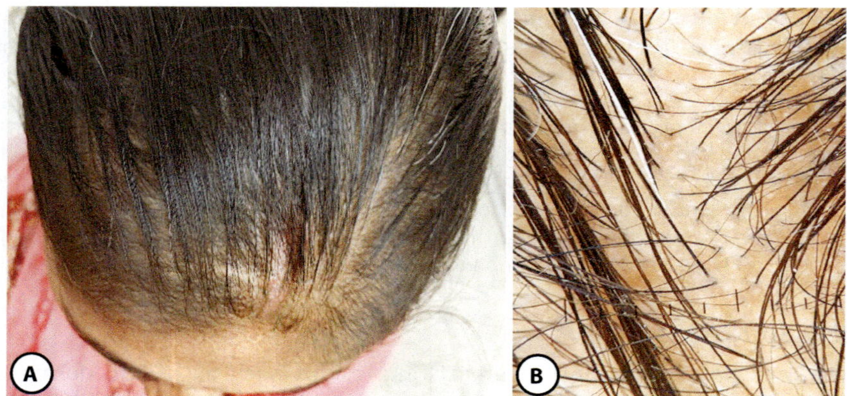

FIGS. 8A AND B: Increased hair shedding in postpartum period, dermoscopy showing decreased hair density with empty follicles.

One of the most noticeable changes is the faster growth rate of nails, driven by enhanced nutrient delivery to the nail matrix. However, nails may also become more brittle, making them prone to breaking or splitting. Some women might find their nails becoming softer and more pliable. Additionally, hormonal changes can lead to the appearance of horizontal or vertical ridges on the nails and occasional color changes, such as a pale or bluish tint due to alterations in blood circulation.

Other common nail issues during pregnancy include onycholysis and increased susceptibility to nail infections like paronychia. These issues can be influenced by elevated levels of estrogen and progesterone, which impact nail growth and strength. Nutritional factors also play a crucial role; deficiencies in essential nutrients such as iron, zinc, and biotin can exacerbate nail problems. None of these findings is very specific and pathological conditions need to be ruled out before labeling them as physiological. After childbirth, as hormone levels stabilize, nail growth and texture generally return to their prepregnancy state, though this normalization process can take several months. Details of nail changes will be dealt with later in this book.

Appendageal Changes

There is excessive sweating during pregnancy. Thyroid enlargement, increased body weight, and increased vasomotor activity leading to alteration in autonomic nervous are the various proposed mechanisms. There is increased incidence of miliaria and dyshidrotic eczema in pregnancy. Palmar sweating is reduced because of increased adrenocorticotropic hormone. Hyperhidrosis though temporary if too problematic 20% solution of aluminum chloride hexahydrate in ethyl alcohol can be used.

Sebaceous gland activity has a variable course in pregnancy. Increased sebaceous activity may lead to pregnancy glow. Also at times specifically toward end of pregnancy there may be increased tendency to develop acne. Increased sebaceous activity on the areolae lead to papular lesions and are named as Montgomery's tubercle **(Fig. 3)**.

There is decreased activity of apocrine gland activity. Hidradenitis suppurativa, Fox-Fordyce, etc., apocrine gland diseases improve during pregnancy with a rebound occurring in postpartum period.

- Pregnancy brings about numerous dermatological changes, driven by hormonal fluctuations, increased blood flow, and immunological adjustments.
- These changes may be very common or relatively rare.
- Knowledge of these changes helps in differentiating those patients who require treatment from those in whom counseling is only required.

SUGGESTED READINGS

1. Motosko CC, Bieber AK, Pomeranz MK, Stein JA, Martires KJ. Physiologic changes of pregnancy: A review of the literature. Int J Womens Dermatol. 2017;3(4):219-24.
2. Chandran V, Kurien G, Mohan V. Pigmentary Demarcation Lines in Pregnancy. Indian J Dermatol. 2016;61(1):127.
3. da Silva JON, e Silva RR, Schneider MG, Selbach MCM, Guisso MES, Neumann DA, et al. Characteristics of physiological changes in pregnancy in a public maternity in Southern Brazil. J Dermatol Res Ther. 2022;7:117.
4. Gondivkar SM, Gadbail A, Chole R. Oral pregnancy tumor. Contemp Clin Dent. 2010;1(3): 190-2.
5. Barankin B, Silver SG, Carruthers A. The skin in pregnancy. J Cutan Med Surg. 2002;6:236-40.
6. Kroumpouzos G, Cohen LM. Dermatoses of pregnancy. J Am Acad Dermatol. 2001;45(1): 1-19.
7. Gupta M. Dermatological complications. In: Sharma A (Ed). A Practical Guide to Third Trimester of Pregnancy and Puerperium, 1st edition. New Delhi: Jaypee Brothers Medical Publishers (P) Ltd.; 2016. pp. 570-85.
8. Ingber A, Lebwohl M. Obstetric Dermatology: A Practical Guide. Berlin, Heidelberg: Springer; 2009. pp. 7-25.

CHAPTER 3

Psoriasis and Skin

Reena Kumari Sharma, Mudita Gupta

INTRODUCTION

Psoriasis is a common, genetically determined, and immune-mediated systemic inflammatory skin disease characterized by T-cell-driven inflammation and excessive keratinocyte proliferation. The occurrence of psoriasis ranges from 1 to 3%, exhibiting significant geographic differences. It is broadly classified into plaque and pustular forms depending upon the morphology of lesions and these forms may even coexist. Chronic plaque psoriasis, also known as psoriasis vulgaris, is the common form and is characterized by erythematous, scaly, and sharply demarcated plaques of variable extent and severity. Pustular psoriasis is marked by sterile pustules and differs from psoriasis vulgaris in terms of genetic predisposition, pathogenesis, clinical presentation, and treatment response. Psoriasis is further divided into two types depending upon the age of onset and genetic predisposition to disease, as most of the patients develop disease during third and fourth decade of life which overlaps with the reproductive period in females. Onset of disease is before 40 years of age in around 75% psoriatic women with an average of 28 years. There are various immunological adaptations during pregnancy leading to improved or worsened outcome of psoriasis during this period. At the same time psoriasis is associated with comorbidities which further influence the management and outcome of the disease. This chapter highlights the immunological changes in pregnancy, its effects on psoriasis and vice versa, safety of treatment modalities used in pregnancy.

- Psoriasis is an immune-mediated disease.
- Broadly classified into two types—chronic plaque and pustular psoriasis.
- Average age of onset is 28 years which corresponds with active reproductive age of females.

IMMUNE AND HORMONAL CHANGES DURING PREGNANCY

As described in the chapter *"Immuno-hormonal Changes in Pregnancy"*, physiological changes occur during pregnancy in maternal immune. These immunological changes may affect the course of psoriasis in pregnancy. A shift in helper T (Th) cell polarization activates the humoral Th2 response and suppresses the cell-mediated Th1 response. Elevated estrogen levels boost the production of specific cytokines [interleukin-2 (IL-2), IL-10, and interferon gamma (IFN-γ)] while inhibiting others, such as tumor necrosis factor-α (TNF-α), in peripheral blood. Progesterone causing reduction in T-cell proliferation, primarily behaves as immunosuppressive. The immune system alterations during pregnancy may be due to changes in the estrogen-progesterone ratio, with progesterone levels rising significantly more than estrogen levels. Additionally, prolactin and human placental lactogen have immune-modulatory effects, although these effects are less well-documented. Th1 cell cytokines play a role in cell-mediated tissue damage in autoimmune diseases such as psoriasis, Crohn's disease, and rheumatoid arthritis.

Interferon-gamma, a Th1 cytokine, is directly embryotoxic and inhibits the Th2 response. Conversely, the anti-inflammatory cytokine IL-10 downregulates proinflammatory Th1 cytokines, thereby promoting a Th2 response. The levels of proinflammatory cytokines progressively decrease during the second and third trimesters of pregnancy. In the final weeks of pregnancy, the cytokine milieu shifts back to a predominance of Th1 cells, creating a favorable environment for labor induction and protecting both mother and fetus from infection during and after birth. TNF-α cytokine has a dual and paradoxical role in embryo development, acting as a potent activator of both apoptotic and antiapoptotic pathways. It stimulates protective mechanisms to prevent abnormalities while also promoting embryo destruction in cases of severe structural abnormalities.

- Various immunological changes alter course of psoriasis in pregnancy.
- Predominance of Th1 response compared to Th2.
- Cytokines lie IL-2, IL-10, and IFN-γ increase, while TNF-α decreases.
- These immunological changes are because of estrogen progesterone ratio.

PATHOGENESIS OF PSORIASIS

The pathogenesis of psoriasis is multifaceted, involving a combination of genetic susceptibility and environmental triggers. At the core of this process is an aberrant immune response, with T cells, especially Th1 and Th17 subsets, playing pivotal roles. These T cells secrete proinflammatory cytokines such as IL-17, IL-22, and TNF-α, which lead to the hyperproliferation of keratinocytes, resulting in the formation of psoriatic plaques. Additionally, other immune cells, including dendritic cells and neutrophils, contribute to the chronic inflammatory milieu.

Genetic factors, notably the HLA-Cw0602 allele, heighten the risk of developing psoriasis. Environmental influences such as infections, stress, and certain medications can act as triggers or exacerbating factors.

EFFECT OF PREGNANCY ON PSORIASIS

Sex hormones contribute to fluctuations in disease activity during specific life stages in women, such as menstruation, menopause, and pregnancy. Although the effect of psoriasis on pregnancy is not predictable, around 30–40% women with psoriasis experience improvements in clinical disease, especially during first two trimesters of pregnancy, while only around 10% deteriorate. There is usually postpartum (during 4–6 weeks) worsening of psoriasis (seen in 40–90% of women). Modification in the clinical course of psoriasis during pregnancy is described in 76.7% cases by Vena et al., with improvement reported in 63.3% of them. The amelioration of psoriasis is usually gradual, while postpartum flare which is the most common scenario as reported in a study in around 87.7% of cases is comparatively sudden in onset due to rapid fall of estrogen and progesterone levels.

Shift in the immune response from a Th1/Th17 to a Th2-dominant state during pregnancy reduces the activity of proinflammatory cytokines such as IFN-gamma, IL-17, and TNF-α, which are crucial in the pathogenesis of psoriasis hence leading to improvement.

The sex steroid which causes improvement in psoriasis during pregnancy is debatable. According to some authors increased progesterone levels cause downregulation of T-cell response and have a direct effect on keratinocyte proliferation. Others state that estrogen is responsible for such improvement.

Female carriers of the HLA-Cw0602 allele are more likely to experience significant improvement in psoriasis symptoms during pregnancy, whereas remission is uncommon in noncarriers.

Worsening of psoriasis which is seen in few patients may be due to inadequate suppression of the Th1/Th17 immune pathways, complex hormonal influences, and environmental stressors, all contributing to increased inflammatory activity in predisposed individuals.

Available data suggest that pregnancy generally does not negatively impact the course and severity of psoriasis. If changes do occur during pregnancy, they are more often improvements rather than worsening in most cases. However, this assumption convincingly holds true for plaque psoriasis. An exception to the earlier-mentioned notion is generalized pustular psoriasis of pregnancy (GPPP), showing sudden flare during late trimesters of pregnancy and postpartum period.

- Improvement in psoriasis in 30–40% cases in pregnancy.
- Postpartum flare in 40–90% cases.
- Skewed Th1 to Th2 balance is responsible for improvement of psoriasis during pregnancy.
- Female carriers of HLA-CW0602 have a more significant improvement during pregnancy.
- Generalized pustular psoriasis may worsen during pregnancy.

IMPACT OF PSORIASIS ON PREGNANCY

Psoriasis and Infertility

Psoriasis is not just a disease of skin it also effects multiple other organs, e.g., cardiac and ophthalmic. Metabolic syndrome and polycystic ovarian disease are common associations of psoriasis. Studies have shown decreased fertility rate in women with moderate-to-severe psoriasis, elevated follicle-stimulating hormone (FSH) levels, FSH/luteinizing hormone (LH) ratio, and decreased antral follicle count. Similarly in males also decrease in sperm count, motility, and decreased percentage of normal morphology sperms were reported in various studies, however, decreased fertility rate was not observed in males treated with biologics.

Recently, Johansen et al. reported that women with moderate-to-severe psoriasis have a higher risk of ectopic pregnancy compared to women without psoriasis.

- Psoriasis decreases fertility in females.
- Decrease in sperm count and mobility in males.
- Psoriasis increases risk of ectopic pregnancy.

Course of Pregnancy in Psoriasis

Risk of complications increases during pregnancy in psoriatic females. Although there were conflicting findings in some studies which dealt mainly with mild psoriasis cases, stating little effects on the outcome of pregnancy. However, a significant association is reported between moderate-to-severe psoriasis and pregnancy complications, thus increasing the maternal and fetal morbidity as well as mortality. Maternal complications reported were pregnancy-induced hypertensive diseases, such as gestational hypertension and preeclampsia. Women with hypertensive diseases of pregnancy shared common risk factors for future development of cardiovascular diseases. Some studies have highlighted association of low birth weight in newborn with severe forms of psoriasis in mother.

Comorbidities such as hypertension, obesity, dyslipidemia, psychiatric disorders, alcohol consumption, and smoking may also contribute to adverse pregnancy outcome. However, mothers who received systemic therapy for severe psoriasis during pregnancy did not have a higher risk of low birth weight suggesting that the risk might be due to the disease itself.

- Mild psoriasis—unaffected pregnancy outcome.
- Moderate-to-severe psoriasis—pregnancy-related complications (gestational hypertension and preeclampsia) and poor pregnancy outcome (low birth weight fetus).

GENERALIZED PUSTULAR PSORIASIS OF PREGNANCY

Generalized pustular psoriasis of pregnancy is a rare variant of pustular psoriasis. It is also known as impetigo herpetiformis because of its presentation in the

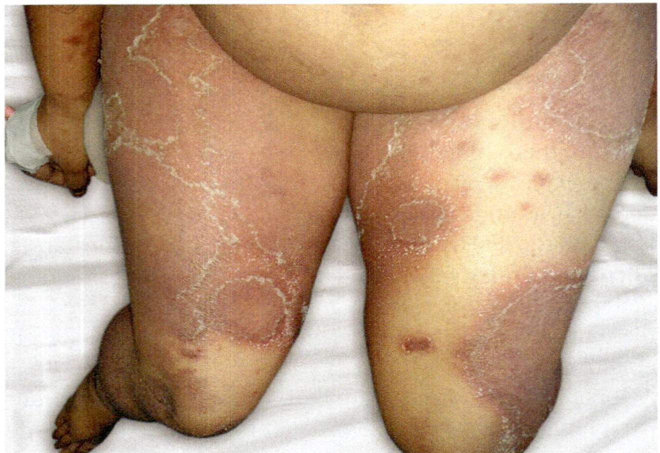

FIG. 1: Centrifugally spreading pustular lesions in groins and on thighs.

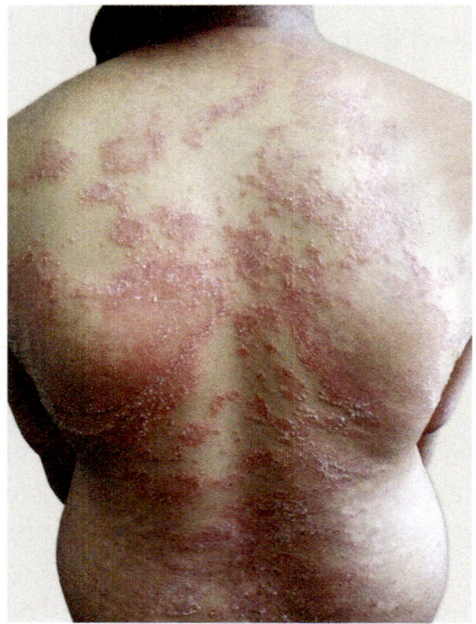

FIG. 2: Disseminated pustular lesions in generalized pustular psoriasis of pregnancy.

form of generalized grouped symmetrical pustules with a tendency of flexural predominance.

The onset of disease is usually in the third trimester of pregnancy with resolution after parturition; however, it may occasionally persist long afterward.

The eruption generally starts over flexures as minute pustules arising on an acutely inflamed skin. These lesions extend centrifugally, drying in the center and forming crusted plaques. These plaques heal with brownish pigmentation **(Figs. 1 and 2)**. Mucosal involvement of tongue, buccal cavity, and even the esophagus may also be seen. Geographic tongue with superficial erosions following short-lived pustules is the most common finding. Severe complications such as maternal death and miscarriages are associated with GPPP in about 50% cases each. Greater risks of placental insufficiency lead to stillbirth, neonatal death, and fetal abnormalities. Increased chances of hypocalcemia in pregnancy due to increased activity of parathyroid hormone in pregnancy aggravate the condition. Constitutional disturbance may be severe. It may be associated with erythroderma and fever. Delirium, diarrhea, vomiting, and death have been described attributable to cardiac and renal failure. Recurrence in subsequent pregnancies shows characteristic recurrence with earlier onset of disease and increased severity.

Generalized pustular psoriasis of pregnancy must be differentiated from its closest differential acute generalized exanthematous pustulosis which typically have temporal correlation with the culprit drug.

- Flare of pustular psoriasis in late third trimester or early postpartum period.
- Pustular psoriasis starts in flexures with sterile pustules at margin.
- Tongue, esophagus, and buccal mucosa may also be involved.
- Poor fetal outcome—still births, neonatal death, and fetal abnormality.
- Maternal—constitutional symptoms, erythroderma, delirium, diarrhea, renal, hypocalcemia, and cardiac failure.

TREATMENT

General Aspects

Psoriatic woman is advised to plan a pregnancy, while in remission and off from all medications or is on minimum effective dose of medications. Medicines can be discontinued in mild disease or in women experiencing an improvement in psoriasis during pregnancy. However, this does not hold true for moderate-to-severe psoriasis where safe and effective treatment is explicitly required.

Change in Psoriasis Treatment during Pregnancy

Treatment of psoriasis is changed during pregnancy. Generally patients stop all medications during pregnancy. In a study it was observed that 52% women were using topical treatment, which was reduced to 9.4% in the third trimester. Similarly, the use of systemic drugs was also reduced from 5.9% before pregnancy to 2.5% in the third trimester.

Effect of Psoriasis Treatment on Pregnancy

Inadvertent fetal exposure to psoriasis therapies depends upon the treatment taken, duration, and period of pregnancy during the treatment. As teratogenic drugs such as acitretin and methotrexate even for shorter duration can lead to various fetal malformations, while relatively safe drugs such as corticosteroids, ciclosporin, and biologics given for longer duration can lead to prematurity and low birth weight babies. So, moderate-to-severe psoriasis in pregnancy need to be managed meticulously.

Effect of Psoriasis on Mode of Delivery

Timing or mode of delivery is not usually affected by presence of psoriasis. However psoriasis can localize into scars or incision site (Koebner's phenomenon). The risk of infection is theoretically higher due to staphylococcal colonization of psoriatic plaques without any clinical signs of infection and wound healing of cesarean section is also delayed; however, no studies have assessed this risk.

- Pregnancy should be planned when psoriasis is mild and systemic drugs have been withdrawn.
- Treatment of psoriasis need to be changed in pregnancy depending upon the safety of drugs.
- Some psoriatic drugs are teratogenic while others can lead to prematurity and low birth weight babies.
- Psoriasis does not affect mode and time of delivery.

Treatment of psoriasis during pregnancy and the Food and Drug Administration (FDA) category of drugs **(Table 1)** are described here.

TABLE 1: The Food and Drug Administration (FDA) pregnancy categories of antipsoriatic agents.

Recommended minimum systemic drug-free interval before conception
Methotrexate: 3 months (men and women)
Retinoids: 2 years (women only)

Category	Antipsoriatic drugs	Description
A	Moisturizers and emollients	Adequate and well-controlled studies have failed to demonstrate a risk to the fetus in the first or later trimesters of pregnancy
B	Systemic biologic drugs: Infliximab, adalimumab, etanercept, ustekinumab	Animal studies have failed to demonstrate a risk to the fetus, but no adequate and well-controlled studies in pregnant women
C	• Topical drugs: Anthralin, calcipotriene, corticosteroids, tretinoin • Systemic drugs: Cyclosporine, corticosteroids • Psoralens plus ultraviolet A (PUVA) phototherapy	Animal studies have shown an adverse effect on the fetus, however, no adequate and well-controlled studies in humans, but potential benefits may warrant use of the drug in pregnancy despite potential risks
D	—	Positive evidence of human fetal risk based on adverse reaction data from studies in humans, but potential benefits may warrant use of the drug in pregnant women despite potential risks
X	• Topical drugs: Tazarotene • Systemic drugs: Acitretin and methotrexate	Positive evidence of human fetal risk based on adverse reaction data and demonstration of fetal abnormalities; the risks involved in use of the drug in pregnancy clearly outweigh potential benefits
N	Coal tar and narrowband ultraviolet B (NB-UVB) phototherapy	FDA has not classified the drug

Topical Therapy

Topical therapy is recommended as the first-line treatment option during pregnancy. It is prudent to use emollients and moisturizers for limited disease being safest and well tolerated.

Topical Corticosteroids (FDA Category C)

Low- to moderate-potency corticosteroids are the preferred over high-potency during second and third trimesters. As the risks associated with high-potency topical steroids if applied on large body surface area (BSA) may parallel to those observed with oral steroids due to increased chances of systemic absorption. In pregnancy, there is an alteration in skin hydration and blood flow, thus changing the bioavailability of topical corticosteroids.

Cutaneous absorption of corticosteroids also depends on various factors, including dosage, surface area to be treated, vehicle used, site of application, duration of treatment, occlusive dressings, and frequency of applications. The extent of absorption also increases in inflamed and/or damaged skin. Hydrocortisone, the lowest-strength corticosteroid, can even cause adrenal suppression if applied over inflamed skin.

Fetal effects of corticosteroids depend upon transplacental passage which is further dependent on activity of enzyme 11-hydroxy dehydrogenase. This enzyme is expressed in large quantities in the placenta and inactivates the topical corticosteroid. Fluorinated corticosteroids such as fluticasone propionate and betamethasone are not metabolized by this enzyme, thus reach the fetus in high concentrations. Cleft lip and growth restriction has been associated with the use of very high potency corticosteroids; however, some authors have suggested inconclusive evidence of cleft lip after corticosteroid application, regardless of potency.

Nevertheless, guidelines recommend use of high potency corticosteroids for as short a time as possible with appropriate monitoring.

Other Topical Agents

Topical Salicylic Acid (FDA Pregnancy Category C)

No studies demonstrated the use of topical salicylic acid in pregnancy. Premature ductus arteriosus constriction and agnathia-otocephaly syndrome was associated with topical salicylic acid use in pregnancy.

Anthralin (FDA Category C)

No animals or humans studies have been conducted with anthralin in pregnancy. Anthralin should be stopped 4 weeks before conception.

Tazarotene (FDA Category X)

Tazarotene is effective in mild-to-moderate plaque psoriasis when used in concentration between 0.05 and 0.1%. Adapalene or tretinoin are classified as category C drugs, while tazarotene is labeled as category X. Bioavailability of tazarotene after topical application is 1–5%, which is much lower and hence the teratogenicity is less compared to oral retinoids, reaching blood levels up to 100 times higher.

Calcipotriol (FDA Category C)

There is increased incidence of skeletal abnormalities and incomplete ossification of fetal bones exposed to calcipotriol.

Coal Tar (No FDA Pregnancy Category)

Studies have reported increased risk of spontaneous abortions and some risk of congenital malformation after coal tar use in pregnancy, so coal tar use should be limited during second and third trimesters and avoided in first trimester of pregnancy.

Tacrolimus (FDA Category C)

Tacrolimus is an immunosuppressive agent but no tendency to cause skin atrophy, so it has become a key corticosteroid-sparing agent. It is mainly used in facial and intertriginous forms of the psoriasis. Safety of tacrolimus in pregnancy is still understudied. Absorption of tacrolimus is less as compared to corticosteroids as seen in atopic dermatitis patients, and even repeated use over extensive areas showed undetectable levels in the blood and even the systemic use of tacrolimus in transplant patients who later become pregnant did not showed evidence of congenital malformation. The earlier-mentioned findings suggest that topical tacrolimus is a safe in pregnancy particularly over facial and intertriginous lesions.

Phototherapy Ultraviolet B Radiation (No FDA Pregnancy Category)

Narrowband ultraviolet B (NB-UVB) phototherapy has immunosuppressive and antiproliferative effect. Though NB-UVB (311–313 nm) has slightly inferior results in psoriasis as compared to psoralen plus ultraviolet A (PUVA) therapy; however, NB-UVB is safer modality. Psoralens have been enlisted as the FDA pregnancy category C drug. Ferreira et al. reported reduction in serum folate levels in psoriatic women treated with NB-UVB therapy. This reduction in folate levels is associated with NB-UVB induced hyperthermia and so, it is better avoided during the first 28 days of gestation. NB-UVB doubles the risk of low folate levels and thereby increased chances of neural tube defects. So it is recommended to measure serum folate levels before initiation of NB-UVB phototherapy and monitoring serum folate levels throughout treatment along with supplementation of folic acid at 5 mg daily dose. Studies have shown good response to NB-UVB in generalized pustular psoriasis in third trimester not responding to topical corticosteroids.

Systemic Traditional Medications

Systemic Corticosteroids (FDA Category C)

The use of systemic corticosteroids during pregnancy has been associated with certain congenital abnormalities and premature birth. Various studies have shown a statistically significant association of prednisone exposure during first trimester of pregnancy with premature birth, low birth weight, and various congenital abnormalities. Use of weekly doses of betamethasone during second trimester of pregnancy has been associated with higher rates of low birth weight babies and attention problems at 2 years of age.

Acitretin (FDA Category X)

Acitretin use in pregnancy is found to be associated with various fetal malformations including cardiovascular anomalies, cranial and vertebral defects, meningomyelocele, facial, ankle, and shoulder and pelvic deformations, syndactyly, and phalangeal defects.

Ciclosporin (FDA Category C)

Ciclosporin is one of the first-line treatment modality of choice in pregnancy for moderate-to-severe psoriasis. Women exposed to ciclosporin during pregnancy observed no significant differences with the control population in terms of congenital malformations and fetal death; however, there are chances of increased rate of low birth weight and premature babies. Ciclosporin can also result in fetal damage due to adverse effects such as hypertension and nephrotoxicity. As ciclosporin affects T-cell development, children exposed to ciclosporin in utero may have malfunctioning of T, B, and natural killer cell which may last up to the first year of life. So, cyclosporine should be prohibited during pregnancy unless potential maternal benefits outweigh the fetal risks.

Methotrexate (FDA Category X)

Exposure to methotrexate during pregnancy may lead to transplacental passage from mother and damage to embryo. Minimum weekly dose of 10 mg/week is sufficient to cause fetal methotrexate syndrome during 6–8 weeks of pregnancy.

Apremilast (FDA Category C)

Human data regarding the use of apremilast in pregnancy is not present till date. However, animal studies have shown dose-related abortions and low birth weight. Currently, apremilast use is prohibited during pregnancy.

Hydroxyurea

There is limited data available on the use of hydroxyurea in pregnancy so, its use in pregnancy is advised to be prohibited by manufacturers.

Fumaric Acid Esters

Fumaric acid esters are widely used in Europe particularly Germany as systemic treatment for psoriasis. There are no studies in pregnancy so they should be used cautiously on a case by case basis.

Biologic Therapy (FDA Category B)

The use of biologic therapy during pregnancy is still enigmatic, as data obtained is mainly from case reports and retrospective, observational studies in the absence of clinical trial in pregnancy due to ethical reasons.

The US FDA and the European Medicines Agency have not yet demonstrated the safety profile of biologic therapy in pregnancy. There is very little experience of biologics in psoriasis during pregnancy and most of the data available is obtained from rheumatoid arthritis and inflammatory bowel disease.

Exposure to biologic treatment can be unintentional in early pregnancy or intentional occurring due to severe refractory disease.

Maternal immunoglobulin G (IgG) antibodies transport is established via Fc receptors (FcRn) on the syncytiotrophoblast, which are expressed in the second trimester of pregnancy (not <14 weeks) and rapidly increases during the third trimester. Transport is dependent on the IgG subtype in the following sequence: IgG1 > IgG4 > IgG3 > IgG2. IgG1 subtype which include infliximab, adalimumab, secukinumab, ustekinumab, guselkumab, risankizumab, tildrakizumab, and bimekizumab is the most easily transported, followed in sequence by IgG4 (ixekizumab), IgG3, and IgG2 (brodalumab). Etanercept, a fusion protein is exception due to its low affinity to FcRn. Certolizumab pegol (CZP), a PEGylated humanized IgG1 antibody, in which the Fab fragment is linked to polyethylene glycol (PEG), hampers placental transfer.

As explained earlier, TNF-α may have dual and paradoxical role in prevention of structural anomalies during embryogenesis. Apparently, TNF-α inhibitors during pregnancy may raise concerns to the fetus. However, no substantial adverse effect to fetus is reported after use of etanercept, infliximab, and adalimumab.

According to the Centers for Disease Control and Prevention (CDC) guidelines administration of live-attenuated vaccines should be delayed to full-term infants exposed to biologics during pregnancy until circulating drug levels were no longer detectable (at least 6 months of age). Disseminated tuberculosis is reported in a 3 months aged child after administration of Bacillus Calmette-Guérin (BCG) whose mother received infliximab for Crohn's disease. The long-term consequences of biologic exposure on the immune systems of newborns are currently unknown. Therefore, it is recommended to stop biologic therapy at 30 weeks of gestation.

Anti-tumor Necrosis Factor Biologic Agents

Tumor necrosis factor being a multifunctional cytokine is responsible for the regulation of hormone synthesis, placenta, and embryo development. Increased levels of TNF-α is known to play a significant role in inflammation and hormone mediated fetal damage and infertility. Two recently published observational cohort studies found anti-TNF agents to be effective and reliable in patients with recurrent miscarriages and infertility. As explained earlier, TNF plays an important role in the immune system development; there are chances of it being interfered by anti-TNF-α agents in newborns exposed to these agents during pregnancy.

Infliximab

No cases of congenital malformations or intrauterine growth restriction are seen with infliximab; however, premature birth and low birth weight are reported.

Adalimumab

No evidence of congenital malformations or pregnancy-related complications is reported in adalimumab use in isolated cases in pregnancy.

Etanercept

No evidence of congenital malformation or maternal or fetal toxicity is reported in patients treated with etanercept during pregnancy.

Certolizumab

Certolizumab pegol having unique structure due to absence of Fc portion is not transferred through placenta causing lower fetal exposure as compared to other TNF-α inhibitors. Pregnancies exposed to CZP during all three trimesters, delivered live births with no discernible major congenital malformations or other pregnancy-associated complications.

IL-12/23 Inhibitors

There is very little information on ustekinumab use during pregnancy in psoriasis. No fetal adverse effects were reported in animal studies; however, contradictory data on humans shows increase in spontaneous abortion after exposure to ustekinumab.

IL-17 and IL-23 Inhibitors

Secukinumab (FDA pregnancy category B) and ixekizumab (FDA category N) target cytokine IL-17A, whilst brodalumab is IL-17 receptor blocker (FDA category N). Tildrakizumab and guselkumab acts by selectively inhibiting IL-23 (FDA category N).

Isolated case reports have shown no adverse effects of secukinumab in pustular psoriasis in pregnancy. Till date, no controlled trials are done to demonstrate the safety of these agents on pregnancy.

So, among the earlier-mentioned treatment options during pregnancy for psoriasis, topical therapies should be the first line for mild disease with preference to emollients and moisturizers. Mild-to-moderate topical corticosteroids are used in limited disease, while in generalized moderate-to-severe psoriasis phototherapy with NV-UVB is the treatment of choice during pregnancy. Patients, refractory to topical therapies and phototherapy, may require systemic agents to achieve disease control. Anti-TNF-α treatment, being the FDA category B drugs, appears to be the safest considering lack of evidence of teratogenicity, embryotoxicity, or foetotoxicity. However, understudies or under reported domain of long-term effects of these agents on the immune system need further clarification. So, in this scenario systemic corticosteroids remains the systemic agent of choice, especially in case of generalized pustular psoriasis followed by cyclosporine in nonresponders and biologics to be given in resistant cases only. Treatment can usually be quickly tapered postpartum.

- Mild psoriasis—topical corticosteroids.
- Moderate-to-severe psoriasis—NB-UVB is the first-line agent.
- Biologics though category B drugs but long-term safety in newborn not known.
- Corticosteroid and cyclosporine in nonresponders are the systemic agents of choice.

SUGGESTED READINGS

1. Vena GA, Cassano N, Bellia G, Colombo D. Psoriasis in pregnancy: challenges and solutions. Psoriasis (Auckl). 2015;5:83-95.
2. Ferrer-Alcala MA, Sánchez-Díaz M, Arias-Santiago S, Molina-Leyva A. Impact of psoriasis and hidradenitis suppurativa in pregnancy, a systematic review. J Clin Med. 2021;10:5894.
3. Kimball AB, Guenther L, Kalia S, Elkem G, Jong J, Lafferty KP, et al. Pregnancy outcomes in women with moderate-to-severe psoriasis from the psoriasis longitudinal assessment and registry (PSOLAR). JAMA Dermatol. 2021;157(3):301-6.
4. Broms G, Haerskjold A, Granath F, Kieler H, Pedersen L, Berglind IA. Effect of maternal psoriasis on pregnancy and birth outcomes: A population-based cohort study from Denmark and Sweden. Acta Derm Venereol. 2018;98:728-34.
5. Ferreira C, Azevedo A, Nogueira M, Torres T. Management of psoriasis in pregnancy—a review of the evidence to date. Drugs Context. 2020;9:2019-11-6.
6. Weatherhead S, Robson SC, Reynolds NJ. Management of psoriasis in pregnancy. BMJ. 2007;334:1218-20.
7. Ceovic R, Lipozencic J, Aida Pasic A, Kostovic K. Psoriasis in Pregnancy: A review of most important literature data. Acta Dermatovenerol Croat. 2009;17(3):193-7.
8. Ruiz V, Manubens E, Puig L. Psoriasis in pregnancy: A review (II). Actas Dermosifiliogr. 2014;105(9):813-21.
9. Owczarek W, Walecka I, Lesiak A, Czajkowski R, Reich A, Zerda I, et al. The use of biological drugs in psoriasis patients prior to pregnancy, during pregnancy and lactation: a review of current clinical guidelines. Postepy Dermatol Alergol. 2020;37:821-30.
10. Sanchez-Garcia V, Hernandez-Quiles R, de-Miguel-Balsa E, Gimenez-Richarte A, Ramos-Rincon JM, Belinchon-Romero I. Exposure to biologic therapy before and during pregnancy in patients with psoriasis: Systematic review and meta-analysis. J EurAcad Dermatol Venereol. 2023;37:1971-90.

CHAPTER 4

Autoimmune Connective Tissue Diseases and Pregnancy

4.1 Systemic Lupus Erythematosus in Pregnancy

Sanjeev Gupta, Nikita Gupta, Sunita Gupta

INTRODUCTION

Systemic lupus erythematosus (SLE) is a chronic inflammatory autoimmune disease affecting multiple organs and tissues which is characterized by period of relapse and remission. Multiple organs may be involved but musculoskeletal system, renal, and skin are most frequently affected system. Immunologic irregularities, such as the production of antinuclear antibodies (ANA), are also characteristic of the SLE. The accumulation of antigen-antibody complexes and impaired adaptive immune response are thought to be the main pathological abnormalities of SLE, leading to severe autoimmune reactions and organ damage. SLE primarily affects females more frequently than males, and due to its onset usually in young individuals, pregnancy is commonly encountered among patients with the condition. It has been noted that SLE does not decrease the fertility rate in female, but reduces the chances of successful pregnancy.

Pregnant women diagnosed with SLE are at increased risk for experiencing adverse pregnancy outcomes (APOs), which includes both maternal and fetal-neonatal complications. Maternal complications include occurrences such as lupus aggravated kidney injury, preeclampsia, hypertension, and venous embolism. Fetal complications associated with SLE pregnancies include abortion, preterm birth, intrauterine growth retardation (IUGR) of neonate, heart block, and neonatal lupus erythematosus. These conditions collectively contribute to the increased challenges and risks faced by pregnant women with SLE, necessitating close monitoring and specialized care throughout pregnancy. Advancements in medicine have led to improved pregnancy outcomes, achieving successful live births. Effective management requires a coordinated multidisciplinary approach involving the expertise of various healthcare professionals and vigilant monitoring throughout pregnancy. This chapter focuses on addressing critical issues and guiding principles for physicians managing pregnant women diagnosed with SLE.

EPIDEMIOLOGY

Systemic lupus erythematosus complicates around 1 in 250 to 1 in 1,500 pregnancies, depending on the population studied. The overall prevalence of SLE in women of reproductive age ranges from 20 to 150 per 100,000 women.

IMMUNOPATHOPHYSOLOGICAL CHANGES OF PREGNANCY DURING SLE

There is complex interplay of physiological and immunological changes and also heterogeneity of disease in SLE pregnancy **(Fig. 1)**.

There are some genes associated with increased susceptibility to SLE that have been identified on the chromosome X which include TLR7, Foxp3, IRAK1, and CD40 ligand. Additionally, estrogen influences various immune responses such as B cell development, antibody generation, Th2 responses, and the persistence of autoreactive cells.

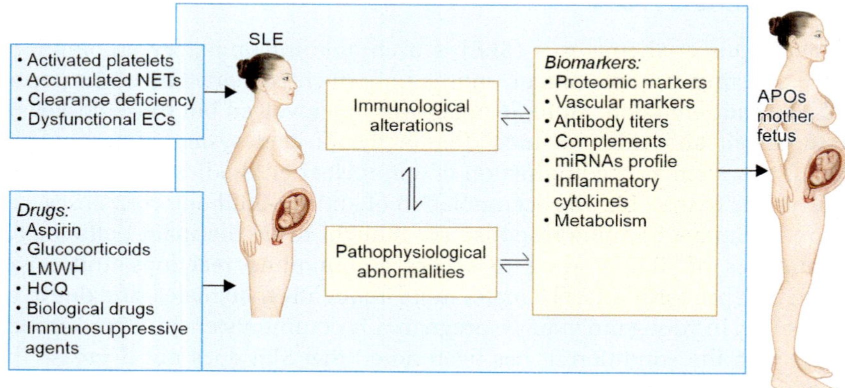

FIG. 1: Etiopathogenesis of systemic lupus erythematosus (SLE). SLE triggers specific immunologic and pathophysiological changes that generate biomarkers useful for predicting adverse pregnancy outcomes (APOs) in both the mother and fetus. Key predictors often include metabolic markers, antibody levels, miRNA profiles, complement levels, angiogenic and antiangiogenic biomarkers, proteomic markers, and inflammatory cytokines. These predictors, along with pathological and immunological abnormalities, can accelerate SLE progression and worsen APOs. During pregnancy with lupus, issues such as impaired clearance of dead cells, accumulation of neutrophil extracellular traps (NETs), activated platelets, and dysfunctional endothelial cells can further exacerbate APOs. Currently, treatments such as hydroxychloroquine (HCQ), immunosuppressive agents, aspirin, glucocorticoids, low-molecular-weight heparin (LMWH), and biologic drugs targeting B cells are commonly used to manage SLE activity and mitigate related APOs.

PHYSIOLOGICAL CHANGES IN SLE PREGNANCY

Normal pregnancy causes an increase in intravascular volume in women, which can result in hypercoagulability, the development of thromboembolism, and the release of cytokines and fibrinogen during inflammation. On the other hand, SLE-associated APOs are initiated by these changes.

Key pathophysiological changes associated with SLE during pregnancy include symptoms such as ulcers in the nasal or oral mucosa, photosensitive skin rashes, and hematological abnormalities like hemolytic anemia, leukopenia, lymphopenia, and thrombocytopenia. Additionally, inflammatory arthritis, elevated anti-dsDNA antibodies, proteinuria, active urinary sediment, fluctuating complement levels, and serositis are observed during this period. Among above listed factors, fluctuating level of serum complement and increased anti-dsDNA antibody levels represent serum markers of disease aggravation in SLE pregnant female. Specifically, there are similarities in the symptoms of SLE flares, preeclampsia, eclampsia, hemolysis, elevated liver enzymes, and low platelet count (HELLP) syndrome. As a result, it is unreliable to differentiate between SLE flares based only on the pathophysiological abnormalities mentioned above.

IMMUNOLOGICAL CHANGES IN SLE PREGNANCY

During pregnancy, achieving immune homeostasis is crucial to protect the fetus from maternal immune responses. A key immunological change is the shift in T helper cell polarization toward either of Th1 or Th2 cells, which is influenced by elevated level of estrogen.

The Th-1 cells predominantly produce proinflammatory cytokines such as interferon-gamma (IFN-γ), interleukin-12 (IL-12), tumor necrosis factor-alpha (TNF-α), and interleukin-2 (IL-2), which are initially important for placental development but may become detrimental later, potentially leading to pregnancy loss. In pregnant women with SLE, increased estrogen levels promote IFN-γ secretion while suppressing TNF-α production.

The Th2 cells, on the other hand, secrete anti-inflammatory cytokines like IL-4, IL-10, and IL-13, supporting humoral immunity. IL-10, in particular, suppresses proinflammatory cytokine production by Th1 cells and macrophages during pregnancy.

Regulatory T cells (Treg), crucial for immune suppression and tolerance maintenance, are elevated in early stage of pregnancy to prevent maternal immune responses. However, in female with SLE pregnancy and dysbiosis of the gut microbiome, there is a decrease in Treg cells and an increase in Th17 cells, exacerbating autoimmune activation and contributing to APOs and recurrent pregnancy loss. Overall, it is important to maintain a balance among Th1/Th2 and Th17/Treg cells, along with normal immune cell functions, to mitigate autoimmunity-mediated inflammation and decrease the incidence of SLE-related APOs during pregnancy **(Fig. 2)**.

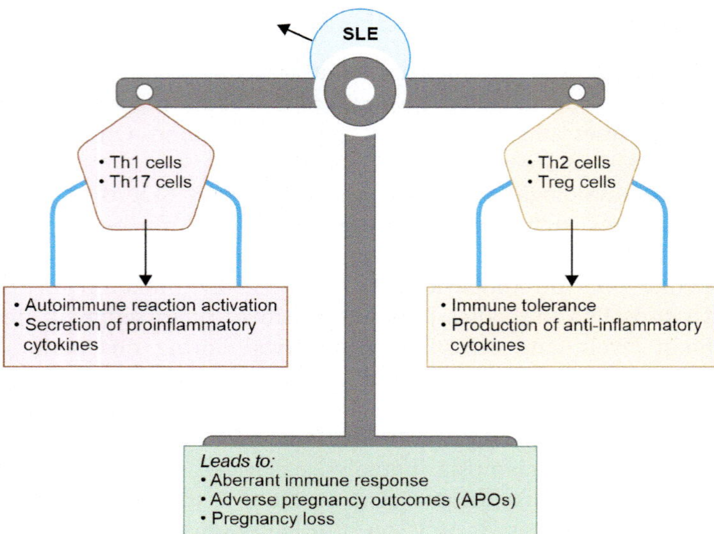

FIG. 2: In systemic lupus erythematosus, there is an imbalance in immune cell populations. Specifically, Th1 and Th17 cells are elevated, while Th2 and Treg cells are decreased as the disease progresses. The increase in Th1 and Th17 cells leads to heightened autoimmune activation and the release of proinflammatory cytokines. Conversely, the reduction in Th2 and Treg cells impairs immune tolerance and decreases the production of anti-inflammatory cytokines. This imbalance exacerbates abnormal immune responses, accelerates adverse pregnancy outcomes (APOs), and can contribute to pregnancy loss.

(SLE: systemic lupus erythematosus)

DISEASE ACTIVITY DURING PREGNANCY

Effect of SLE on Fertility

The fertility of couples, defined as their ability to conceive, is generally estimated to be between 20 and 30% per month in humans. Unexplained infertility affects 10% of infertile couples on average. One of the many reasons for the same may be due to autoimmune illness (SLE and antiphospholipid syndrome). SLE presents significant challenges during pregnancy, as noted by studies emphasizing the importance of family planning soon after diagnosis. While many women with SLE can have successful pregnancies with careful management, the condition unpredictably complicates maternal and fetal outcomes, as highlighted by obstetric data indicating increased risks of miscarriage, preterm birth, and cesarean delivery among SLE patients. Research underscores the emotional and physical toll of navigating pregnancies with SLE, including increased risks of hypertension, arthritis, and lupus flares, which contribute to prolonged hospital stays and personal distress. Understanding and support from partners are crucial for patients managing both fertility issues and the complexities of SLE-related pregnancies, as they face ongoing challenges that impact their quality of life and emotional well-being.

Effect of Pregnancy on SLE

The likelihood of SLE exacerbation increases during pregnancy, with reported flare rates ranging from 25 to 65%. There are various risk factors associated with flare during pregnancy like:

- Active SLE disease within the 6 months prior to conception
- Active lupus nephritis (LN)
- Serious underlying medical disease
- Cessation of drug hydroxychloroquine (HCQ)

Various organ systems respond differently to pregnancy; for instance, musculoskeletal flares are less frequent, whereas hematologic and renal flares are more prevalent. The majority of pregnancy-related flares in SLE are mild-to-moderate in severity, with only a small percentage of patients experiencing severe flares. Physiological pregnancy changes that may mimic exacerbation of disease flare. In order to manage flare of SLE in pregnancy, we need to recognize features of pregnancy and SLE as they are quite overlapping **(Table 1)**.

So, pregnancy can affect the activity of SLE while concurrently, SLE can impact outcomes of pregnancy.

MATERNAL AND FETAL COMPLICATIONS OF SLE IN PREGNANCY

Systemic lupus erythematosus poses significant risks during pregnancy, impacting both maternal health and fetal outcomes. It can lead to fertility issues

TABLE 1: Differentiation of physiological pregnancy changes from SLE flare.

Characteristic findings	Changes related to pregnancy	Flare in SLE
Cutaneous	• Facial flushing • Palmar erythema • Postpartum loss of hair	• Photosensitive rash • Nasal or oral ulcer
Musculoskeletal	• Myalgia • Arthralgia	Arthritis (inflammatory)
Immunological	Level of complement is high	• Complement levels falls • Anti-DNA levels rise
Hematologic	• Anemia (mild) • Thrombocytopenia (mild)	• Immune hemolytic anemia • Thrombocytopenia • Leukopenia • Lymphopenia
Renal	Proteinuria (physiologic) <300 mg/day	• Proteinuria >300 mg/day • Active urinary sediment
Other findings	• Edema (mild) • Resting dyspnea (mild) • Fatigue	• Pleuritis • Lymphadenopathy • Fever

(SLE: systemic lupus erythematosus)

and complicate pregnancies, resulting in complications such as preterm labor, preeclampsia, placental insufficiency, abortion, stillbirth, whereas in neonate, there are increased mortality risks and preterm birth. Additionally, SLE-related antibodies can cause neonatal lupus in babies, a condition that may contribute to structural abnormalities. Overall, SLE presents serious risks for both the mother and fetus, potentially leading to fatal outcomes and numerous complications.

Maternal Complication

Pre-eclampsia

Preeclampsia affects 16–30% of pregnancies in women with SLE, presenting a 3–5 times higher risk compared to the general population. It is one of most common complications in SLE. Risk factors for preeclampsia include old maternal age, preexisting comorbidities like hypertension, obesity or diabetes, and family history of the disease. In SLE, additional specific risk factors include past history or present active LN, presence of antiphospholipid antibodies, decreasing complement levels, and thrombocytopenia.

One of the significant clinical challenges is distinguishing between a flare of SLE and preeclampsia, especially given that up to 20% of pregnancies in women with lupus are affected by preeclampsia. This differentiation is crucial because preeclampsia requires immediate delivery, while an SLE flare necessitates immunosuppressive treatment. Although both conditions can lead to hypertension and proteinuria, urinalysis findings in preeclampsia typically show less active sediment compared to SLE flares. Thrombocytopenia is common in both conditions, but elevated liver function tests are indicative of preeclampsia **(Table 2)**. Ultrasonography, particularly assessing abnormal uterine artery waveforms, has proven to be a valuable diagnostic tool for early identification.

TABLE 2: Differences between lupus nephritis and preeclampsia.

Laboratory and clinical features	Preeclampsia	Lupus nephritis
Platelets	Low to normal	Low to normal
Complements	Normal to low	Low
Anti-dsDNA antibody	Absent or remain unchanged	Increasing levels
Hypertension	After 20W of pregnancy	Can occur at any time
Serum creatinine	Normal to elevated	Normal to elevated
Serum uric acid	Increased (>5.5 mg/dL)	Normal
Urinary sediments	Inactive	Active
24-hour urinary calcium	Below 195 mg/dL	Above 195 mg/dL
Other organs involvement	Sometimes CNS or HELLP syndrome	Evidence of active nonrenal SLE
Response to steroids therapy	No	Yes

(HELLP: hemolysis, elevated liver enzymes, and low platelets; SLE: systemic lupus erythematosus)

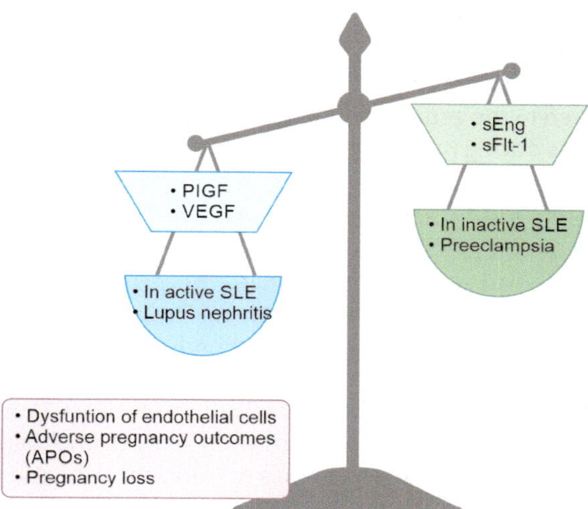

FIG. 3: In systemic lupus erythematosus (SLE), angiogenic factor levels exhibit specific alterations. In active SLE and lupus nephritis (LN), there is an increase in VEGF and PlGF, while sFlt-1 and sEng levels are decreased. Conversely, elevated levels of sFlt-1 and sEng are typically seen in preeclampsia and inactive SLE. These variations in serum levels of VEGF, PlGF, sEng, and sFlt-1 can lead to endothelial cell dysfunction, contribute to the development of adverse pregnancy outcomes (APOs), and even result in pregnancy loss.

(VEGF: vascular endothelial growth factor; sFlt-1: soluble fms-like tyrosinekinase-1; PlGF: placental growth factor; sEng: soluble endoglin)

During pregnancy, distinguishing between preeclampsia and active LN can be achieved by assessing specific biomarkers. Pregnant women with active LN typically exhibit elevated levels of vascular endothelial growth factor (VEGF), whereas those with preeclampsia show an increased ratio of soluble fms-like tyrosine kinase-1 (sFlt-1) to placental growth factor (PlGF). This distinction highlights the utility of serum VEGF, PlGF, and sFlt-1 levels as diagnostic markers to differentiate between these two conditions in pregnant women **(Fig. 3)**.

Hypothyroidism

There are many studies that have linked subclinical hypothyroidism and thyroid antibody positivity in euthyroid women to miscarriage and premature birth. Elevated thyroid-stimulating hormone (TSH) levels within the normal range during pregnancy increase the likelihood of unfavorable outcomes, including abortion and fetal or neonatal death. Minor thyroid function changes have been associated with breech presentations at term, higher rates of cesarean sections, and potential impacts on offspring intelligence. Treatment with levothyroxine in thyroid peroxidase antibody-positive pregnant women with elevated TSH levels has shown to decrease adverse outcomes. Postpartum thyroiditis affects a significant proportion of women, especially those with type 1 diabetes mellitus. In SLE-affected women, active disease and presence of antiphospholipid antibodies further elevate the risk of miscarriage and preterm delivery, with children often requiring intensive care due to complications like heart block. Mortality rates are also higher among pregnant women with SLE. Additionally, hypothyroidism and autoimmune thyroid disease are more prevalent in women with SLE compared to the general population, highlighting the complex interplay of these conditions during pregnancy and the need for vigilant management.

Neurological Complications

Central nervous system (CNS) complications in pregnant women with SLE are infrequent but can lead to severe outcomes. The neurological manifestations of SLE are complex and multifaceted, involving diverse pathogenic processes. These include the presence of various autoantibodies such as antiphospholipid, antineuronal, anti-P, antiendothelial, and others, as well as inflammatory byproducts like complement or platelet activation products. Antiphospholipid antibodies, known for their role in thrombosis in arteries and veins, particularly affect cerebral circulation, leading to strokes or transient ischemic attacks (TIAs). Neurological symptoms in SLE span a spectrum from mild issues like headaches and cognitive impairment to severe conditions such as memory loss, seizures, and stroke, which can be life-threatening. Treatment options for neurologic manifestations often target coagulopathy-related symptoms, yet the cognitive and emotional dimensions remain poorly understood. Diagnostic approaches for CNS disorders typically involve brain imaging and also evaluating cerebrospinal fluid and performing electroencephalography.

Lupus Nephritis

Lupus nephritis represents a critical complication of SLE, with substantial implications for pregnancy. It is one of the most prevalent and potentially fatal side effects of SLE, which impairs fertility and raises mortality rates. Clinical manifestations can include proteinuria, microscopic hematuria, and renal failure. Active renal disease is characterized by >500 milligram of proteinuria per day or a glomerular filtration rate (GFR) below 60 mL/min/1.73 m^2 in nonpregnant individuals. Kidney involvement is present in about one-third of patients when SLE is diagnosed, and eventually, renal issues affect 50% of those with SLE. Inflammation, complement activation, and deposition of immune complexes contribute to kidney damage in this condition. Women who already have kidney disease before pregnancy face about a 16% risk of developing active nephritis during pregnancy.

Laboratory features of LN include:

- Elevated level of anti-dsDNA antibodies
- Decreased complement level
- Increased level of serum creatinine
- Urinary red cell cast present

Gold standard test for diagnosis of LN is renal biopsy.

Hematological Complications

Blood-related complications include anemia, leukopenia, and thrombocytopenia.

Anemia can be iron deficiency, hemolytic or anemia of chronic disease. Leukopenia occurs secondary to lymphopenia or neutropenia. It may be due to disease activity, infection, or due to drug toxicity of immunosuppressant drugs. Thrombocytopenia occurs in approximately 25% of pregnancies in women with SLE and arises from the immune-mediated breakdown of platelets. Risk factors include prior history of low platelet count, the presence of antiphospholipid (aPL) antibodies, and increased activity of disease.

Antiphospholipid Syndrome

Antiphospholipid syndrome (APS) can occur independently or alongside SLE or other autoimmune disorders. It is characterized by persistent presence of antiphospholipid antibodies (such as anti-β2 glycoprotein I, anticardiolipin antibodies, and lupus anticoagulant) with previous history of thromboembolic events.

It manifests in two main forms—thrombotic APS (T-APS) and obstetric APS (OB-APS).

Thrombotic APS is characterized by recurrent arterial or venous thromboses occurring in any tissue or organ.

Obstetric APS, on the other hand, includes specific obstetric complications:

- Three or more consecutive spontaneous abortions before 10 weeks of gestation.
- One or more unexplained fetal losses occurring after 10 weeks of gestation.
- One or more premature births of a morphologically normal neonate before 34 weeks of gestation due to eclampsia or preeclampsia. Diagnosis requires the presence of aPL on more than two occasions, separated by at least 12 weeks.

Antiphospholipid syndrome management in SLE:

- The ACR Reproductive Health Guidelines state that healthy individuals without SLE, who have antiphospholipid antibodies (aPL) but no history of thrombosis or pregnancy complications, do not require prophylactic therapy to prevent pregnancy loss. However, the guidelines conditionally recommend daily low-dose aspirin (81–100 mg) in such cases.
- For women diagnosed with obstetric antiphospholipid syndrome (APS), the guidelines recommend combining low-dose aspirin with prophylactic doses of heparin (low-molecular weight heparin).
- During the vulnerable postpartum period (6–12 weeks), anticoagulation therapy is continued due to the increased risk of clotting. Pregnant women diagnosed with thrombotic APS (T-APS) should receive aspirin and therapeutic dose heparin throughout pregnancy and the postpartum period.
- Hydroxychloroquine may potentially lower the risk of thrombosis and improve pregnancy outcomes associated with APS.

Fetal Outcomes

Adverse Pregnancy Outcome

In pregnancies among women with SLE, the most common issues are preterm births and their associated health challenges. Thyroid disorders further increase the risk of preterm delivery in these pregnancies. Additionally, approximately 10–30% of pregnancies in women with SLE experience complications such as fetal growth restriction and babies born small for their gestational age.

There are biomarkers for predicting APOs in patients with SLE. These biomarkers encompass immunological, metabolic, angiogenic, complement-related, inflammatory, proteomic, and miRNA-related factors that contribute to predicting adverse outcomes in pregnant women with SLE **(Table 3)**.

Fetal Mortality

Most prevalent complication is pregnancy loss which affects about 16.5% pregnancies. There could be an association between SLE activity, kidney disease, antiphospholipid antibodies, and the chances of fetal loss in SLE. Pregnancy outcomes are poor in people with active nephritis. Although pregnancy loss is only 10% common in people with mild renal illness, it is around 60% more in people with moderate-to-severe nephritis.

Preterm Birth

Preterm birth is defined as delivery before 37 weeks of gestation and presents significant risks in pregnancies complicated by SLE. Studies indicate that SLE patients experience higher rates of preterm birth compared to the general population, with percentages varying depending on factors such as LN and disease activity during conception. Contributing factors include systemic inflammation and inadequate placental development, which can be exacerbated by conditions like LN. Hormonal imbalances, particularly lower levels of estradiol in SLE patients, also play a role in triggering premature labor. Additionally, medications such as oral prednisone used to manage SLE may contribute to the

TABLE 3: Biomarkers for prediction of APO.

Biomarker category	Biomarkers included	Role in prediction of APOs
Antibody levels	Anti-La/SSB, anti-Ro/SSA, anti-C1q, anti-dsDNA antiphospholipid antibodies (aPL)	Correlate with pregnancy hypertension, premature birth
Metabolic changes	Lysophosphatidylcholine (lysoPC) C22:5, tryptophan, bile acids	Reflect metabolic dysregulation in SLE and APOs
Angiogenic and antiangiogenic factors	sFlt-1, PlGF, soluble endoglin (sEng), VEGF, IFN-α	Indicators of placental dysfunction and cardiovascular risk
Complement activation	C3, C4, sC5b-9, Bb	Reflects complement system dysregulation in SLE
Inflammatory cytokines	Interleukin-8 (IL-8), IP-10, IL-10, IL-1β, IFN-β, MIG	Elevated levels associated with SLE-related APOs
miRNAs pattern	miRNA-150, miRNA-145, miRNA-142-5p, miRNA-7, miRNA-155, miRNA-224	Dysregulated expression associated with SLE flares

(APO: adverse pregnancy outcome; PlGF: placental growth factor; sFlt-1: soluble fms-like tyrosinekinase-1; SLE: systemic lupus erythematosus; VEGF: vascular endothelial growth factor)

risk of preterm delivery, independent of their anti-inflammatory effects. Overall, the complex interplay of clinical and subclinical inflammation, autoimmune responses, hormonal disruptions, and therapeutic interventions underscores the increased vulnerability of SLE patients to preterm births.

Intrauterine Growth Retardation and Small for Gestational Age

Research found that the incidence of small for gestation age (SGA) was higher in the SLE pregnant group. However, birth weight and gestational age were lower in this group of SLE pregnant females because the pregnancy was carried to full-term with prenatal care for a variety of obstetric issues.

Mothers with lupus experience a worse perinatal outcome than healthy pregnant women. As a result, careful assessment of neonate and treatment of the baby is required, even if the pregnancy can be maintained until full-term by avoiding obstetrical complications that may arise during pregnancy and delivery.

Neonatal Lupus Erythematosus

- Neonatal lupus syndrome (NLS) results from passive transfer of maternal antibodies like anti-Ro and anti-La to the fetus, leading to symptoms like rash, liver issues, and blood abnormalities, all reflecting the presence of maternal antibodies in the neonate circulation. The rash in neonatal lupus is often described as erythematous and annular or plaque-like. The rash typically appears on the face, especially around the eyes, where it can create a "raccoon-eye" appearance or periorbital erythema. It can also affect the scalp, neck, and other sun-exposed areas of the body, such as the arms and upper torso. These symptoms typically resolve as the antibodies are cleared from the infant's system by 6–8 months of age. However, cardiac complications, caused by maternal antibodies affecting the fetal heart's conduction system, can result in permanent damage.
- In neonatal lupus, cardiac complications include conduction abnormalities, structural defects, cardiomyopathy, and congestive heart failure. The most common issue is congenital heart block (CHB), occurring in around 2% of infants born to mothers with anti-Ro antibodies during their first pregnancy. Subsequent pregnancies after the birth of an affected child have a significantly increased risk, increasing to approximately 16–20%.
- Given the serious risks associated with neonatal lupus, it is essential to educate pregnant women who test positive for anti-Ro/SSA antibodies about the potential complications.
- Additional risk factors include maternal hypothyroidism, higher levels of maternal antibodies, and fetal genetic variations.
- Fetal Doppler echocardiography is commonly used for monitoring, with recommended weekly assessments from 16 to 26 weeks of gestation due to the increased vulnerability during this period, followed by biweekly checks thereafter.
- Hydroxychloroquine is highly recommended for preventing APOs in SLE patients. It reduces the risk of neonatal lupus triggered by anti-Ro/SSA and anti-La/SSB antibodies, particularly transient rash and life-threatening

CHB. Intravenous immunoglobulin (IVIG) has shown promise in preventing antibody-mediated CHB by affecting multiple pathological processes. Type I interferons (IFNs) are crucial in CHB pathogenesis, promoting inflammatory responses and cardiac tissue damage in the fetus, suggesting potential for type I IFN inhibitors as a therapeutic strategy.

MANAGEMENT OF SLE IN PREGNANCY

Women with SLE disease still face high risk during pregnancy but due to recent advances, these patients can have successful pregnancies. Successful pregnancy outcomes benefit from thorough planning and vigilant monitoring of the patient throughout the entire process. It is crucial to adopt a multidisciplinary team approach involving obstetricians, rheumatologists, and neonatologists, ensuring comprehensive care from before conception to childbirth. EULAR recommendations for effective management of pregnant SLE female **(Table 4)**.

TABLE 4: EULAR recommendations.

Recommendation	
1. Preconception counseling and risk stratification	Counsel on SLE activity, lupus nephritis, serological activity, previous history of adverse pregnancy outcomes, aPL profile, history of vascular thrombosis in past SLE diagnosis, anti-Ro/SSA and/or anti-La/SSB and end-stage organ damage/comorbidities
2. Contraceptive measures	• Use effective contraception (oral, subcutaneous or IUDs) based on disease activity and risk of thrombosis • For all patients with SLE and/or APS who do not have any other gynecological contraindications, intrauterine devices can be recommended • In individuals with stable or inactive systemic lupus erythematosus (SLE) and negative antiphospholipid antibodies (aPL), combined hormonal contraceptives may be considered as a contraceptive option • Hormonal contraception (progesterone only) for pregnant women with positive aPL, whether or not they have a definitive APS, needs to be carefully considered against the risk of thrombosis
3 and 4. Fertility preservation	Discuss fertility issues; consider GnRH analogs for menstruating women receiving alkylating agents; safe use of assisted reproduction techniques
5. Assisted reproduction techniques (ARTs)	Assisted reproduction techniques (ARTs), such as ovulation induction treatments and in vitro fertilization protocols, were found to have comparable efficacy in women with SLE and/or APS as compared in the general population, and can be safely used in patients with stable/inactive disease
6. Predictive biomarkers for maternal disease activity	Evaluate disease activity; monitor renal function and serological markers during pregnancy

Continued

Continued

Recommendation	
7. Pregnancy monitoring	Use Doppler ultrasonography and biometric parameters in the third trimester for fetal surveillance; consider fetal echocardiography for suspected dysrhythmias
8. Drugs for prevention and management of SLE flares	HCQs, azathioprine, oral steroid, cyclosporine-A, and tacrolimus can be used to prevent or manage SLE flares during pregnancy. Moderate-to-severe flares of SLE pregnancy are managed with glucocorticoids IV pulse therapy, IVIG, and plasmapheresis. Mycophenolic acid (MMF) cyclophosphamide, leflunomide, and methotrexate are avoided
9 Adjunct treatment during pregnancy	• For patients with systemic lupus erythematosus (SLE), hydroxychloroquine is advised before conception and throughout pregnancy. Low-dose aspirin (LDA) is utilized to manage the risk of preeclampsia • Women with systemic lupus erythematosus (SLE) associated with antiphospholipid syndrome (APS) or primary APS are recommended to undergo combination therapy involving low-dose aspirin and heparin to reduce the likelihood of adverse pregnancy outcomes • Calcium, vitamin D, and folic acid should be offered as supplementation in the general population
10. Menopause	Consider hormone replacement therapy (HRT) for severe menopausal symptoms in stable/inactive disease; weigh risks in positive aPL cases
11. Screening for malignancies	Screen for malignancies similar to the general population; monitor cervical lesions; consider HPV immunization in stable/inactive disease
(GnRH: gonadotropin-releasing hormone; HCQ: hydroxychloroquine)	

Preconception evaluation and counseling are important part of management of SLE pregnancy **(Table 5)**.

There are some conditions which are high risk for pregnant mothers with SLE.

Pregnancy is not advisable in following situations:

Absolute contraindications:

- Severe pulmonary hypertension (systolic pulmonary artery pressure above 50 mm Hg)
- Advanced renal insufficiency (creatinine level greater than 2.8 mg/dL)
- Advanced heart failure
- Severe restrictive lung disease (forced vital capacity less than 1 L)
- History of previous severe preeclampsia or HELLP syndrome (hemolysis, elevated liver enzyme levels, low platelet count) despite treatment

Relative contraindications:

- Recent episode of stroke in the past 6 months
- Severe disease flare-up within last 6 months

TABLE 5: Preconception counseling and evaluation.	
Key question to be asked	Are you planning to become pregnant in the coming year?
Birth control discussion	Contraceptive methods are discussed if pregnancy is not wanted
Disease control measures	Ensure systemic lupus erythematosus is stable for at least last 6 months; pregnancy is delayed if disease remains moderate-to-severe in degree and birth control measures are discussed
Biomarker evaluation	Assess for antibodies like anti-Ro/SSA, anti-La/SSB, and lupus anticoagulant and antiphospholipid antibodies
Thyroid function testing	Perform thyroid function tests
Medication assessment	Review current medications for compatibility with pregnancy
Comorbidity assessment and management	Evaluate and manage concurrent conditions such as diabetes, hypertension, and renal disease
Multidisciplinary team assembly	Form a comprehensive team including maternal–fetal medicine specialists, rheumatologists, neonatologists or pediatric cardiologists, and nephrologists as needed

Monitoring of SLE Pregnancy

Pregnancies in women with SLE are considered high-risk, necessitating a coordinated monitoring approach. Regular assessments throughout pregnancy are crucial to detect and manage potential complications as soon as possible. Physiological changes during pregnancy, such as fatigue, joint pain, skin rashes, and swelling, can mimic symptoms of lupus disease activity. Additionally, certain laboratory changes are typical in healthy pregnancies. So, vigilant monitoring of pregnant female with SLE is required from conception to child birth **(Table 6)**.

Medications Use during Pregnancy

An essential component of management involves use of suitable medications during the pregnancy considering potential risk to developing fetus. There should be safety considerations for common medications used in the treatment of SLE during preconception, pregnancy, and breastfeeding periods **(Table 7)**.

Drugs

Hydroxychloroquine

Hydroxychloroquine is an FDA-approved autophagy inhibitor widely used in the management of SLE due to its diverse therapeutic benefits **(Fig. 4)**. HCQs are effective in treating SLE flares and APOs:

- *Lipid profile regulation*: Patients with SLE often exhibit elevated levels of very low-density lipoprotein particles (VLDL-P), low-density lipoprotein (LDL), and triglycerides (TGs), along with decreased levels of large high-density lipoprotein particles (HDL-P), particularly during SLE flares. These lipid abnormalities are associated with increased risk of atherothrombosis and worsened APOs. HCQ therapy has been shown to decrease VLDL, LDL, and

TABLE 6: Antenatal monitoring and management plan.

Timeline of pregnancy	Monitoring	Management
Preconception evaluation and counseling	• Monitor blood pressure • Clinical evaluation of SLE • Routine laboratory tests including antiphospholipid antibodies, lupus anticoagulant and anti-Ro/SSA, anti-La/SSB antibodies	• Discuss birth control options if pregnancy is not desired • For females wanting pregnancy: Switch to medications which are safe in pregnancy and low activity of disease or remission for at least 6 months is ensured • Start or continue hydroxychloroquine (HCQ) if not contraindicated • Discontinue NSAIDs if conception is difficult
First trimester of pregnancy	• Monitor blood pressure (BP) • SLE clinical evaluations • Routine laboratory tests	• Begin aspirin in low dose (81 mg/day) • Review medication compliance • Watch for disease flares
	• Fetal ultrasound to confirm intrauterine pregnancy and establish gestational age of fetus	• Start prophylactic heparin for females with obstetric antiphospholipid syndrome (APS) • Begin full-dose heparin for patients with thrombotic APS • For active SLE, increase or add pregnancy-compatible DMARD (disease-modifying antirheumatic drug)
Second trimester of pregnancy	• Monitor BP • SLE clinical evaluations • Routine laboratory tests, including genetic screening and gestational diabetes if applicable • Fetal echocardiogram from week 16 to 25 for mothers with +anti-Ro/SSA or +anti-La/SSB • Ultrasound to evaluate fetal anatomy, growth, placental sufficiency	• Monitor for disease aggravation • Review medication compliance • Steroid—start oral dexamethasone (4 mg daily) for fetuses with evidence of 1st or 2nd degree heart block and then response is assessed • Dexamethasone for fetuses with 3rd degree heart block without cardiac inflammation is avoided • Avoid NSAIDs after 20 weeks of gestation

Continued

Continued

Timeline of pregnancy	Monitoring	Management
Third trimester of pregnancy	• Monitor blood pressure • SLE clinical evaluations • Routine laboratory tests • Regular ultrasounds to evaluate fetal growth, amniotic fluid adequacy, and placental sufficiency	• Monitor for disease flares • Review medication adherence • Prepare for labor and delivery
Postpartum period and lactation	• Monitor blood pressure • SLE clinical evaluations • Routine laboratory tests	• Monitor for disease flares • Switch to lactation-safe medications if breastfeeding • For prednisone doses ≥20 mg/day, avoid breastfeeding for 4 hours after taking the medication

Notes: The following laboratory tests should be conducted—complete blood count (CBC), comprehensive metabolic profile (CMP), urinalysis, serum uric acid level, morning urine protein to creatinine ratio (UPCR), anti-double stranded DNA (dsDNA) antibodies, and measurement of complement levels (CH50, or C3 and C4).

(NSAID: nonsteroidal anti-inflammatory drug; SLE: systemic lupus erythematosus)

TABLE 7: Safety profile of common drugs during preconception, during pregnancy, and lactation.

Drugs	Before pregnancy	During pregnancy	Breastfeeding
Hydroxychloroquine (HCQs)	Safe	Safe	Safe
Tacrolimus	Safe	Safe	Safe
Cyclosporine A (Cyc-A)	Safe	Safe	Safe
Azathioprine	Safe	Safe	Safe
Sulfasalazine	Safe	Safe	Safe
Prednisolone	Maintain dose <20 mg/day	Maintain dose <20 mg/day	Maintain dose <20 mg/day
NSAIDs	Discontinue with difficulty in conceiving	Stop at week 20	Safe
Drugs to be stopped at conception			
Rituximab	Stop with positive pregnancy test		Safe
Abatacept	Stop with pregnancy test positive		Safe
Belimumab	Stop with positive pregnancy test		Safe
Not safe			
Cyclophosphamide	Stop 3 month before conception	Not recommended for use	Not recommended

Continued

Continued

Drugs	Before pregnancy	During pregnancy	Breastfeeding
Mycophenolic acid (MMF)	Stop 6 weeks before conception	Not recommended for use	Not recommended
Leflunomide	Stop with cholestyramine washout	Not recommended for use	Not recommended
Methotrexate	Stop ~1–3 month before conception	Not recommended for use	Not recom-mended—low transfer into breast milk
(NSAID: nonsteroidal anti-inflammatory drug)			

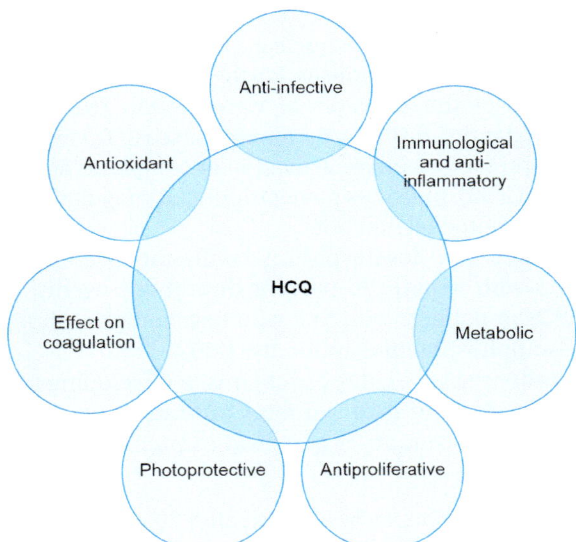

FIG. 4: Mechanism of action of hydroxychloroquine (HCQ) sulfate.

triglyceride levels, while increasing HDL levels and HDL particle size, thereby mitigating SLE flare severity and reducing the progression of APOs.

- *CD154/CD40 pathway inhibition*: HCQ inhibits the interaction between CD154 (CD40 ligand) and CD40 receptors, which is crucial for T cell-mediated B cell activation and autoantibody production in SLE. By blocking this pathway, HCQ helps in controlling LN and mitigating the severity of APOs.
- *NOX2 inhibition*: Endosomal NADPH oxidase 2 (NOX2) is involved in proinflammatory and prothrombotic signaling cascades that contribute to APOs in patients with SLE. HCQ effectively inhibits NOX2-mediated thrombus formation and reduces inflammatory cytokine secretion, thereby alleviating APOs.

- *Downregulation of proinflammatory chemokines*: Hydroxychloroquine in combination with other medications like prednisone downregulates the secretion of inflammatory chemokines such as CXCL10 and CCL2, which are significantly elevated in SLE. This anti-inflammatory effect helps in managing SLE flares and improving pregnancy outcomes.

Hydroxychloroquine plays a pivotal role in the treatment of SLE by regulating lipid metabolism, inhibiting autoimmune pathways, reducing thrombotic risks, and modulating inflammatory responses. Its ability to improve pregnancy outcomes underscores its importance as a safe and effective therapy recommended for continuous use throughout pregnancy in women with lupus.

Aspirin

Aspirin, a commonly used NSAID, reduces inflammation by inhibiting the activation of the proinflammatory nuclear factor-kappa B (NF-kB) signaling pathway during inflammatory responses. Furthermore, it regulates inflammation through modulation of the activator of transcription (STAT3) pathway and inhibition of prostaglandin-E (PGE)/cyclooxygenase (COX) signaling pathways. Additionally, it suppresses excessive activation of complement levels and serum thromboxane-B2 (sTXB2), mitigates platelet-induced coagulation processes, and enhances vascular endothelial function.

In clinical practice, low-dose aspirin is commonly prescribed either alone or in combination with heparin to prevent thrombotic events, cardiovascular diseases, and APOs in patients with SLE who have antiphospholipid syndrome (APS) or positive antiphospholipid antibodies (aPL).

It may rarely induce severe kidney problems in developing fetus which may lead to oligohydramnios and death of fetus around 20 weeks of gestation or later. After 30 weeks of gestation, it may lead to premature closure of ductus arteriosus.

Recommendation: NSAIDs should be stopped after 20 week of gestation but low-dose aspirin can be continued for duration of pregnancy.

Steroids

Glucocorticoids, such as prednisone and prednisolone, are widely used steroidal anti-inflammatory drugs recommended for treating SLE. They are crucial for managing acute SLE, where high-dose glucocorticoids can rapidly suppress severe disease activity and maintain remission. However, prolonged use of high-dose glucocorticoids, whether orally or intravenously, can lead to irreversible body damage. Current research indicates that high-dose glucocorticoids inhibit autoreactive T cells and alter T cell receptor (TCR) CDR3 repertoires, although these effects vary among individuals. This highlights the need for personalized therapeutic approaches in SLE to mitigate adverse outcome.

The gut microbiota plays a significant role as a driver of autoimmune and proinflammatory processes in SLE. Glucocorticoid therapy has been shown to downregulate inflammatory markers such as IFN-γ, IL-2R, IL-10, IL-35, and

TNF-α. It also helps restore normal gut microbiota and metabolic signaling, thereby inhibiting the development of SLE-associated APOs.

Despite their benefits in preventing various complications of acute SLE, glucocorticoids should be used cautiously due to their potential side effects. They exert their therapeutic effects by enhancing the expression of tumor necrosis factor receptor family-related protein (GITR) on resting responder T lymphocytes (Tresp) rather than on regulatory T cells (Treg). Additionally, glucocorticoids induce apoptosis in Tresp cells among patients with SLE.

Recommendations: Keep prednisone dose as low as possible during pregnancy.

Anticoagulant Drugs

Low-molecular weight heparin (LMWH) is the preferred anticoagulant for preventing thrombosis, a significant contributor to APOs. LMWH acts by enhancing the activity of antithrombin III, thereby inhibiting thrombin formation. It also prevents platelet adhesion and aggregation, inactivates thrombin, and inhibits the activation of factors V and XIII induced by thrombin.

Presently, LMWH is utilized alone or in conjunction with prednisone or aspirin to address pregnancy complications and enhance the live birth rate in individuals diagnosed with SLE complicated by antiphospholipid syndrome (APS) or positive antiphospholipid antibodies (aPL). Importantly, LMWH treatment has been found to have no adverse effects on neonatal bone health.

Immunosuppressants

- In the treatment of SLE, immunosuppressive drugs such as cyclosporine, azathioprine, and tacrolimus play crucial roles. Azathioprine is commonly used for severe and refractory cases of SLE. A novel drug delivery system involving biocompatible polyhydroxyalkanoate (PHA) nanoparticles conjugated with azathioprine has been developed to increase therapeutic efficacy and minimize the side effects.
- Macrophage activation syndrome (MAS) is a rare complications of SLE. Treatment of MAS include combination of dexamethasone sodium phosphate and IVIG with cyclosporine. This combination helps alleviate MAS symptoms, suppress inflammatory cytokine production, and improve outcomes, including fetal outcomes.
- Tacrolimus is another effective immunosuppressive agent in SLE treatment. It promotes regulatory T (Treg) cell activity, inhibits Th17 cells, and upregulates molecules like indoleamine-2,3-dioxygenase and interleukin-10 (IL-10), which suppress autoimmune inflammation. Tacrolimus achieves this by inhibiting the calcineurin pathway in T cells and reducing inflammatory cytokine production. A low daily dose (2–3 mg) is both effective and safe for treating LN.
- While these immunosuppressive drugs offer promising therapeutic benefits for SLE and associated complications, their potential side effects must be carefully managed and monitored during treatment.
- Leflunomide, methotrexate, and cyclophosphamide are teratogenic medications that can cause birth defect and should be discontinued before

conception. Methotrexate and cyclophosphamide should be stopped 1–3 months before conception.

- Mycophenolate mofetil/mycophenolic acid (MMF), commonly used for LN, is teratogenic and increases the risk of pregnancy loss in the first trimester. It should be stopped 6 weeks before conception.

Biological Drugs Targeting B Cells

B cells play a crucial role in the pathogenesis of SLE and APOs. Inhibitors that target B cells, such as belimumab, work by binding to B cell stimulating factor (BSF), preventing its interaction with B cells and promoting B cell apoptosis. However, belimumab is not recommended during pregnancy due to a higher incidence of abortions and congenital malformations. Instead, immunosuppressants compatible with pregnancy are preferred alternatives.

Rituximab (RTX) is another biological agent that targets CD20 on B cells and is conditionally recommended for patients with refractory SLE. However, its use is associated with an increased risk of abortions due to depletion of neonatal B cells. While these drugs effectively manage SLE flares and various APOs, their potential adverse effects on both mother and fetus need careful consideration.

CONCLUSION

- Systemic lupus erythematosus is an autoimmune multiorgan disorder primarily affecting female of reproductive age group. So, it has been reported that SLE has effect on pregnancy outcomes and also pregnancy has effect on disease activity.
- Systemic lupus erythematosus pregnancy is associated with APOs like preeclampsia, lupus flare, preterm birth, IUGR, and antiphospholipid syndrome.
- One of the fetal complication is neonatal lupus which is characterized by CHB. So, it is essential to educate pregnant women about the potential complications and to test for anti-Ro/SSA antibodies before conception.
- Use of effective contraception (oral, subcutaneous, or IUDs) is based on disease activity and risk of thrombosis is considered if pregnancy is not desired.
- Pregnant women diagnosed with SLE should maintain their use of hydroxychloroquine throughout pregnancy. To mitigate the risk of preeclampsia, low-dose aspirin is recommended starting at the end of the first trimester.
- Prednisolone should be administered at the lowest possible dose for managing nonrenal flares during pregnancy.
- Many medications used to manage SLE are safe for breastfeeding mothers. These include hydroxychloroquine, sulfasalazine, NSAIDs, and immunosuppressive agents like azathioprine, cyclosporine, and tacrolimus. Biologic medications such as rituximab, belimumab, and abatacept are also compatible with breastfeeding. However, lactating women should avoid methotrexate, mycophenolate mofetil, cyclophosphamide, and leflunomide.

KEY POINTS

- Systemic lupus erythematosus is very common autoimmune connective tissue disorder which affects pregnancy outcome and concurrently pregnancy has effect on disease activity as it may cause flare of disease.
- Systemic lupus erythematosus may affect newborn baby, so proper counseling regarding nature of disease and effect on newborn is essential part of management.
- Hydroxychloroquine (HCQ) is safe drug and should be continued throughout pregnancy and lactation.
- Oral contraceptive to be avoided as method of contraception in SLE females.

SUGGESTED READINGS

1. Tan Y, Yang S, Liu Q, Li Z, Mu R, Qiao J, et al. Pregnancy-related complications in systemic lupus erythematosus. J Autoimmun. 2022;132:102864.
2. Dao KH, Bermas BL. Systemic lupus erythematosus management in pregnancy. Int J Women's Health. 2022;14:199-211.
3. Lateef A, Petri M. Managing lupus patients during pregnancy. Best Pract Res Clin Rheumatol. 2013;27(3):435-47.
4. Sangah AB, Jabeen S, Hunde MZ, Devi S, Mumtaz H, Shaikh SS. Maternal and fetal outcomes of SLE in pregnancy: a literature review. J Obstet Gynaecol. 2023;43(1):2205513.
5. Lateef A, Petri M. Systemic lupus erythematosus and pregnancy. Rheumat Dis Clin. 2017;43(2):215-26.
6. Silver R, Craigo S, Porter F, Osmundson SS, Kuller JA, Norton ME; Society for Maternal-Fetal Medicine (SMFM). Society for Maternal-Fetal Medicine Consult Series# 64: systemic lupus erythematosus in pregnancy. Am J Obstet Gynecol. 2023;228(3):B41-60.

4.2 Scleroderma in Pregnancy

Sunil Kumar Gupta, Swati Suman

INTRODUCTION

Overview of Scleroderma

The term "scleroderma" originates from the Greek terms skleros (meaning hard) and derma (meaning skin), and it refers to a condition marked by the gradual hardening and thickening of the skin. Scleroderma is a long-lasting, systemic, and connective tissue illness of unknown cause that is distinguished by fibrous and degenerative alterations in the skin and internal organs. It sometimes can affect joints, heart, muscles, lungs, kidneys, blood vessels, or intestines. Scleroderma is characterized by changes in the skin, including thickness, tightness, induration, and consequent loss of mobility and rigidity.

Clinical presentation: Clinical presentations of scleroderma are described in **Table 1 and Boxes 1 to 3**.

TABLE 1: Classification of systemic sclerosis.

Limited cutaneous systemic sclerosis (lcSSc)	Also known as CREST (Calcinosis, Raynaud's phenomenon, Esophageal dysmotility, Sclerodactyly, Telangiectasia) syndrome
Diffuse cutaneous systemic sclerosis (dcSSc)	Characterized by bilateral symmetrical diffuse scleroderma of face, upper limbs, and lower limbs
Systemic sclerosis sine scleroderma	Typical systemic features of systemic sclerosis but no cutaneous involvement
Overlap syndrome	Features of systemic sclerosis associated with features of other autoimmune collagen disorders

BOX 1 Diffuse cutaneous scleroderma and pregnancy.

Diffuse cutaneous scleroderma (dcSSc):

- Greater severity and acuteness of skin involvement compared to lcSSc
- Characterized by symmetry and diffusion
- Affects the face, proximal extremities, and trunk; fingers occasionally spared
- Higher frequency of complications like prematurity and late pregnancy losses in dcSSc
- SRC commonly seen in early and rapidly progressing dcSSc patients
- Postpartum skin thickening reported in women with diffuse SSc
- Early dcSSc with antitopoisomerase or RNA polymerase III antibodies suggests higher risk of progression
- Pregnancy in diffuse SSc should be considered 3–5 years after symptom onset and after 6 months of stable disease

(lcSSc: limited cutaneous systemic sclerosis; SRC: scleroderma renal crisis)

BOX 2 Limited cutaneous scleroderma and pregnancy.

Limited cutaneous scleroderma (CREST syndrome):

- CREST syndrome includes Calcinosis, Raynaud phenomenon, Esophageal dysmotility, Sclerodactyly, and Telangiectasia
- Cutaneous manifestations on the face and distal regions of the upper and lower extremities
- Outcome of pregnancy is better than in dcSSc
- Less frequent elective termination of pregnancy in lcSSc
- PAH can occur in both limited and diffuse SSc, possibly more prevalent in lcSSc
- PAH is associated with lcSSc, anticentromere antibodies, anti-TH/To, and anti-U3 RN antibodies

(dcSSc: diffuse cutaneous systemic sclerosis; lcSSc: limited cutaneous systemic sclerosis; PAH: pulmonary arterial hypertension)

Importance of Pregnancy Considerations in Scleroderma

Similar to many autoimmune diseases, systemic sclerosis (SSc) has a strong female prevalence and affects women of childbearing age at least 4× than men. Many physiological changes are triggered by pregnancy, such as elevated blood supply, fibrinogen levels, and exposure to immunological factors. The occurrence of maternal complications around the time of childbirth, such as pregnancy-induced high blood pressure, and complications affecting the fetus, like

BOX 3 Overlap syndrome and pregnancy.

Overlap syndromes:
- Exhibits symptoms of SSc and other systemic connective tissue disorders, including rheumatoid arthritis, dermatomyositis, systemic lupus erythematosus, or mixed connective tissue disease
- Muscle involvement in SSc includes idiopathic inflammatory myopathies (IIM) like polymyositis (PM), with a reported incidence of 5–10% and associated autoantibodies
- Differential diagnosis is crucial in cases with hypertensive complications
- Must distinguish the origin of hypertensive complications to determine if they are secondary to SRC, an obstetric event (preeclampsia), or overlap with another rheumatic condition
- Distinguishing hypertensive complications, especially in cases of lupus erythematosus with kidney involvement, can be clinically challenging

(SRC: scleroderma renal crisis; SSc: systemic sclerosis)

premature birth and low birth weights (LBWs), have been documented in brief observational studies. Pregnancy, if not properly managed, presents a significant risk to both the mother and the baby. A multidisciplinary team should work with patients with scleroderma to determine the ideal time to get pregnant and to provide appropriate supportive care for the duration of the pregnancy in order to reduce risks.

EPIDEMIOLOGY OF SCLERODERMA IN PREGNANCY

Prevalence and Incidence

The frequency is 2–10 cases per million, and it is 3–5 times more prevalent in women than in men. This higher occurrence in females is even more pronounced during the reproductive years (15–50 years), during which women are 15 times more likely to be affected compared to men. Connective tissue disease used to typically impact individuals in their late reproductive and postreproductive years. Over the past few decades, a growing number of women have delayed childbirth until their 30s or 40s. Consequently, it is anticipated that the incidence of SSc among women and the likelihood of them becoming pregnant will increase.

Demographic Variations

Although SSc is a global condition, reports of its incidence vary greatly between nations; for instance, larger rates are recorded in Europe, North America, and South America than in East Asia. About one-third of individuals have scleroderma in its systemic form. The likelihood of developing scleroderma, the age at which it first manifests, and the pattern or degree of internal organ involvement may all be influenced by other variables, such as race and ethnic origin.

Comparative Analysis with General Population

A Swedish study found that parous women who gave birth at a younger age (under 20 years old) had a higher risk of scleroderma, similar to nulliparous women.

A French study suggests that the number of pregnancies before the onset of SSc may impact the age at which the disease begins. It indicates that women who have never been pregnant are younger at the onset of SSc and may experience a more severe clinical course. Therefore, women with a history of pregnancy typically experience SSc onset at around the age of 44, whereas women in whom SSc developed before or during pregnancy typically experience onset at around 26 years of age.

- Systemic sclerosis is more common in females especially in fourth decade
- Previously, pregnancies were more common in 20–30 years age group but now the trend has shifted to 30–40 years age group
- The incidence of SSc in pregnancy is thus expected to increase
- Incidence also depends on ethnicity
- Younger age of onset of SSC during pregnancy has a worse prognosis

IMMUNOPATHOGENESIS OF SCLERODERMA IN THE CONTEXT OF PREGNANCY

Immunological Changes during Pregnancy

The mother's immune system undergoes significant changes throughout pregnancy in order to defend against infections and prevent harmful immunological reactions against the allogeneic fetus. During pregnancy, the mother's body experiences hormonal fluctuations that are essential for sustaining the pregnancy and ensuring the survival of the fetus. As the pregnancy progresses, the levels of cortisol, estrogens, and progesterone in the bloodstream increase steadily. Furthermore, immunoregulatory substances released by the placenta inhibit the growth of T-cells and promote tolerance in the T-cells of the mother. There is no generalized reduction in immunity brought on by pregnancy. Normal responses to both active and passive immunization are observed, while the maternal defense mechanisms remain undisturbed, showing tolerance to fetal antigens. Changes are seen in both innate and adaptive immunity.

Autoimmune Mechanisms in Scleroderma

Lesional scleroderma skin has higher concentrations of T lymphocytes, macrophages, and mast cells, either activated or in an increased quantity. These cells release growth factors, cytokines/chemokines, and other mediators that actively contribute to the pathophysiology of the disease. Furthermore, SSc patients have unusually high levels of activated peripheral B lymphocytes. B cells support the generation of diverse cytokines, T cell activation and differentiation, and antibody production.

Interaction between Pregnancy-related Immune Modulation and Scleroderma

Pregnancy-related changes in hormone profiles cause significant immunomodulatory alterations that, if not properly handled, may interact negatively with scleroderma. For the majority of women (63–72%) who have SSc, pregnancy does not appear to have an impact on disease activity. On the other hand, preeclampsia and other hypertension problems during pregnancy may be more common in women with SSc. Because pregnancy causes a natural vasodilation, symptoms of Raynaud's phenomenon (RP) often go better, whereas symptoms of reflux illness get worse. Skin involvement might increase after giving birth, although it typically stays steady or gets better. Pregnancy does not increase the likelihood of renal crises. SSc is linked to a higher risk of intrauterine growth restriction (IUGR), prolonged hospital stays, premature birth (14–29%), and miscarriages in women with diffuse scleroderma for an extended period of time.

Pregnancy does not usually affect course of SSc:
- *Manifestations of SSc improving during pregnancy*: Raynaud's phenomenon
- *Manifestations of SSc worsening during pregnancy*: Reflux esophagitis and other upper gastrointestinal symptoms hypertension, skin tightening
- *Remain same*: Risk of renal crisis, interstitial lung disease
- SSc-associated PAH increases pregnancy complications
- Risk of abortions and preterm birth are not increased in SSc
- Intrauterine growth retardation may be seen

CLINICAL MANIFESTATIONS OF SCLERODERMA IN PREGNANT PATIENTS

Skin and Musculoskeletal Involvement

Pregnancy frequently causes cutaneous presentation to remain constant. On the other hand, those who stop receiving therapy have been known to get worse. During pregnancy, the majority of expectant mothers experience a gradual thickening of their skin, while around 15% of women with both diffuse cutaneous systemic sclerosis (dcSSc) and limited cutaneous systemic sclerosis (lcSSc) may notice a worsening of their skin condition following childbirth.

In patients with SSc, muscle involvement can be caused by idiopathic inflammatory myopathies (IIM), which include polymyositis (PM), dermatomyositis, and seldom, fibrosing myopathy, necrotizing myopathy, and sarcopenia. The reported incidence ranges for SSc-associated PM (SSc-PM) is 5–10%. Pregnancy and IIM are uncommon. Myositis can occur prior to pregnancy in pregnant women with pre-existing SSc, with a risk of flare-up during the postpartum period, particularly in those who conceive with active illness. De novo presentations can happen both during and after childbirth.

Gastrointestinal Manifestations

In up to 80% of cases with SSc, gastrointestinal tract problems occur. Nearly all involve the esophagus. Pregnancy results in longer small and large bowel transit durations, delayed stomach emptying, and reduced peristalsis. As pregnancy progresses, reflux symptoms may worsen, although constipation, nausea, and vomiting are typical throughout SSc and pregnancy. For up to 20% of SSc women, pregnancy exacerbates upper gastrointestinal symptoms.

Cardiopulmonary Complications

The most typical cardiac symptom of SSc is pulmonary arterial hypertension (PAH). It is the primary cause of mortality, affecting around 10% of women with SSc. Even in the absence of the additional physiological strain of pregnancy, women with SSc and PAH had a poorer prognosis than those with idiopathic PAH. With high rates of maternal death (from 17 to 33%) and newborn mortality (from 11 to 13%), PAH continues to be a major pregnancy concern. Pregnancy and the first 2 months postpartum have the highest risk of mortality or severe decompensation. Pregnancy advice is essential for individuals with PAH diagnoses, emphasizing the serious dangers associated with getting pregnant.

Up to 90–100% of women with SSc have some degree of parenchymal lung involvement, which is frequent in interstitial lung disease (ILD). Pregnant women with SSc report stable ILD most of the time, but limited research indicates that they are more likely to experience type 1 or type 2 respiratory failure.

Renal Involvement

The most significant renal consequence, known as scleroderma renal crisis (SRC), affects 5–20% of people with SSc. The use of glucocorticoids (≥15 mg/day of prednisone or equivalent), diffuse skin involvement, the existence of anti-RNA polymerase III antibodies, and the lack of anticentromere antibodies are risk factors. The risk of SRC is not increased by pregnancy per se, and the rates of dcSSc are similar to those that do not occur during pregnancy. Pregnancy-related SRC incidence is estimated to be 2%, peaking between weeks 16 and 28 of gestation. If a pregnancy is planned within 3–5 years following the beginning of symptoms, the chance of SRC is reduced.

Vascular Involvement

According to published research, the symptoms of RP and digital ulcer disease (DU) often become better during pregnancy (32% and 20%, respectively), with just 1% and 4% of women having worsening symptoms, respectively. Following childbirth, symptoms often deteriorate. Improvement is linked to an increase in cardiac output and a decrease in peripheral vascular resistance during pregnancy.

PREGNANCY OUTCOMES IN WOMEN WITH SCLERODERMA

Maternity Outcomes

In most recent investigations, a significant stability in disease activity during pregnancy and puerperium has been noted. According to a prospective research, 20% of patients had improvement, 20% had a deterioration of their condition, and 60% of patients had stable disease. Particularly RP can become better, while other symptoms like acid reflux, thicker skin, and arthritis can get worse. According to one of the studies' findings, there did not seem to be a significant difference in long-term renal, pulmonary, or global function outcomes between pregnancies with $\lesssim 1$ following SSc diagnosis. Nevertheless, a number of publications proposed that women who have dcSSc, with a beginning occurring before 4 years of age, and who test positive for anti-topoisomerase antibodies may be more susceptible to the disease's advancement. SRC causes high mortality and morbidity. As with other main organ issues in SSc, it develops in the first few years of the disease, hence pregnancy is avoided during this period. Women with PAH should avoid pregnancy due to the increased risk of maternal death.

Obstetric Complications

Spontaneous Abortion

After the disease begins, 15% of patients experience this, but the rate of miscarriages in SSc is not greater than that in the overall population.

Pregnant women with late-stage dcSSc have been found to be at an increased risk. The early miscarriages (<10 weeks) in all SSc subgroups were found to be similar to the overall obstetric population, according to research conducted more recently by Taraborelli et al.

Preeclampsia

It can be challenging to differentiate SRC from preeclampsia in pregnant women with SSc; both disorders pose a significant risk of severe complications for both the mother and the fetus if not aggressively treated. Cases of preeclampsia, however, were isolated as per most studies.

Fetal Outcomes: Growth Restriction, Neonatal Complications

Prematurity

Preterm births have been documented in 11–40% of SSc pregnancies, especially in early dcSSc. But when compared to healthy women, it does not seem that SSc women have a noticeably increased risk of premature birth. Therefore, while preterm births are known to occur in pregnancies with SSc, it is possible that these births are caused by a chronic illness rather than SSc itself.

Intrauterine Growth Restriction

Pregnant women with SSc have a sixfold higher risk of IUGR and LBW infants than healthy controls. Thus, it is recommended to have further fetal growth scans while pregnant. Despite the fact that LBW and preterm delivery are linked to higher steroid usage, these findings are complicated by the fact that higher corticosteroid use is frequently linked to higher disease activity. The rates of preeclampsia and other maternal-placental problems are raised by this alone.

Other Considerations

The presence of anti-Ro and/or anti-La autoantibodies increases the risk of congenital heart block in the fetus by 2%, a risk that escalates with multiple affected pregnancies (up to 10 times higher). In those with SSc, the frequency of anti-Ro and anti-La autoantibodies is up to 37% and 4%, respectively.

DIAGNOSTIC CHALLENGES IN PREGNANCY WITH SCLERODERMA

Differential Diagnosis

Disorders which may present clinical similarities with SSc and pose difficulty during pregnancy are given in **Table 2**.

Biomarkers and Imaging Techniques

Table 3 describes the biomarkers and imaging techniques.

TABLE 2: Differential diagnosis of diffuse cutaneous systemic sclerosis.

• Nephrogenic systemic fibrosis • Eosinophilic fasciitis • Eosinophilia–myalgia syndrome • Graft versus host disease • Reflex sympathetic dystrophy • Generalized morphea • Diabetic cheiroarthropathy • Porphyria cutanea tarda	• Morphea • Linear scleroderma • Radiation exposure • Scleromyxedema (generalized lichen myxedematosus) • Scleroderma adultorum of Buschke • Scleroderma diabeticorum

TABLE 3: Biomarkers and imaging techniques.

Prepregnancy	Antepartum	Delivery	Postnatal
• Complete blood counts • Kidney function test • Oral glucose tolerance test • Urine routine and microscopy • Blood pressure • Lung function test • ECG/ echocardiogram	• Increased fetal monitoring and obstetric ultrasounds especially early dcSSc and anti-Ro/anti-La (1–2 weekly fetal heart rate auscultation between 16 and 28 weeks with fetal echocardiography at 20–24 weeks and at 28 weeks) • Home BP monitoring in high-risk groups • Review GI symptoms • Echocardiography for PAH	• Early anesthetic review • Mode of delivery taking into account contractures • Check if on maintenance oral steroids	Blood film, LDH, Cr screening for SRC

(dcSSc: diffuse cutaneous systemic sclerosis; GI: gastrointestinal; PAH: pulmonary arterial hypertension; SRC: scleroderma renal crisis)

PHARMACOLOGICAL MANAGEMENT DURING PREGNANCY

Safety and Efficacy of Common Medications

Recently, a commission of the European League Against Rheumatism (EULAR) drafted a consensus statement regarding the use of antirheumatic drugs during pregnancy and lactation. It is important to discontinue drugs with teratogenic potential, such as mycophenolate, methotrexate, or bosentan, preferably at least 3 months before planning to conceive **(Table 4)**. ACE-inhibitors should be administered to manage renal crises. While calcium channel blockers can be used cautiously, they are generally not deemed necessary. In case of gastrointestinal issues, proton pump inhibitors and histamine blockers are considered safe and can be used.

Adjustments in Immunosuppressive Therapy

When pregnant, it is not recommended to use immunosuppressants like cyclophosphamide or mycophenolate mofetil, although they have occasionally been administered in an attempt to halt the advancement of pulmonary

TABLE 4: Safety of various systemic therapies in dcSSc in pregnancy.

Drug	First trimester	Second and third trimester
Mycophenolate Mofetil	Teratogenic potential	Teratogenic potential
Methotrexate	Teratogenic potential	Teratogenic potential
Bosentan	Teratogenic potential	Teratogenic potential
Macitentan	Teratogenic potential	Teratogenic potential
ACE-inhibitors	Teratogenic potential	• The use of these medications is acceptable during a renal crisis, despite their teratogenic potential • During the latter part of pregnancy, the risk of pulmonary hypoplasia, anhydramnios, or renal atresia is increased
Nifedipine	No contraindications	No contraindications
Proton pump inhibitors and histamine blockers	No contraindications	No contraindications
Corticosteroids	Avoid/lowest dose possible	Avoid/lowest dose possible
Low-dose aspirin	No contraindications (it may reduce pre-eclampsia risk in high-risk pregnancies)	No contraindications
Folic acid	Recommended	Recommended
Hydroxychloroquine	No contraindications	No contraindications

(ACE: angiotensin-converting enzyme; dcSSc: diffuse cutaneous systemic sclerosis)

fibrosis. Consideration may be given to the use of low-dose corticosteroids and immunosuppressive treatment in the immediate postpartum period.

One study mentioned that azathioprine should only be used for pregnant women with severe or life-threatening conditions. Lowering the azathioprine dosage during the 32nd week of pregnancy could help avoid severe neonatal leukopenia and thrombocytopenia. It is crucial to closely monitor prenatal growth and conduct long-term assessments of the children's health.

Use of Biologics and Therapeutics

There is insufficient evidence as of now on the usage of biologics, although multiple trials of biologics in early dcSSc and antifibrotics in progressive SSc-associated ILD have been reported during pregnancy **(Table 5)**.

NONPHARMACOLOGICAL MANAGEMENT STRATEGIES

Recently, EULAR published evidence-based recommendations for the non-pharmacological management of SSc.

Lifestyle Modifications

Nondrug treatments should focus on enhancing the quality of life for SSc patients. Patients should receive information about their condition and guidance on self-care techniques. Assessing smoking habits and introducing ways to quit should be a priority. Considering the avoidance of cold exposure may help prevent RP.

Nutritional Support

The GI tract is frequently affected in SSc and can result in substantial malnutrition. Consideration of home nutritional support in patients with SSc has been suggested in a study when the disease is relatively stable, and there is no major organ failure present.

Physical Therapy and Rehabilitation

Choosing the right physical exercise should be considered for people with SSc after considering health, cardiorespiratory status, and any potential risks or

TABLE 5: Safety of biologics in dcSSc in pregnancy.

Agent	Indication	Pregnancy category	US	EU
Nintedanib	SSc-ILD	D	Approved	Approved
Tocilizumab	SSc-ILD	Not assigned	Approved	Not approved
Rituximab	SSc	C	Not approved	Not approved

(SSc-ILD: scleroderma-associated interstitial lung disease)

medical considerations. Information and guidance on how to alleviate symptoms related to the hands and mouth, and enhance the capacity to engage in daily tasks. Mouth, face, and hand movements, as well as aerobic and resistance exercise should be considered. In case of puffy hands, patients may be offered manual lymph drainage.

MULTIDISCIPLINARY CARE MODELS

Collaborative Care Protocols

Obstetrician in collaboration with dermatologists, rheumatologists, and other specialists, along with physicians and other health professionals like specialized nurses and physical therapists, forms multidisciplinary teams (MDTs). These teams can efficiently address various aspects of the disease that affect the prognosis and quality of life of SSc patients with pregnancy, enhancing communication and empowering patients.

A comprehensive approach involving multiple disciplines and thorough prenatal monitoring are essential for treating pregnant women with complications.

Case Coordination and Communication

Rheumatologists ranked clear delineations of roles and responsibilities, treatment strategy alignment, and patient communication in multidisciplinary cooperation as their top areas of improvement. Therefore, it is very important to have clear coordination and communication among MDTs for an effective management of the patients with SSc during pregnancy.

ETHICAL AND PSYCHOSOCIAL CONSIDERATIONS

Counseling and Support for Patients and Families

Counseling and multidisciplinary management is mandatory. Pregnancy counseling is essential and should cover risks of pregnancy loss, morbidity, and mortality as well as organ evaluation (including lung function and echocardiography) before conception. It is important to carefully assess the impact of medications, especially immunosuppressants, on both the mother and the fetus. Women with SSc who are of childbearing age should have a discussion about contraception. Patients with early onset of dcSSc or positive anti-topoisomerase or RNA polymerase III antibodies are at a higher risk of developing more aggressive disease compared to those with long-standing disease and anti-centromere antibodies.

Systemic sclerosis-affected pregnant individuals should be considered at high risk for premature delivery and complications associated with the condition. As such, they should undergo thorough monitoring by a dedicated pregnancy team comprised of a rheumatologist, dermatologists, obstetrician, and neonatologist. It is crucial to keep a check on blood pressure and perform routine assessments of fetal development. Additionally, it is important to conduct Doppler velocimetry of uterine and/or umbilical arteries as part of regular evaluations.

Reproductive Planning and Ethical Issues

For women with early stage diffuse SSc, there might be an increased risk of progression during pregnancy or after giving birth, so it may be advisable to delay pregnancy or have frequent monitoring. If there is significant organ damage (such as PAH, severe restrictive lung disease, renal failure, or cardiomyopathy), it may be necessary to think about avoiding or ending the pregnancy. Patients who have previously experienced renal crisis and are reliant on ACE inhibitors may also need to steer clear of becoming pregnant.

Quality of Life and Psychosocial Impact

People with SSc frequently encounter increased levels of psychological distress due to alterations in their physical appearance, pain, fatigue, and challenges in everyday activities. Individuals with SSc may experience an impact on their perceived quality of life due to different aspects of the condition. Research has indicated that the primary factor leading to poor QoL in SSc patients is restrictions in performing daily activities. Management of the disease focuses on enhancing the quality of life for individuals with SSc. EULAR has also published nonpharmacological interventions some of which are aimed toward improvement of QoL through targeted exercises and physical therapies.

- Systemic sclerosis does not carry much risk during pregnancy
- Some risk of prematurity and low birth weight baby is seen
- Risk factors for increased maternal morbidity are:
    - Diffuse cutaneous systemic sclerosis
    - Late stage of disease
    - Severe organ damage
    - Duration of disease <4 years
    - Anti-topoisomerase I or anti-RNA polymerase III
    - Antibodies
    - Active disease at conception

CONCLUSION

Systemic sclerosis patients can experience successful pregnancies with low risk of serious complications by having candid conversations with their physicians and strategically planning their pregnancies, while receiving attentive care from obstetricians.

Pregnancy should be considered high risk for women with SSc from the beginning, as they are more likely to experience premature delivery and deliver babies with LBW.

In the initial stages of pregnancy, it is important for the doctor to conduct a comprehensive assessment of each patient to identify the particular disease being addressed (whether it is diffuse or limited), the stage (early or late), and the degree and seriousness of organ damage.

Individuals experiencing symptoms for <4 years (early stage SSc), those with the diffuse subtype, or those possessing anti-topoisomerase I or anti-RNA polymerase III antibodies, face increased obstetric risks and should consider delaying pregnancy until they progress to a later stage with reduced disease activity.

The final trimester of pregnancy is the most crucial time, as it can lead to the development of problems like hypertension, renal failure, pulmonary hypertension, ILD, or heart failure.

Research suggests that SSc patients do not experience fertility issues as a result of their condition.

SUGGESTED READINGS

1. Clark KE, Etomi O, Ong VH. Systemic sclerosis in pregnancy. Obstet Med. 2020;13(3):105-11.
2. de León Aguirre AR, Calvo JA, Reyna TS. Comprehensive approach to systemic sclerosis patients during pregnancy. Reumatología Clínica (English Edition). 2015;11(2):99-107.
3. Chung M, Chung L. Pregnancy. Scleroderma: From Pathogenesis to Comprehensive Management. Cham: Springer International Publishing AG; 2024. pp. 613-23.
4. Yoshizaki A. B lymphocytes in systemic sclerosis: Abnormalities and therapeutic targets. J Dermatol. 2016;43(1):39-45.
5. Lazzaroni MG, Crisafulli F, Moschetti L, Semeraro P, Cunha AR, Neto A, et al. Reproductive issues and pregnancy implications in systemic sclerosis. Clin Rev Allerg Immunol. 2023;64(3):321-42.
6. Yuvienco C, Batra K. The Care and Management of Rheumatologic Disease in Pregnancy. Medical Management of the Pregnant Patient: A Clinician's Handbook. New York: Springer; 2015. pp. 275-317.
7. Andreoli L, Gerardi MC, Fernandes M, Bortoluzzi A, Bellando-Randone S, Brucato A, et al. Disease activity assessment of rheumatic diseases during pregnancy: a comprehensive review of indices used in clinical studies. Autoimmun Rev. 2019;18(2):164-76.
8. Grant-Orser A, Metcalfe A, Pope JE, Johannson KA. Pregnancy considerations for patients with interstitial lung disease. Chest. 2022;162(5):1093-105.
9. Sobanski V, Launay D, Depret S, Ducloy-Bouthors AS, Hachulla E. Special considerations in pregnant systemic sclerosis patients. Expert Rev Clin Immunol. 2016;12(11):1161-73.
10. Chakravarty EF. Vascular complications of systemic sclerosis during pregnancy. Int J Rheumatol. 2010;2010(1):287248.
11. Betelli M, Breda S, Ramoni V, Parisi F, Rampello S, Limonta M, et al. Pregnancy in systemic sclerosis. J Scleroderma Relat Disord. 2018;3(1):21-9.
12. Olsson KM, Channick R. Pregnancy in pulmonary arterial hypertension. Eur Respirat Rev. 2016;25(142):431-7.
13. Lidar M, Langevitz P. Pregnancy issues in scleroderma. Autoimmun Rev. 2012;11(6-7):A515-9.
14. Doss BJ, Jacques SM, Mayes MD, Qureshi F. Maternal scleroderma: placental findings and perinatal outcome. Human Pathol. 1998;29(12):1524-30.
15. Skorpen CG, Hoeltzenbein M, Tincani A, Fischer-Betz R, Elefant E, Chambers C, et al. The EULAR points to consider for use of antirheumatic drugs before pregnancy, and during pregnancy and lactation. Ann Rheum Dis. 2016;75(5):795-810.
16. Parodis I, Girard-Guyonvarc'h C, Arnaud L, Distler O, Domján A, Van den Ende CH, et al. EULAR recommendations for the non-pharmacological management of systemic lupus erythematosus and systemic sclerosis. Ann Rheum Dis. 2024;83(6):720-9.

4.3 Miscellaneous Connective Tissue Disorders in Pregnancy

Sanjeev Gupta, Nikita Gupta, Sunita Gupta

INTRODUCTION

Autoimmune connective tissue diseases (CTDs) are more prevalent in women, especially during childbearing years. The relationship between these diseases and reproduction is reciprocal: autoimmune conditions can impact women's reproductive health, and pregnancy can influence the course of the disease. Traditionally, concerns about disease flares and adverse pregnancy outcomes (APOs) have led to caution among women with autoimmune disorders regarding pregnancy. However, the effect of pregnancy on disease progression and vice versa varies depending on the specific autoimmune condition. Women with CTDs are known to face increased risks of pregnancy complications such as miscarriage, preeclampsia, fetal growth restriction, and preterm birth. With appropriate preconception counseling, effective disease management before conception, and comprehensive medical care during pregnancy, women with CTDs can often achieve safe and successful pregnancies.

DERMATOMYOSITIS

Dermatomyositis (DM) and polymyositis (PM) are autoimmune inflammatory muscle disorders characterized by symmetric weakness in proximal muscles. DM is further distinguished by distinctive skin manifestations.

Epidemiology

Women are twice as likely to be affected as men, and this ratio may increase from 1.5–2:1 to 5:1 during childbearing years. There are about 14% patients of DM who present during pregnancy.

Effect of Pregnancy on Dermatomyositis/Polymyositis

Exact effect of pregnancy on DM/PM is not well studied. While few studies report an improvement, others have observed increase in activity of disease. These conditions can be exacerbated by complications affecting the lungs, metabolism, and heart. Pulmonary issues, particularly interstitial lung disease, are the most common. Cardiovascular complications such as arrhythmias, coronary artery disease, and congestive heart failure are also observed, along with a heightened risk of hypertension and diabetes. Adverse fetal outcomes such as intrauterine growth restriction (IUGR), fetal loss, and premature birth may be seen. In a study, 42.9% of pregnancies with active disease ended in fetal death.

Risk factors for aggravation of DM/PM during pregnancy and poor fetal outcome are:

- *Type of antibodies and relation to aggravation in pregnancy*: Oya et al. reported association of anti-transcriptional intermediary factor-1 gamma (anti-TIF-1γ) with aggravation of DM/PM during pregnancy. Akiyama et al. observed aggravation of DM and PM during pregnancy to be associated with various myositis-specific antibodies including anti-ARS, anti-Mi-2, anti-TIF-1γ, and anti-MDA-5.
- Delays in commencing treatment
- Poor response to corticosteroids
- Elevation of muscle enzymes
- Lung involvement
- High disease activity
- Associated comorbidities

SJÖGREN'S SYNDROME

Primary Sjögren's syndrome (PSS) is an autoimmune CTD. Clinically, it manifests as dryness of the main mucosal surfaces to systemic involvement (extraglandular manifestations).

Epidemiology

It affects approximately 0.1–0.6% of the general population globally. It is more commonly seen in females. The female-to-male ratio is approximately 9:1. It typically occurs between the ages of 40 and 60 years, but can occur in reproductive age group.

Effects of Sjögren's disease on pregnancy and vice versa:

- *Pregnancy outcomes*: Women with Sjögren's disease generally have good pregnancy outcomes, especially when the disease is well-controlled. However, the presence of certain autoantibodies (anti-Ro/SSA and anti-La/SSB) increases the risk of complications.
- *Neonatal lupus*: Infants born to mothers with Sjögren's disease, particularly those with anti-Ro/SSA and anti-La/SSB antibodies, are at risk for neonatal lupus, which can cause skin rashes, liver abnormalities, or hematologic issues. The most serious complication is congenital heart block (CHB), a potentially life-threatening condition that may require pacemaker implantation.
- *Risk of miscarriage and preterm birth*: There may be a slightly increased risk of miscarriage and preterm birth in women with Sjögren's disease, particularly in those with active disease or severe systemic involvement.
- *Exacerbation of symptoms*: Sjögren's symptoms, such as dryness of the eyes and mouth, may either improve, worsen, or remain unchanged during pregnancy.

- Sjögren syndrome is likely to worsen during pregnancy and more so in the postpartum period.
- Postpartum flares of the disease are common and may require medical management. This is because the disease is sometimes complicated by pulmonary hypertension, which frequently worsens during the postpartum period.
- Several studies have reported an increased rate of spontaneous abortion and fetal loss associated with Sjögren's syndrome.

Research on pregnancy outcomes in PSS, however, remains limited compared to systemic lupus erythematosus (SLE) or antiphospholipid syndrome (APS). Notably, screening for neonatal lupus is crucial in managing pregnancy for patients with primary or secondary SS and anti-Ro/La antibodies.

The rationales for treatment to reduce maternal autoantibodies, decrease the inflammation once it occurs before it leads to permanent fibrosis and irreversible CHB.

RHEUMATOID ARTHRITIS

Rheumatoid arthritis (RA) is a chronic autoimmune disease characterized by inflammation of the joints and surrounding tissues. It primarily affects the synovium, the lining of the joints, leading to pain, swelling, stiffness, and eventual joint destruction. RA can also cause systemic symptoms and affect other organs.

Epidemiology

Rheumatoid arthritis affects approximately 0.5–1% of the global population. It is seen in age group of 40 and 60 years. The incidence increases with age, particularly in women after menopause. Women are 2–3 times more likely to develop RA than men. RA may affect females in childbearing age. As a result, managing RA during conception and pregnancy presents a frequent challenge for both rheumatologists and obstetricians.

Effects of RA on pregnancy and vice versa:

- Traditional belief about RA patients was that it often improves spontaneously during pregnancy, with a flare-up likely within 3–4 months postpartum but recent studies with objective measures offer a detailed view of RA activity during and after pregnancy.
- Pregnancy outcomes for women with well-managed RA are generally similar to those in the general population. However, women with active RA may face a higher risk of adverse obstetric outcomes, these risks include IUGR, hypertensive disorders, and cesarean delivery.
  Standard assessment tools like Global Health Scale and ESR are influenced by pregnancy; modified tools such as DAS28-CRP (excluding Global Health and ESR) and HAQ are suggested for pregnancy studies.
- During pregnancy, around 50–70% of women with RA experience an improvement in their condition. This reduction in disease activity typically begins in the first trimester and continues throughout pregnancy. Despite

these improvements, about half of these women still have moderately to severely active RA during pregnancy.

- The likelihood of disease remission during pregnancy does not seem to be influenced by factors such as the duration of the disease or the functional class of the patient. However, some evidence indicates that patients who test negative for both rheumatoid factor (RF) and anti-citrullinated peptide antibodies (ACPAs) are more likely to see improvement compared to those who are positive for one or both autoantibodies. Additionally, the degree of human leukocyte antigen (HLA) class II disparity between the mother and fetus may also affect disease activity.
- Postpartum disease flares in RA are frequent, affecting nearly half of patients.
- Furthermore, research has indicated that the risk of developing RA for the first time is significantly elevated in the first 3 months after a woman's initial pregnancy.
- Pregnancies complicated by RA are also linked to higher rates of cesarean deliveries. The reasons for this increased rate may be due to patient preference, provider recommendations, obstetric factors, or medical indications.
- Long-term use of nonsteroidal anti-inflammatory drugs (NSAIDs) in RA has been linked to anovulation and reduced fertility. By inhibiting prostaglandin production, NSAIDs can impede the release of a mature egg, resulting in ovulation failure. Additionally, NSAIDs may interfere with the implantation of the blastocyst.

UNDIFFERENTIATED CONNECTIVE TISSUE DISORDER

The diagnostic criteria for undifferentiated connective tissue disease (UCTD) were initially proposed in 1999 and remain a topic of ongoing debate. According to these criteria, UCTD is typically diagnosed when the following conditions are met:

- Symptoms suggestive of a CTD without meeting specific criteria for a defined CTD.
- Positive antinuclear antibodies (ANA) detected on two separate occasions.
- Disease duration of at least 3 years.

However, patients with recent symptom onset, shorter follow-up periods, or an unclear clinical profile should also be considered as having UCTD. In such cases, this undifferentiated state may represent an early phase of a CTD, highlighting the importance of recognizing and monitoring these conditions to guide appropriate treatment decisions. Early identification of CTDs like SLE is crucial to prevent irreversible organ damage.

Epidemiology

The annual incidence of UCTD ranges from 41 to 149 per 100,000 adults. Women make up the majority of UCTD cases, accounting for up to 90%, with the condition most commonly occurring in individuals aged 32–44 years.

Clinical Features

- Pericarditis
- Thyroid disease
- Interstitial lung disease
- Skin lesions like telangiectasia, urticaria, and purpura
- Raynaud phenomenon
- Hematological disorders (leukopenia, anemia, and thrombocytopenia)
- Arthritis/myositis

- It has been estimated that approximately 30% of patients diagnosed with UCTD will eventually develop a specific defined CTD.
- Conversely, a significant percentage, ranging from 21 to 87%, may remain in the undifferentiated state over time. Among those who transition to a defined CTD, SLE is frequently reported.
- The risk of developing a specific CTD appears to be higher in the initial years following symptom onset and in patients with multiple positive autoantibodies, including anti-double-stranded DNA (dsDNA), antiphospholipid antibodies (aPL), anti-Ro/SSA, and anti-La/SSB, based on the finding.
- Regular follow-up is crucial, particularly during the early stages of symptoms or under conditions that could influence the course of autoimmune diseases, such as pregnancy. Notably, UCTD has been reported as the most frequently diagnosed systemic rheumatic disorder during the first trimester of pregnancy, with a prevalence of 2.5%.

Effect of Pregnancy on Undifferentiated Connective Tissue Disease

- During pregnancy, the female immune system undergoes significant changes to support the developing fetus and ensure its successful implantation, growth, and birth. These changes, however, do not compromise the maternal immune response or increase susceptibility to infections.
- A shift toward a Th2-type cytokine profile is crucial for maintaining tolerance to the fetal antigens. During pregnancy, specific Th2, Th17/Th2, and Treg cells accumulate in the decidua and maternal bloodstream, helping to modulate autoimmune responses. This generally results in improved outcomes for Th1/Th17-type autoimmune diseases, such as rheumatoid arthritis, multiple sclerosis, Graves' disease, and Hashimoto's thyroiditis, but can exacerbate Th2-type autoimmune diseases like SLE and systemic sclerosis.
- Research has also indicated that an imbalance between Th17 and Treg cells may contribute to the progression of UCTDs to more definitive CTDs.
- In women with stable disease at conception, fetal and maternal outcomes are favorable. So, women with UCTD pregnancy should be counseled to conceive during stable or inactive disease to reduce the risk of flare of disease and APOs.
- On the contrary, pregnant female with serological and clinical disease activity have increased risk of disease flare as well as APOs **(Fig. 1)**.

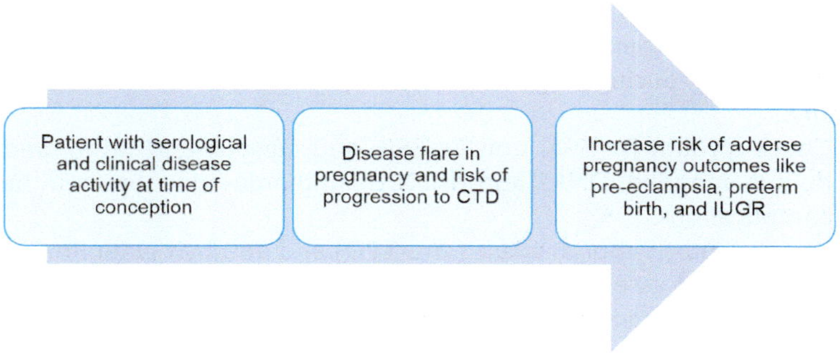

Patient with serological and clinical disease activity at time of conception

Disease flare in pregnancy and risk of progression to CTD

Increase risk of adverse pregnancy outcomes like pre-eclampsia, preterm birth, and IUGR

FIG. 1: Pregnancy implications on active UCTD.

(CTD: connective tissue disease; IUGR: intrauterine growth retardation; UCTD: undifferentiated connective tissue disease)

Effect of Undifferentiated Connective Tissue Disease on Pregnancy Outcomes

- *Obstetric complications*: 29% of UCTD pregnancies experienced complications, including preterm birth, small for gestational age infants, intrahepatic cholestasis of pregnancy, preterm premature rupture of membranes, gestational diabetes, and preeclampsia.
- *Anti-Ro (SSA) antibodies*: These antibodies, present in some UCTD patients, are linked to higher complication rates (50%) and risks such as CHB and neonatal lupus.
- *Antiphospholipid and ENA antibodies*: Increased risk of miscarriages and stillbirths.
- *Uterine artery notching*: More common in UCTD patients and associated with adverse outcomes, possibly due to inadequate trophoblast invasion.
- *Antinuclear antibodies (ANAs)*: May impact placental function, oocyte quality, embryo development, uterine blood flow, and endometrial receptivity, contributing to poor outcomes.
- *Endothelial dysfunction and cytokine imbalances*: Observed in UCTD, potentially leading to preeclampsia, fetal growth restriction, small for gestational age infants, recurrent pregnancy loss, and impaired spiral artery remodeling.

MANAGEMENT OF PREGNANT FEMALE WITH CONNECTIVE TISSUE DISEASE

Preconception Counseling and Evaluation

Women with UCTD should be referred to a high-risk pregnancy center for preconception counseling and ongoing care. Better maternal and fetal outcomes are associated with well-controlled disease prior to conception.

Preconception evaluation: Assess disease activity and major organ involvement.

- *Medication management*: Review and adjust medications before conception to ensure safety during pregnancy.
- *Testing*:
  - Check for anti-Ro/SSA, anti-La/SSB, antiphospholipid (aPL), and anti-double-stranded DNA (anti-dsDNA) antibodies due to their links to complications.
  - Test for anti-thyroperoxidase (anti-TPO) and antithyroglobulin (anti-TG) antibodies to assess risks for recurrent pregnancy loss and other issues.
- *Past obstetric outcomes*: Consider history of adverse outcomes (e.g., fetal growth restriction, preeclampsia) for monitoring and prophylactic treatments.
- *Monitoring*:
  - Frequent rheumatologic evaluations every 4–8 weeks
  - Monthly obstetric assessments
  - Adjust timing for ultrasound scans and Doppler assessments based on autoantibody positivity and disease severity
  - Perform fetal echocardiography in anti-Ro/SSA-positive patients.

Timing of Pregnancy and Contraception

Planning for pregnancy is crucial for women with CTDs to minimize risks. Specifically, for women with active diseases like lupus nephritis, it is recommended to wait for at least 6 months of inactive disease before attempting to conceive to improve both maternal and fetal outcomes.

Effective contraception is crucial for managing pregnancy timing, especially in women with rheumatic diseases who have an increased risk of thrombosis. While hormonal contraceptives carry thrombotic risks, they can be used with caution.

Contraception for pregnant female with UCTD:
For aPL-negative patients:

- *Combined hormonal methods*: Safe to use
- *Progestin-only options*: Safe to use
- *Long-acting reversible contraceptives (LARCs)*: Preferred; includes IUDs and implants
- *Depot medroxyprogesterone acetate (DMPA)*: Effective for 3 months, but long-term use may increase osteoporosis risk, especially in those with significant corticosteroid use

For aPL-positive patients:

- *Combined hormonal methods*: Contraindicated (CDC Category 4)
- *Progestin-only methods*: Classified as Category 3 (risks may outweigh benefits); includes progestin-only pills, injections, implants, and IUDs
- *Copper IUD*: Safe for aPL-positive patients but not recommended for those with severe thrombocytopenia due to increased menstrual bleeding
- *Levonorgestrel (LNg) IUD*: Category 3; reduces menstrual bleeding after initial 3 months and may be suitable for some, but use with caution, particularly in patients on warfarin

Treatment of Connective Tissue Disease

There are different types of drugs used in pregnancy which are discussed in **Table 1**.

TABLE 1: Drugs compatible with pregnancy.

Medication/ therapy	Use in pregnancy	Safety and recommendations
Hydroxy-chloroquine (HCQ)	Used in women with rheumatic diseases; may improve disease course and pregnancy outcomes	Generally safe, though recent study suggests a potential increase in congenital malformations. Compatible with breastfeeding
Aspirin	Used for management of antiphospholipid syndrome (APS), prevention of preeclampsia (PE), and rheumatic disease	Low-dose aspirin is safe; high-dose should be avoided. Compatible with breastfeeding
Corticosteroids	Used to manage rheumatic diseases and other inflammatory disorders	Safe in each trimester; use lowest effective dose. May increase risk of PROM, FGR, and maternal complications. Potential risk of fetal cleft palate, but evidence is mixed
Azathioprine (AZA)	Used as an immunosuppressant in severe cases	Generally considered safe but associated with some risks. More recent data do not confirm previous concerns. Further studies needed
Sulfasalazine (SSZ)	Used for its anti-inflammatory and antibacterial properties	Safe with no reported increase in miscarriage or malformations. Recommended to take folic acid supplements. Compatible with breastfeeding except in certain conditions
Tacrolimus	Used as an immunosuppressant; calcineurin inhibitor	Compatible with pregnancy, but use the lowest effective dose and monitor levels
Cyclosporine (CSA)	Used as an immunosuppressant; calcineurin inhibitor	Generally safe during pregnancy; monitor maternal blood pressure and renal function
Biologic agents	Includes TNF inhibitors, rituximab, anakinra, ustekinumab, tocilizumab, abatacept, and belimumab	TNF inhibitors are generally safe except in the third trimester. Certolizumab is compatible throughout pregnancy. Rituximab has potential neonatal effects
Vitamin D	Regulates calcium metabolism and immune function	Deficiency linked to adverse pregnancy outcomes. Further studies are needed to confirm benefits of supplementation
Aspirin and low molecular weight heparin (LMWH)	Aspirin used for APS and potential benefits in other autoimmune diseases. LMWH has anticoagulant, anti-inflammatory, and immunomodulatory properties	LMWH is used to improve outcomes in APS; potential benefits in UCTD but insufficient evidence for standard use

(FGR: fetal growth restriction; PROM: premature rupture of membrane; TNF: tumor necrosis factor)

KEY POINTS

- The autoimmune CTDs predominantly affect women and the majority of them are in the childbearing age group.
- The relationship between autoimmune CTD and reproduction is reciprocal: autoimmune conditions can impact women's reproductive health, and pregnancy can influence the course of the disease.
- Rheumatoid arthritis improves during pregnancy and flare up during the postpartum period.
- Undifferentiated connective tissue disease often presents with milder symptoms during pregnancy and favorable outcomes are associated with low disease activity at conception, while high disease activity increases the risk of disease flares, progression to a specific CTD, and obstetric complications.
- Preconception counseling should be an integral part of routine care for women with UCTD. It should focus on safe and effective contraception, careful pregnancy planning, and medications compatible with pregnancy.

SUGGESTED READINGS

1. Serena C, Clemenza S, Simeone S, Zullino S, Ottanelli S, Rambaldi MP, et al. Undifferentiated connective tissue disease in pregnancy: a topic yet to be explored. Front Pharmacol. 2022;13:820760.
2. Marder W, Littlejohn EA, Somers EC. Corrigendum to "Pregnancy and autoimmune connective tissue diseaes" [Best Practice & Research Clinical Rheumatology 30 (2016) 63-80]. Clin Rheumatol. 2020;34(6):101490.
3. Ateka-Barrutia O, Nelson-Piercy C. Connective tissue disease in pregnancy. Clin Med. 2013;13(6):580-4.
4. Kolstad KD, Fiorentino D, Li S, Chakravarty EF, Chung L. Pregnancy outcomes in adult patients with dermatomyositis and polymyositis. Semin Arthritis Rheum. 2018;47(6):865-9.
5. Arese V, Murabito P, Ribero S, Panzone M, Tonella L, Fierro MT, et al. Autoimmune connective tissue diseases and pregnancy. G Ital Dermatol Venereol. 2019;154(3):263-76.
6. Akiyama C, Shirai T, Sato H, Fujii H, Ishii T, Harigae H. Association of various myositis-specific autoantibodies with dermatomyositis and polymyositis triggered by pregnancy. Rheumatol Int. 2022;42:1271-80.

CHAPTER 5

Acne and Rosacea in Pregnancy

Sanjeev Gupta, Meghna Khatri, Namya Gupta

ACNE IN PREGNANCY

INTRODUCTION

Acne vulgaris is a prevalent and persistent inflammatory disorder of the pilosebaceous unit affecting teenagers and young adults but can affect any age group, including expectant mothers. It represents the most often reported primary concern in routine dermatological clinics, affecting up to 85% of teenagers. Hispanic women and blacks are more likely to develop acne in comparison to women of white, Asian, or continental Indian descent.

Pregnancy and acne interact in diverse ways. Because of the sebosuppressive influence of estrogens, pregnancy generally has a positive impact on acne activity. However, a small percentage of cases experience acne flare-ups that have to be treated aggressively, particularly if scarring is a concern. Pregnancy can cause acne to appear for the first time, as it is an early characteristic of certain pregnancies; it can also aggravate preexisting acne, or sometimes it may resolve completely. However, pregnant women with acne throughout adolescence are more likely to have acne flare-ups during pregnancy. Below are shown factors associated with an increased likelihood of developing acne during pregnancy.

Factors associated with an increased likelihood of developing acne during pregnancy:

- Females with a history of irregular menstrual cycles
- Females 25 years of age
- Females with a prior history of PCOS (polycystic ovarian syndrome)
- Females having higher BMI (body mass index)
- Primigravida females

PATHOPHYSIOLOGY

The pathophysiology of acne during pregnancy involves the complex interaction of various host factors, including increased keratinization of the follicular epithelium, dysbiosis of facial microbiome such as overgrowth of *Cutibacterium acnes* (*C. acnes*) (formerly *Propionibacterium acnes*), genetic and dietary influences and excess androgen production leading to sebaceous gland stimulation. Although the precise mechanisms accountable for the aggravation of acne during pregnancy are unclear, it is believed that physiologic and hormonal alterations, especially during the second and third trimesters, can induce the development of inflammatory acne.

Pregnancy-related hormonal changes significantly impact sebaceous gland activity and the pathophysiologic mechanisms of acne vulgaris have been linked to variations in sebum production. The amount of sebum production and the growth of sebaceous gland acini are closely attributed to androgen production, particularly 5α-dihydrotestosterone (5α-DHT). Higher androgen (testosterone) levels within the pilosebaceous unit, as well as increased sensitivity, might result in sebum production and the aggravation of acne. Further details are elaborated in the chapter on "Hormonal and immunological changes during pregnancy".

Cutaneous changes are most noticeable during the first and third trimesters due to the effects of human chorionic gonadotropin (hCG), estrogen, and progesterone. The noticeable spike in beta-hCG during the first trimester, which resembles the endogenous luteinizing hormone (LH), increases the synthesis of estrogen and progesterone, both of which rise until the time of delivery and may cause acne. Progesterone and estrogen levels increase throughout the second and third trimesters, surpassing the premenstrual spike. Although the sebosuppressive impact of estrogens is not proven, they are thought to lessen acne by opposing the effect of androgens. High levels of progesterone are thought to exacerbate acne by promoting the proliferation of keratinocytes and sebum production. The most frequent association between progesterone and acne during pregnancy has been seen in females with polycystic ovarian syndrome (PCOS) and a history of diabetes, as well as in women with higher insulin resistance. High prolactin levels during the third trimester might also enhance sebum secretion in the skin, resulting in acne through androgen-dependent mechanisms, either directly or indirectly.

Additionally, high insulin levels enhance the maturation and development of sebaceous glands, which is facilitated via the overexpression of growth hormone (GH) receptors on sebocytes. Insulin also plays a role in decreasing the production of SHBG (sex hormone binding globulin) in the liver, which in turn increases the levels of free sex hormones, particularly androgens, which positively impact ovarian and adrenal androgen synthesis. Overall, elevated insulin levels during pregnancy may contribute to acne by potentially leading to excess sebum and androgen production.

- Pregnancy-related hormonal alterations, especially in the second and third trimesters, lead to an increase in androgens such as 5α-dihydrotestosterone (5α-DHT)
- Elevated androgen levels → growth of sebaceous gland acini and increased sebum production
- High progesterone levels promote keratinocyte proliferation and increase sebum production, potentially worsening acne
- Estrogen is thought to oppose androgen effects
- High insulin levels during pregnancy increase sebaceous gland activity by upregulating growth hormone receptors on sebocytes, leading to excess sebum production, and exacerbating acne

CLINICAL PRESENTATION AND DIAGNOSIS

Acne during pregnancy can occur with varying degrees of severity. Physiological and hormonal changes during pregnancy can lead to the development of inflammatory acne lesions, especially during the second and third trimesters. Acne affects up to 43% of pregnant women. The most commonly involved areas in the face during pregnancy were the perioral areas, cheeks, and forehead. However, a substantial number of women are prone to involve the temples, nose, areas between the eyebrows, and the neck. Rarely chest, upper and lower back can be affected by acne.

Patients present with blackheads (open comedones), whiteheads (closed comedones), hyperpigmented cicatricial macules, pustules, papules, cysts, and nodules. Other clinical symptoms include a flare-up of truncal acne and new or worsened postinflammatory pigment alterations. Some women develop new-onset acne during the postpartum period, such as acne conglobata "postgestational acne".

The diagnosis of acne is made by physical examination rather than laboratory tests. Bacterial cultures are often negative, although a gram-negative bacterium may be detected occasionally, particularly in individuals not responding to antibiotic therapy. Serologic testing is typically not conducted for acne patients unless PCOS is suspected or if patients have a history of hirsutism, oligomenorrhea, a family history of hyperandrogenism, or acanthosis nigricans. In these patients, androstenedione, free and total testosterone, luteinizing hormone, follicle-stimulating hormone, and dehydroepiandrosterone sulfate (DHEAS), as well as a glucose and insulin levels, lipid panel can be obtained.

DIFFERENTIAL DIAGNOSIS

Differential diagnosis of acne vulgaris includes milia, rosacea, perioral dermatitis, demodex folliculitis, sebaceous hyperplasia, and keratosis pilaris rubra faceii.

TREATMENT

Treatment of acne during the reproductive period in females and pregnancy have to be tailored according to severity of disease, as mentioned in **Tables 1 to 3**.

TABLE 1: Treatment of acne during pregnancy planning and preconception period.

Contraindicated	Pregnancy Food and Drug Administration (FDA) category	Not recommended Especially in first trimester	Pregnancy FDA category
Tazarotene	X	Amoxicillin	B
Isotretinoin	X	Oral metronidazole	B
Trimethoprim/ sulfamethoxazole	C	Oral corticosteroids	C
Spironolactone	C	Oral erythromycins	B
		Other topical retinoids (tretinoin, trifarotene, and adapalene)	C

TABLE 2: Treatment of acne during pregnancy.

Severity of acne	Drug class	Food and Drug Administration (FDA) pregnancy category
Mild-to-moderate acne	Benzoyl peroxide	C
	Azelaic acid	B
	Topical clindamycin/metronidazole/ dapsone + BPO	B
	Glycolic/salicylic acids	–
	Topical sodium sulfacetamide ± sulfur	C
Moderate-to-severe acne	Oral cephalexin/erythromycins/ amoxicillin/clindamycin/azithromycin	B
Fulminant/recurrent acne	Oral/intralesional corticosteroids	C
	Light and laser therapies	–
	Oral metronidazole	B
	Oral tetracyclines	D
Contraindicated drugs	Isotretinoin, tazarotene, and clascoterone	X
	Topical retinoids, trimethoprim/ sulfamethoxazole, and spironolactone	C

TABLE 3: Treatment of acne during lactation.

Severity of acne	Drug class	Hale's lactation risk categories
Mild-to-moderate acne	Benzoyl peroxide	L2
	Azelaic acid	L3
	Topical metronidazole + BPO	L3
	Topical clindamycin + BPO	L2

Continued

Continued

Severity of acne	Drug class	Hale's lactation risk categories
	Glycolic/salicylic acids	L3
	Topical retinoids	L3
	Topical sodium sulfacetamide ± sulfur	L2
Moderate-to-severe acne	Oral cephalexin/azithromycin/ clindamycin/spironolactone	L2
	Oral amoxicillin	L1
	Oral erythromycin/trimethoprim/ sulfamethoxazole	L3
Fulminant/recurrent acne	Oral/intralesional corticosteroids	L3/L2
	Light and laser therapies	–
	Oral metronidazole	L2
	Oral tetracyclines	L3–L4
	Isotretinoin	L5
	Topical dapsone	L4
	Clascoterone	–
(L1: compatible; L2: probably compatible; L3: presumed compatible; L4: potentially hazardous; L5: hazardous)		

OVERVIEW OF TREATMENTS FOR ACNE DURING PREGNANCY

Topical Treatments

For mild-to-moderate acne, topical treatments are typically the primary approach. They also play a crucial role in the treatment of more severe acne, working together with oral medications. When using topical anti-acne agents during pregnancy, it is important to consider their measurable systemic absorption.

Azelaic Acid

Azelaic acid, a pregnancy category B drug, is considered safe during pregnancy and lactation. This naturally occurring dicarboxylic acid has anti-inflammatory, comedolytic, and antimicrobial properties, effectively treating inflammatory and noninflammatory acne, as well as postinflammatory hyperpigmentation. It is minimally absorbed through the skin (4–8%) and is found in foods such as rye, wheat, barley, and milk. It can be used twice daily at up to 20% strength. Azelaic acid is a suitable alternative for those who cannot tolerate benzoyl peroxide or need treatment for hyperpigmentation.

Benzoyl Peroxide

Benzoyl peroxide (BPO), a pregnancy category C topical preparation with keratolytic and antimicrobial properties, is generally considered safe during pregnancy. It is absorbed systemically at low rates (about 5%) and metabolized into benzoic acid, a food additive. BPO poses minimal risk of congenital malformations as it rarely reaches maternal or fetal circulation because of rapid renal clearance. It is often used as a first-line treatment for mild-to-moderate acne and can be combined with azelaic acid or other agents to prevent antibiotic resistance. Despite limited safety data, BPO up to 5% strength is recommended for pregnant patients.

Salicylic Acid

Salicylic acid, a pregnancy category C keratolytic agent, is considered safe for limited use in small areas during pregnancy. Although high concentrations or widespread application could lead to salicylate toxicity, such issues have not been reported with acne treatments. For mild-to-moderate acne, salicylic acid is a second-line option, with minimal systemic absorption when used topically. It should be avoided over large areas or with occlusive dressings to prevent increased absorption. Overall, topical salicylic acid and similar acids, such as glycolic acid, are deemed safe during pregnancy and breastfeeding.

Glycolic Acid

Glycolic and lactic acid are generally considered safe during pregnancy and lactation due to their minimal dermal penetration. Glycolic acid, an α-hydroxy acid, helps reduce sebum production and is used for its keratolytic and comedolytic properties. Although there is no Food and Drug Administration (FDA) pregnancy rating and limited safety data, no birth complications have been reported. Animal studies with high oral doses have shown fetal issues, but these doses are much higher than those used topically. Topical glycolic acid is unlikely to reach significant fetal levels and is considered likely safe for use.

Sodium Sulfacetamide

Topical sodium sulfacetamide, classified as FDA pregnancy category C, is an anti-inflammatory and bacteriostatic agent used to treat acne by inhibiting bacterial folic acid synthesis. While safety data during pregnancy is limited, no fetal anomalies have been reported, and it is generally considered safe due to minimal systemic absorption. It is also safe during lactation, though caution is advised for breastfeeding infants with hyperbilirubinemia or G6PD (glucose-6-phosphate dehydrogenase) deficiency due to potential risks of kernicterus and jaundice. Sodium sulfacetamide is often combined with sulfur, which is also deemed safe during pregnancy and lactation.

Topical Antibiotics

Topical antibiotics with anti-inflammatory and bactericidal properties are used during pregnancy to target *C. acnes*, a primary cause of acne. These antibiotics have a long history of treating inflammatory acne by decreasing *C. acnes* on the skin. To minimize the risk of developing antibiotic resistance, combining topical antibiotics with another antimicrobial agent, such as BPO, is recommended.

Clindamycin

Topical clindamycin phosphate, FDA pregnancy category B, is effective for mild-to-moderate acne and safe throughout pregnancy and lactation due to minimal systemic absorption. It is commonly combined with BPO to enhance efficacy and reduce bacterial resistance. Caution is advised for individuals with a history of gastrointestinal issues due to pseudomembranous colitis and potential *Clostridium difficile* diarrhea. While generally safe, avoid applying it to the chest area of lactating women to prevent potential diarrhea in breastfed infants.

Erythromycin

Topical erythromycin, FDA pregnancy category B, is safe for all pregnancy trimesters and shows minimal systemic absorption. It is a widely used treatment for mild-to-moderate acne. However, its effectiveness is decreasing due to rising antibiotic resistance, therefore alternative topical antibiotics may be preferred. As with clindamycin, it should not be applied to the breast area in lactating women to avoid potential issues in breastfeeding infants.

Metronidazole

Metronidazole, formerly classified as FDA category B, is a second-line topical treatment for acne that is safe for use during pregnancy and lactation. It has antimicrobial, immunosuppressive, and anti-inflammatory effects. While studies are limited, topical metronidazole is associated with negligible systemic absorption and no adverse fetal effects have been reported. It is considered safe throughout all trimesters of pregnancy and during breastfeeding.

Minocycline Foam

Minocycline foam 4% is approved for treating inflammatory, nonnodular moderate-to-severe acne. It has minimal systemic absorption and low bioavailability, making significant fetal exposure unlikely. Despite this, it is wise to avoid its use during the second and third trimesters due to the potential risk of tooth discoloration in the fetus.

Topical Dapsone

Topical dapsone, previously classified as FDA pregnancy category C, is a second-line treatment for mild-to-moderate acne. It is generally safe during the first and second trimesters but should be discontinued 1 month before delivery due to a theoretical risk of neonatal hyperbilirubinemia. It is not recommended during the third trimester or lactation as it can transfer into breast milk.

Topical Retinoids

Topical retinoids, including tretinoin, adapalene, and tazarotene, are used for acne treatment, but their use during pregnancy is controversial due to potential risks. As the level of exposure that could lead to teratogenicity in humans is unknown, avoidance of both tretinoin and tazarotene is recommended in pregnant women.

- *Tretinoin:* Previously classified as FDA category C, tretinoin has been associated with rare reports of fetal abnormalities. Though its percutaneous absorption is minimal, it can cross the placenta, so its use is generally avoided during pregnancy due to potential risks.
- *Adapalene:* Also classified as FDA category C, adapalene has been linked to rare cases of teratogenicity in early pregnancy. However, a large trial indicates it has a reassuring safety profile, and it is generally considered safe in later pregnancy trimesters.
- *Tazarotene:* Assigned FDA category X due to teratogenic effects in animal studies, it is contraindicated during pregnancy and lactation.
- *Trifarotene:* The newest FDA-approved topical retinoid trifarotene did not identify any maternal or fetal risks among pregnant participants in clinical trials.

While topical retinoids are effective for acne due to their anti-inflammatory and comedolytic properties, their safety during pregnancy remains uncertain. Despite limited absorption and some reassuring studies, the potential risks of congenital malformations lead to a general recommendation to avoid these medications during pregnancy.

Topical Antiandrogen: Clascoterone

Clascoterone cream (1%) is a new topical antiandrogen for moderate-to-severe inflammatory and hormonal acne, offering a lower risk of systemic side effects than oral treatments. Limited human data during pregnancy show no adverse outcomes from a Phase 3 trial, but animal studies suggest potential dose-dependent malformations. Due to these concerns and limited safety data, clascoterone is generally avoided during pregnancy. Despite its rapid metabolism and minimal systemic absorption, alternative treatments are recommended for pregnant and lactating individuals.

Systemic Treatments

Topical therapies alone may not provide sufficient improvement for some patients. Oral treatments are generally recommended for those with moderate-to-severe inflammatory acne or for cases that do not respond well to extended use of topical agents. During pregnancy, preferred oral antibiotics are penicillins/aminopenicillins, followed by cephalosporins and macrolides. To combat bacterial resistance, it is advised to (1) combine topical BPO with oral antibiotics, (2) use oral antibiotics for the shortest duration necessary, and (3) avoid them for long-term acne maintenance.

Oral Antibiotics

Doxycycline/Minocycline

Tetracyclines, including doxycycline and minocycline, are often used for moderate-to-severe acne but should generally be avoided during pregnancy.

Doxycycline may be considered for severe conditions in the first trimester, but tetracyclines pose risks such as tooth discoloration, bone growth inhibition, infantile inguinal hernia, hypospadias, limb hypoplasia, and other adverse outcomes after the 15th week of gestation. Classified as pregnancy category D, they can also cause enamel hypoplasia and maternal liver toxicity in the third trimester. While minimally transferred through breast milk, rare cases of black galactorrhea have been reported.

Sarecycline

Sarecycline, a newer narrow-spectrum tetracycline approved for moderate-to-severe inflammatory acne, may offer a better safety profile with less impact on the gastrointestinal microbiome and lower risk of bacterial resistance. However, due to limited reproductive data, it is advised to avoid sarecycline during pregnancy. It may still cause developmental issues such as reduced bone growth and tooth discoloration, especially in the second and third trimesters.

Erythromycin

Oral erythromycin, used for moderate-to-severe inflammatory acne, is generally considered safe during pregnancy and is classified as FDA pregnancy category B. While some evidence suggests potential risks such as fetal pyloric stenosis and cardiovascular malformations, these are uncertain, and erythromycin is typically deemed compatible with pregnancy. The erythromycin estolate formulation should be avoided due to a risk of reversible cholestatic liver injury. Erythromycin base or ethylsuccinate are preferred. It crosses the placenta poorly and is safe for short-term use, though long-term effects are less studied. It is also safe during lactation, though some studies suggest avoiding it in the first 2 weeks of breastfeeding due to concerns about infantile pyloric stenosis, a finding not consistently supported by research.

Azithromycin

Azithromycin, an FDA pregnancy category B macrolide, is considered safe for use during pregnancy. It crosses the placenta without adverse effects on the fetus and is a suitable alternative to erythromycin if the latter is poorly tolerated or ineffective. Azithromycin has a longer half-life, allowing for once-daily dosing and fewer gastrointestinal issues compared to erythromycin. It is safe for use throughout pregnancy and lactation.

Beta-lactams

Amoxicillin

Amoxicillin, an FDA pregnancy category B aminopenicillin, can treat acne, particularly in cases resistant to other treatments. Although generally safe, it may increase the risk of oral clefts if used in early pregnancy, so its use should be restricted to the second and third trimesters. It may be used alone or with other medications but can cause gastrointestinal side effects such as nausea and vomiting.

Cephalexin

Cephalexin, a first-generation cephalosporin and pregnancy category B drug, is effective for acne and has not shown fetal defects in animal studies. However, human data are limited, and there are concerns about potential resistance development against *Staphylococcus* species.

Trimethoprim-sulfamethoxazole/Sulfonamides

Trimethoprim, a pregnancy category C folate antagonist, is linked to a doubled miscarriage risk in the first trimester and is generally contraindicated during pregnancy. Trimethoprim-sulfamethoxazole, effective for acne, poses risks including neural tube defects, miscarriage, preterm birth, and neonatal hyperbilirubinemia. It should be used only if no safer alternatives are available and when the benefits outweigh the risks. While it transfers minimally to breast milk and is acceptable for full-term infants, it should be avoided in premature infants or those with G6PD deficiency due to the risk of worsening hyperbilirubinemia.

Clindamycin

Oral clindamycin, a third-line acne treatment, is generally considered safe throughout pregnancy and lactation. It crosses the placenta at about 50% of maternal serum levels without known teratogenic effects. While it is associated with pseudomembranous colitis, this risk does not increase during pregnancy. Clindamycin is also safe during lactation due to minimal transfer to breast milk, though one case of bloody stools in a breastfed infant has been reported without a confirmed link.

Metronidazole

Oral metronidazole, rarely used for acne but often for pregnancy-related infections, is generally considered safe during pregnancy and lactation. It may be an alternative for severe, resistant acne during pregnancy. While generally well tolerated, there have been reports of *Candida* infections, lactose intolerance, and diarrhea in breastfed infants of mothers taking metronidazole.

Spironolactone

Spironolactone, an off-label systemic acne treatment, is a former FDA pregnancy category C medication. It inhibits 5α-reductase and aldosterone but has caused feminization in male fetuses and delayed sexual maturation in female fetuses in animal studies. Due to these risks, it should be avoided during pregnancy, and a washout period of at least 1 month before conception is recommended. It is generally safe during breastfeeding, as it transfers minimally to breast milk and has not shown significant adverse effects or electrolyte imbalances in infants, though it may affect lactation.

Isotretinoin

Isotretinoin, an FDA pregnancy category X medication, is strictly contraindicated during pregnancy and lactation due to severe teratogenic effects, including craniofacial, central nervous system (CNS), cardiovascular, and thymic defects. It is crucial to wait at least 1 month and one menstrual cycle after medication discontinuation before trying to conceive. The I-Pledge program in the US mandates strict contraception and monthly pregnancy testing to prevent fetal exposure. Although highly effective for severe acne, isotretinoin should not be used during lactation due to its high lipid solubility and potential risks, despite no documented adverse effects in breastfed infants.

Hormone Treatment

Hormonal treatments, such as androgen receptor blockers and oral contraceptives, are effective for managing hyperandrogenism in nonpregnant patients. However, these therapies are not advised during pregnancy due to their potential risks. Early pregnancy use of hormonal therapy has been linked to a higher incidence of Down syndrome, as well as risks of feminization and hypospadias in male fetuses.

Systemic Steroids

Prednisone, used for severe acne with scarring, should be carefully managed during pregnancy and only after consulting an obstetrician. It is classified as FDA pregnancy category C and is associated with risks such as reduced head circumference, cleft palate, and decreased brain growth from animal studies, and human studies link it to oral clefts, miscarriage, and preterm births. For severe acne, low-dose prednisone (<20 mg/day) for up to 1 month is generally considered safe after the first trimester. Avoid high doses due to risks of premature labor, intrauterine growth restriction, eclampsia, and gestational diabetes. Prednisone should not be used in the first trimester due to orofacial cleft risks. During lactation, it is safe as it transfers minimally into breast milk; mothers should wait 4 hours postmedication before breastfeeding to reduce exposure.

Zinc

Oral zinc salts, effective for mild-to-moderate acne, either alone or in combination, are used in doses of 30–150 mg/day. Zinc is considered safe for the fetus at doses under 75 mg/day, with no adverse effects reported during lactation. It helps with acne through its antibacterial, anti-inflammatory, and antisebum properties. Zinc sulfate is FDA pregnancy category C, while zinc gluconate lacks formal classification. Studies show no increased risk of fetal abnormalities at doses under 75 mg/day. High doses can cause gastrointestinal issues and hypocupremia, so recommended doses should not be exceeded. The recommended zinc intake during pregnancy is 11 mg, with potential side effects such as nausea generally being temporary and dose dependent.

The safety of different drugs in pregnancy and lactation has been categorized in **Tables 1 to 3**.

Procedural Treatments

Pregnant patients and their healthcare providers might also consider procedural treatments as alternatives or supplements to topical and oral acne medications.

Factors such as cost and limited available data should be taken into account when evaluating these options.

Intralesional Corticosteroids

Intralesional triamcinolone injections can effectively treat inflammatory papules and acne cysts, alleviating symptoms such as pain. Low concentrations of 2.5 mg/mL are generally considered safe during pregnancy. While systemic corticosteroid use in the first trimester has been linked to an increased risk of cleft palate and lip, the minimal systemic absorption of intralesional corticosteroids means they pose a low risk to the fetus. This treatment is also deemed safe during breastfeeding due to its minimal absorption into breast milk.

Chemical Peels/Cosmetic Peels

Glycolic and lactic acid peels, which promote desquamation and epidermolysis, are considered safe for use during pregnancy due to their minimal dermal penetration. In contrast, salicylic acid peels, which also induce desquamation and epidermolysis, can penetrate deeper, particularly when applied to large areas or under occlusion. While not contraindicated, salicylic acid peels should be used on small areas during pregnancy. Glycolic acid, classified as a pregnancy category N drug (not rated), is used topically for acne and effectively treats both comedonal and inflammatory acne, improves postinflammatory changes, and enhances the absorption of other topical treatments, with no reported adverse effects during pregnancy.

LIGHT AND LASER THERAPIES

Light and laser therapies, including photodynamic therapy (PDT), narrowband-ultraviolet B phototherapy (NBUVB), pulse-dye laser treatments, and Nd:YAG laser can be effective for treating refractory acne. These therapies are generally considered safe during pregnancy, as there is no evidence of teratogenic effects. Although data on their use in pregnant patients is limited, they are not known to cause harm to the developing fetus.

Phototherapy

Narrowband UVB (NBUVB) phototherapy is an effective and generally safe option for treating mild-to-moderate acne during pregnancy, as supported by its use in psoriasis patients. However, cumulative NBUVB exposure may reduce serum folic acid levels, which are crucial for fetal nervous system development and preventing neural tube defects. To mitigate this risk, it is advisable to ensure adequate folic acid supplementation and monitor serum levels in pregnant patients undergoing NBUVB therapy. Consulting with obstetricians for appropriate folic acid management is recommended.

Photodynamic Therapy

Photodynamic therapy is an alternative treatment for pregnant patients with acne, using aminolevulinic acid (ALA) as a photosensitizer. However, ALA is classified as pregnancy category C, with limited safety data during pregnancy. Although a case report showed no adverse effects, its safety during pregnancy is not well-established. Consequently, PDT should be performed without ALA during pregnancy. Barriers to PDT include lack of insurance coverage and the need for frequent dermatologist visits.

Lasers

Fractionated CO_2 lasers for acne scarring and vascular lesion lasers (595 nm) are generally considered safe during pregnancy and lactation but are often postponed until after delivery. Studies have shown that CO_2 lasers used for genital condyloma during pregnancy did not result in maternal or fetal complications. In 2022, the FDA approved two new lasers for acne treatment—the AviClear (Cutera) and the Accure (Accure Acne Inc.), both utilizing a 1726-nm wavelength to target sebaceous glands with electrothermolysis. Although these devices show promise, more research and long-term safety data are needed before they can be recommended for use during pregnancy. For lactating patients, laser and light therapies are expected to pose minimal risk due to limited systemic absorption.

ROSACEA AND PREGNANCY

INTRODUCTION

- Rosacea can be particularly challenging during pregnancy due to hormonal and reproductive changes. Around half of the women with preexisting rosacea report worsening symptoms, about one-third see no change and a few experience improvement
- Similar to the treatment of acne, managing rosacea during pregnancy primarily involves using specific oral and topical antibiotics, avoiding triggers, moisturizers, soap-free cleansers, broad-spectrum sunscreens with high sun protection factor (SPF), while harsh or heavy products should be avoided

Rosacea is a prevalent chronic inflammatory skin dermatosis affecting the face, which usually arises in adults, affecting 10–22% of people. It is more frequent in women between the ages of 35 and 50 years and is especially prominent in Caucasians than in individuals with darker skin types. There is a limited data set related to the clinical course and treatment of rosacea during pregnancy.

It is a persistent disease with an unknown cause, but mostly believed to be genetic and multifactorial in origin. The rash often affects the nose, forehead, cheeks, and chin, with at least 20% of individuals developing ocular symptoms such as conjunctival inflammation, dryness of eyes, and others. Rosacea may develop de novo or flare up during pregnancy but does not impact the baby's health or the course of the pregnancy. However, there is minimal research on the clinical course and management of rosacea during pregnancy.

Rosacea may be more prevalent in women due to hormonal and reproductive causes. Premenopausal women are more likely than postmenopausal women to develop rosacea and longer duration of hormonal therapy at menopause as well as oral medications including conjugated estrogen are associated with an increased risk of rosacea. Rosacea is more likely prevalent in females with advanced maternal age and nulliparous women (with a decrease in risk as the number of babies increases).

Pyoderma faciale or rosacea fulminans (RF), a severe and rare subtype of rosacea, may develop or exacerbate during pregnancy probably due to a weakened immune system. The relationship of RF to rosacea is also unclear as a preceding history of rosacea may or may not be present. The significant inflammation of the face, with many pustules and cystic lesions, and coalescing sinuses in RF patients were linked to adverse fetal and maternal outcomes during pregnancy.

Rosacea adversely impacts patients' quality of life, along with their psychological and social well-being. Those affected often expressed anxiety, low mood, shame, self-blame and embarrassment, leading them to hide their condition and "fight" with their skin. This fight encompasses not only the financial burden of treatment but also the social cost of concealing their challenges to fit in and prevent rejection.

PATHOPHYSIOLOGY (FIG. 1)

The precise cause of rosacea is neither clearly defined nor entirely understood. The pathogenesis of rosacea is multifactorial and may involve dysfunction of adaptive and innate immunity, exposure to ultraviolet (UV) radiation, neurovascular

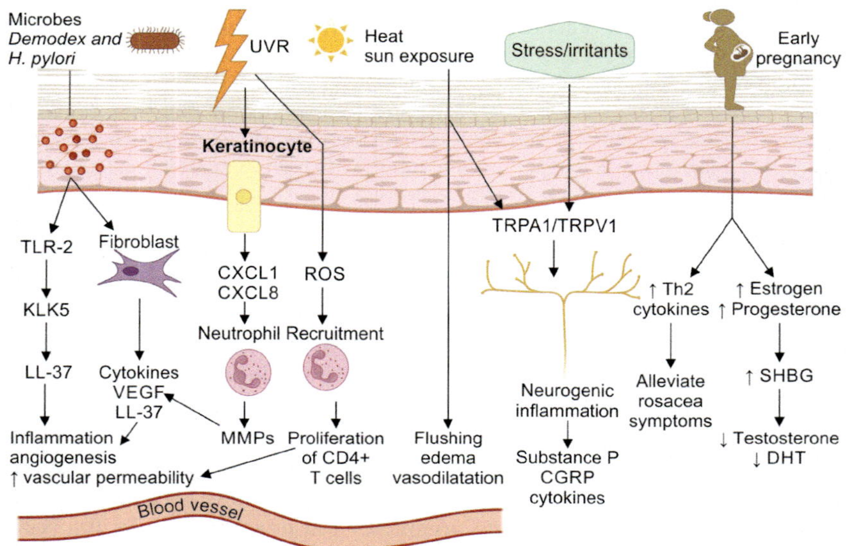

FIG. 1: Various triggers and pathophysiology of rosacea.

(DHT: dihydrotestosterone; MMP: matrix metalloproteinase; ROS: reactive oxygen species; SHBG: sex hormone binding globulin; VEGF: vascular endothelial growth factor)

dysregulation, genetic and hormonal influences, abnormal homeostasis of cutaneous vasculature, neurogenic inflammation and local inflammatory responses to cutaneous microbes. Various triggers of rosacea are listed here.

Common triggers of rosacea:
- Stress
- Ultraviolet radiation
- Spicy foods
- Extreme temperatures
- Alcohol consumption
- Saunas
- Hot baths
- Intense exercise
- Dairy products
- Certain medications and cosmetics

The distinctive phenotype observed in rosacea patients results from an underlying inflammatory process affecting the facial vasculature and pilo-sebaceous unit. The inflammatory cascade of rosacea is linked to a biological network of chemokines and cytokines. TLR-2 (Toll-like receptor 2) signaling triggers the release of IL-1 (interleukin-1) and TNF-α (tumor necrosis factor-α), stimulating keratinocytes and recruiting Th17 and Th1-T helper cells. These cells release various cytokines such as interleukin-17 (IL-17), which facilitates angiogenesis through activation of vascular endothelial growth factor (VEGF). Moreover, exposure to UV radiation stimulates keratinocyte synthesis of chemokines (CXCL8 and CXCL1), thus aiding the recruitment of neutrophils. Exposure to UV-A inhibits the synthesis of collagen and reduces MMP (matrix metalloproteinase) activity, whereas exposure to UV-B increases the production of angiogenic factors and inflammatory cytokines.

Reactive oxygen species (ROS) can cause damage to fibroblasts, endothelial cells, and keratinocytes by releasing TNF-α and interleukin-1. In recent times, microbes such as *Helicobacter pylori* and *Demodex folliculorum* have been known to trigger rosacea, and the latter has also been found in the inflamed hair follicles of individuals with rosacea. Rosacea may also be linked to various metabolic, psychiatric, and neurologic disorders and systemic diseases such as inflammatory bowel disease and obesity as well as certain foods, drugs, and malignancies.

During pregnancy, various physiological alterations occur, which can impact conditions such as rosacea. For instance, a shift from Th1/Th17 to Th2 cytokines during the third trimester may help alleviate rosacea symptoms and this returns to baseline postpartum. This pattern suggests that the improvement of rosacea seen during pregnancy and the recurrence of rosacea postpartum might be due to these physiological changes rather than just the natural progression of rosacea. This shift could be clinically important, as Th1/Th17 cytokines are believed to play a key role in driving inflammation in rosacea. Moreover, hormonal fluctuations and reduced peripheral vascular resistance during pregnancy might exacerbate rosacea.

As the pregnancy advances, serum levels of estrogen and progesterone rise sharply, leading to a significant increase in SHBG (sex-hormone-binding globulin). SHBG has a strong binding affinity for dihydrotestosterone (DHT) and testosterone, which lowers their serum concentrations early in pregnancy. This decrease in hormone levels results in reduced sebum production, follicular hyperplasia, and fewer pustules and papules. During the third trimester, free testosterone levels are roughly twice as high as the baseline, while levels of other androgens such as dehydroepiandrosterone sulfate (DHEAS) and dehydroepiandrosterone (DHEA) either decrease or remain unchanged throughout pregnancy.

The pathophysiology of RF is not clearly known but may be attributed to extreme emotional trauma (such as divorce, an accident, or a family member's death). Pregnancy can be regarded as an aggravating factor for RF, and hormonal changes during pregnancy may be a trigger for RF and in women using oral contraceptives.

DIAGNOSIS

Rosacea is a chronic inflammatory condition affecting the centrofacial skin, with a high concentration of sebaceous glands. The primary characteristics of rosacea include telangiectasias, chronic erythema, transient erythema/flushing, as well as pustules and papules. Secondary characteristics include a dry appearance, plaques, stinging and burning sensations, phymatous changes, or edema. The various subtypes of rosacea are shown in **Flowchart 1**.

Rosacea fulminans is marked by a sudden and severe onset, with a rapidly progressing course, confined exclusively to the face, and absence of acneiform lesions on the back or chest and comedones. The distinctive lesions include intensely inflamed, superficial nodules and papulopustules, with draining sinuses often accompanied by cyanotic erythema. In one documented case, severe ocular involvement by RF led to ocular perforation.

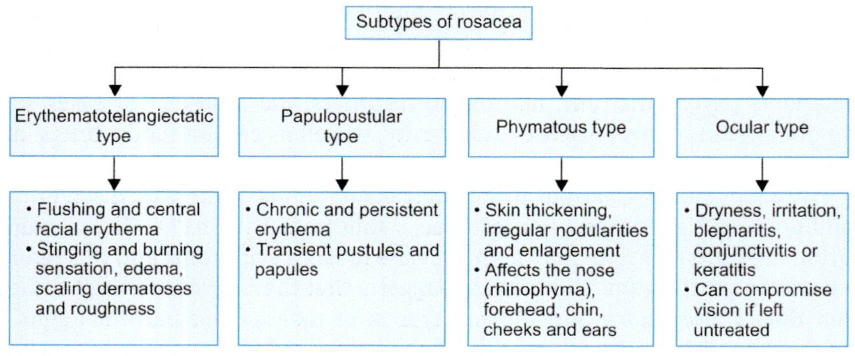

FLOWCHART 1: Subtypes of rosacea.

TREATMENT

Similar to the treatment of acne, managing rosacea during pregnancy primarily involves using specific oral and topical antibiotics. It is obligatory that all patients learn about rosacea and its triggers and avoid them. Given the diverse manifestations and causes of rosacea, treatment should be tailored to each individual, incorporating multiple approaches. All treatment plans should include moisturizers, soap-free cleansers, and broad-spectrum sunscreens with high sun protection factor (SPF), while harsh or heavy products should be avoided. Rosacea cannot be cured, but several therapies are available that can greatly reduce the symptoms and enhance quality of life.

For managing rosacea during pregnancy:

- *Papulopustular rosacea:* Topical treatments such as azelaic acid, metronidazole, and clindamycin are commonly used and considered safe. These treatments help reduce inflammation and improve symptoms.
- *Erythematotelangiectatic rosacea:* Vascular lesion lasers (595 nm) are effective but typically postponed until after pregnancy due to a lack of extensive safety data.
- *Ocular rosacea:* Treated with erythromycin ophthalmic ointment and sulfa eye drops.
- *Rosacea fulminans:* Treatment may involve oral corticosteroids and antibiotics. However, systemic steroids should be used cautiously due to the risks of intrauterine growth restriction, diabetes, and hypertension. Topical and systemic treatments such as metronidazole and azithromycin have been used in severe cases.

Topical Treatments

- *Azelaic acid:* It reduces inflammation and erythema.
- *Metronidazole:* It decreases inflammation by reducing reactive oxygen species.
- *Sodium sulfacetamide/sulfur:* It is anti-inflammatory and reduces papules but not suitable for those with renal issues or drug hypersensitivity.
- *Brimonidine tartrate:* Vasoconstrictor for improving flushing and erythema.
- *Oxymetazoline hydrochloride:* It reduces erythema.
- *Ivermectin:* It is used for papulopustular rosacea; has anti-parasitic and anti-inflammatory effects.

Oral Treatments

- *Tetracyclines:* Effective but not recommended due to potential fetal tooth discoloration.
- *Macrolides (erythromycin and azithromycin):* Safe alternatives.
- *Isotretinoin:* Highly effective but contraindicated due to teratogenic risks.

Laser Therapies

- *Safe options:* Fractionated CO_2 lasers, vascular lesion lasers, and certain newer lasers such as the AviClear and Accure are generally considered safe but require more research.
- *Considerations:* Light-based therapies are effective for vascular symptoms, though the safety profile in pregnancy is still under study.
- *Pregnancy-safe options*: Azelaic acid, brimonidine, and metronidazole are considered relatively safe, while tetracyclines and isotretinoin should be avoided. Light-based therapies may also be safe.

Overall, managing rosacea during pregnancy involves balancing effective treatment with safety for both the mother and fetus, with a preference for topical therapies and cautious use of systemic treatments.

KEY POINTS

- Pregnancy can trigger the onset of acne for the first time, worsen preexisting acne, or occasionally lead to its complete resolution.
- Hormonal and physiologic changes, increased sebum production, and altered immune function during pregnancy can worsen and increase the prevalence of acne across different trimesters.
- For mild-to-moderate acne, start with topical treatments such as BPO, azelaic acid, or keratolytics. Systemic or procedural treatments may be needed for refractory cases, with careful consideration of fetal risks.

SUGGESTED READINGS

1. Tyler KH. Cutaneous Disorders of Pregnancy, 1st edition. Springer International Publishing; 2020.
2. Ingber A, Lebwohl M. Obstetric Dermatology. Springer; 2008.
3. Kutlu Ö, Karadağ AS, Ünal E, Kelekçi KH, Yalçınkaya İyidal A, Topaloğlu Demir F, et al. Acne in pregnancy: A prospective multicenter, cross-sectional study of 295 patients in Turkey. Intern J Dermatol. 2020;59(9):1098-105.
4. Gomolin T, Cline A, Pereira F. Treatment of rosacea during pregnancy. Dermatol Online J. 2021;27(7).
5. Ly S, Kamal K, Manjaly P, Barbieri JS, Mostaghimi A. Treatment of Acne Vulgaris during Pregnancy and Lactation: A Narrative Review. Dermatol Ther (Heidelb). 2023;13(1):115-30.

CHAPTER 6

Melasma and Pregnancy

Sanjeev Gupta, Meghna Khatri, Mudita Gupta

INTRODUCTION

Pregnancy is a period of significant change and stress for a woman. Skin changes during pregnancy can be attributed to hormonal, immunologic, vascular, and metabolic factors. Approximately 90% of pregnant women exhibit some degree of hyperpigmentation, specifically those with darker skin types and hair. Most of the time, they are a source of distress and concern to the patient. Hyperpigmentation may impair quality of life and increase the stress of a pregnant patient. The exact cause is unknown but appears to be related to elevated levels of estrogen, melanocyte-stimulating hormone, and possibly progesterone. It begins as mild widespread hyperpigmentation in the first trimester, accentuating already hyperpigmented areas such as the nipples, areola, axillae, inner thighs, and genital skin. It becomes crucial to rule out hyperthyroidism and genetic predisposition in cases of generalized hyperpigmentation. Secondary areola is produced when the area surrounding the areola darkens, and linea alba darkens to become linea nigra, which is often accompanied by displacement of the umbilicus to the right known as "ligamentum teres sign". Lentigines, nevi, ephelides, and recent onset scars may enlarge and become hyperpigmented.

MELASMA IN PREGNANCY: INTRODUCTION AND EPIDEMIOLOGY

Melasma is an acquired, generally symmetrical, blotchy hyperpigmentation that arises on sun-exposed areas such as the face and neck. It is clinically characterized by irregular, brown to grayish-blue macules and patches with distinctive borders. The term "melasma" is derived from the Greek word melas, meaning "black", referring to its brownish clinical presentation. In pregnancy, it is referred to as "pregnancy mask" or "chloasma gravidarum", which comes from the Greek "chloazein"—green. However, since the resulting pigmentation is gray-brown, the term "melasma" is preferred.

Melasma can arise before or during pregnancy, with typical presentation during the second half of gestation or many years after delivery. The incidence during pregnancy varies from 2.5 to 75%, with a reported higher incidence in dark-skinned individuals (skin types IV–VI). The data on the epidemiology of melasma in Indian women is limited, however, few studies reported a very low incidence of 2.5–8.5%. Wide ethnic variation is noted, with predominance among Asian, African, and Hispanic descendants.

Pigmentation usually undergoes spontaneous remission within 1 year of delivery but may persist in a significant number of cases with some pigmentary sequelae. Recurrences are noted in subsequent pregnancies, and the likelihood of having melasma for the first time during pregnancy increases double to triple-fold with a history of multiple pregnancies. There is an increase of 8% in melasma with each year increase in maternal age of primigravida.

ETIOPATHOGENESIS OF MELASMA IN PREGNANCY

Although the exact cause and pathophysiology of melasma is not clearly understood, various factors are implicated which include:

Risk Factors of Melasma in Pregnancy

Risk factors of melasma in pregnancy:

- Ultraviolet radiation, visible light, and infrared radiation exposure
- Hormonal changes during pregnancy
- Use of hormone replacement therapy (HRT) and oral contraceptives before pregnancy
- Thyroid abnormalities
- Genetic susceptibility
- Racial factors
- Medications, including cosmetics and aesthetic procedures

- *Exposure to UV radiation (UVR):* The course and progression of melasma were directly proportional to the duration of sun exposure. Melasma was more noticeable and darker during summer than winter, when it was less evident, and is more prevalent in intertropical regions suggesting the role of sun exposure in the pathogenesis of melasma. Long-term exposure to UVR triggers melanin synthesis by activating the inflammatory cascade mainly through free radical scavenging and indirectly by activating various melanogenic factors, enhances dermal inflammation, causes basement membrane disruption, and alters the extracellular matrix. UVR acts on melanocytes (increasing melanogenesis and melanosome transfer), keratinocytes [increasing adrenocorticotropic hormone (ACTH), melanocyte stimulating factor (MSH), and β-endorphin], mast cells (releasing histamine), and fibroblasts [keratinocyte growth factor (KGF)], interleukin (IL)-6, tumor necrosis factor (TNF)-α, stem cell factor (SCF), basic fibroblast growth factor (bFGF) leading to increased pigmentation. It also causes degradation of the basement membrane. In addition to this, it causes an increase in vascular endothelial growth factor (VEGF), prostaglandins, endothelin, nitric oxide, leukotrienes, and calcitonin gene-related peptide (CGRP) which contributes to an increase in melanogenesis **(Fig. 1)**. All these processes lead to the activation of tyrosinase, tyrosinase-related protein 1, and dopachrome tautomerase; and secretion of alpha-melanocyte-stimulating hormone (α-MSH), corticotrophin, and the ligand stem-cell factor. UV radiation also triggers erythema, angiogenesis, and oxidative stress.

- *Hormonal factors:* Many cases of melasma are linked to excess estrogen, either produced endogenously during pregnancy and from ovarian tumors or delivered exogenously through the use of oral contraceptive pills (drugs, injectables, and implants) and hormone replacement therapy. Esposito et al. observed the prevalence of melasma in pregnant women ranged from 14.5 to 56%, while 11–46% of cases were associated with the use of hormonal contraceptives. Hormones work synergistically with UVR to increase sensitivity to UVR.
    - *Pregnancy:* Concerning pregnancy, melasma is regarded as a common physiologic skin change, exacerbating during pregnancy because of alterations in the placental, ovarian, and pituitary hormones. The sex hormones at various sites **(Fig. 1)** as described below:
        - Pregnancy triggers the production of pituitary hormones such as luteinizing hormone (LH), follicular-stimulating hormone (FSH), and melanocyte-stimulating hormone (MSH), which increase physiologic pigmentation including melasma, primarily during the third trimester acting through transcription of dopachrome, tyrosinase and TRP-2, promoting melanogenesis.

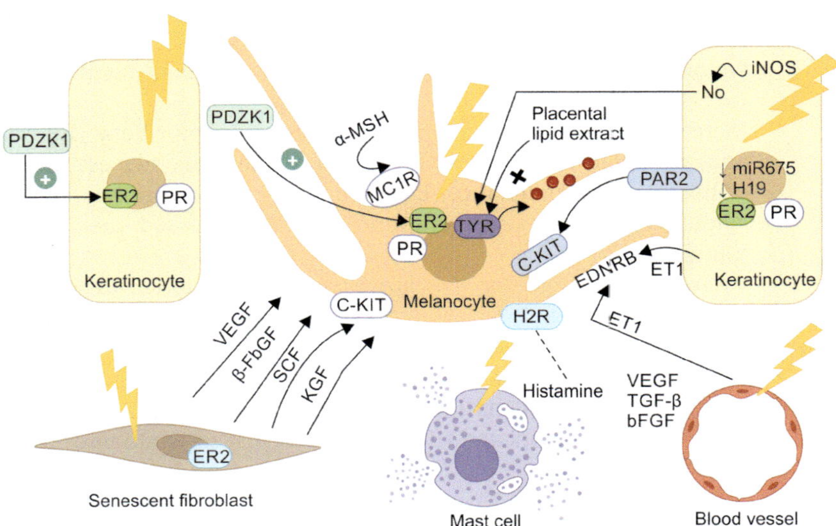

FIG. 1: Pathomechanism of melasma caused by ultraviolet rays and hormonal change in pregnancy.

(KGF: keratinocyte growth factor; MSH: melanocyte stimulating factor; PR: progesterone receptor; SCF: stem cell factor; TGF-β: transforming growth factor-β; VEGF: vascular endothelial growth factor)

- Progesterone levels rise throughout pregnancy, while estrogen production increases from the 8th week and begins to drop after the 30th week. This pattern represents the progression of hyperpigmentation. Elevated estrogen and progesterone levels increase MSH. During the first trimester, circulating immunoreactive α-MSH levels were undetectable in most patients, but significantly higher in late pregnancy, suggesting no pigmentary role of MSH in pregnancy-induced melasma. Progesterone causes melanin to disseminate in the keratinocytes, while estrogen works directly on melanocyte receptors, increasing the quantity of melanin in cells.
- Estrogens also increase the expression of PDZK1 which acts through estrogen receptors (ERs) in both melanocytes and keratinocytes, leading to an increase in tyrosinase, cyclic adenosine monophosphate (c-AMP)-responsive element binding protein and microphthalmia-associated transcription factor (MITF).
- An increase in estradiol in the papillary dermis triggers endothelial cell proliferation, potentially altering estrogen, progesterone, endothelin-1, and SCF levels. Increased endothelial cell count may also induce hyperoxia, stimulating melanogenesis, thereby affecting blood vessel function.
- Recently, it was discovered that a placental lipid extract induces pigmentation both in vivo and in vitro, which was found to be rich in bioactive sphingolipids, which induce melanogenesis by upregulating the expression of various melanogenic enzymes—tyrosinase, TRP-1, and 2 at the translational and transcriptional levels.
- Women carrying a male fetus exhibit a more proinflammatory/proangiogenic (G- CSF, IL-12p70, IL-21, and IL-33) and angiogenic factors (PlGF and VEGF-A). immune environment than women carrying a female fetus.
- Increased protein expression of estrogen receptor-beta (ER-beta) and progesterone receptor (PR) in facial melasma suggest the role of hormones in pregnancy. Estrogen causes downregulation of H19 leading to tyrosinase overexpression and increased melanosome transfer.
- *microRNA as a regulator of melanogenesis:* Expression of an H19 RNA-derived miRNA, miR-675, is reduced in melasma due to decreased expression of tyrosinase.

○ *Hormone replacement therapy (HRT)*: Administration of hormones, including topical estrogens have been linked to melasma. Extrafacial melasma has been associated with hormone replacement therapy during menopause.

○ *Oral contraceptive pills:* Hormonal contraception such as contraception pills, injections, and implants have varying degrees of impact on the onset of melasma since they contain estrogen and progesterone which induce melanogenesis. These processes include the action of c-AMP on cell membranes and are mediated by peptide hormones (peptides and glycoproteins). Melasma has been reported as an adverse reaction of contraceptives containing the synthetic progestin levonorgestrel, with increased expression of PR proteins in hyperpigmented skin. Hence, progesterone may play a role in melasma development, but progesterone in oral contraceptives can prevent melasma by reducing proliferation without significant effects on tyrosinase activity, counteracting estrogen's stimulatory effects in cultured melanocytes. Furthermore, facial hyperpigmentation is linked to uterine and ovarian function abnormalities is known as "chloasma uterine".

- *Hypothyroidism and thyroid autoimmunity:* Hypothyroidism increases estrogen and progesterone levels, hence, predisposing patient for hyperpigmentation. Melasma can be ascribed to conditions associated with skin inflammation, as patients with hyperthyroidism exhibit higher levels of proinflammatory cytokines. Melasma patients are four times more likely to have thyroid disorders, more commonly associated with hormone-associated melasma.
- *Role of visible and infrared light:* Although having lower melanogenic potential than UVR, high-energy visible light (HEVL) (400–450 nm) alone or in combination with infrared light can contribute to pigmentation by the generation of reactive oxygen species, causing indirect DNA damage and increasing expression of matrix metalloproteinase (MMP) and MITF. Moreover, the activation of the photoreceptor Opsin 3 by HEVL can also induce pigmentation by altering the activity of the enzyme tyrosinase and MITF leading to melasma. Iron oxide in tinted sunscreens can mitigate the effect of Opsin 3.
- *Infrared light exposure* also affects matrix metalloproteinase 1 activation, release of proinflammatory cytokines and may cause direct cytotoxicity.
- *Use of laser and light technologies and cosmetic procedures:* Intense pulsed light (IPL) and chemical peels can also aggravate melasma by causing inflammation and rebound hyperpigmentation.
- *Genetic and racial predisposition:* Genetic predisposition in melasma is supported by few reports of familial occurrence in first-degree relatives and identical twins. Patients with darker skin types (IV–VI) are more likely to have a family member with melasma and tend to have a longer duration of disease. Racial predominance is noted among Hispanics, Africans, and Asians with skin types III–IV.
- *Medications*: Hyperpigmentation follows the administration of drugs such as antimalarials, tetracyclines, sulfonylureas, anticonvulsants, and metals such as gold, copper, silver, iron, and bismuth as they stimulate melanin production by accumulation in the stratum corneum.
- *Cosmetics:* Cosmetics containing photosensitizers or irritants, and exposure to oils and crude tars are major causes for the development of melasma. The common practice of applying vegetable (mustard) oils after a bath on the face may also trigger melasma after sun exposure.
- *Vascular factors:* The evidence supporting the involvement of vascular factors in melasma comes from the increased density and size of blood vessels in the

dermis and an increased expression of VEGF in the lesional skin. Moreover, the efficacy of tranexamic acid, a plasminogen inhibitor, and pulsed dye laser (PDL) in reducing vascular proliferation further supported the vascular theory.

CLINICAL FEATURES

Melasma is seen as a blotchy macular pigmentation which can be classified depending on the region on face involved as shown in **Flowchart 1**.

Melasma can be classified depending on the depth of hyperpigmentation into epidermal, dermal, or mixed.

Clinical, dermoscopic features, and histopathology of these lesions help in classifying melasma and hence help in determining the response to treatment **(Flowchart 2)**.

PATHOLOGY

Hyperactive melanocytes with singly dispersed melanosomes and increased dendrites are seen. There may be damage in the basement membrane due to matrix metalloproteinases 2 and 9 which increases the risk of dermal melasma. Inflammatory cells, such as $CD4^+$ T cells, $CD68^+$ macrophages, mast cells, and increased levels of the inflammatory cytokine interleukin 17 (IL-17) and enzyme cyclooxygenase 2 (COX-2) are seen in the inflammatory type of melasma. These lead to increased prostaglandins. Persistence of this inflammatory infiltrate is responsible for recurrences of melasma even after pregnancy. Mast cells in the infiltrate may not only lead to a breach in the basement membrane but histamine release leads to proliferation and migration of melanocytes **(Fig. 1)**. Associated dermal elastosis, vascularization, and senescent fibroblasts are seen in chronically photodamaged skin. Increased bFGF, VEGF, and nitric oxide stimulate melanogenesis through tyrosinase **(Fig. 1)**.

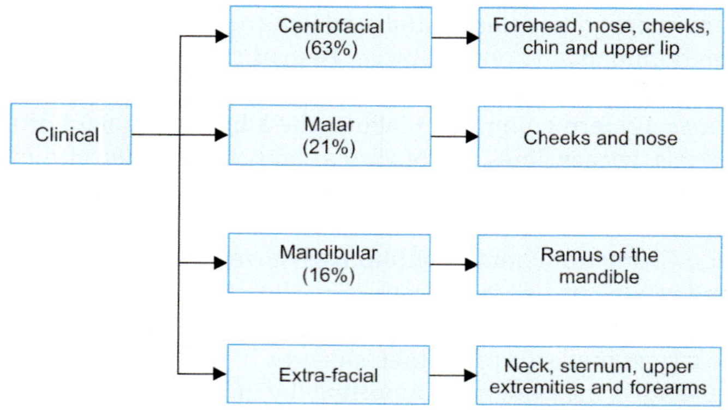

FLOWCHART 1: Classification of melasma depending on the site involved.

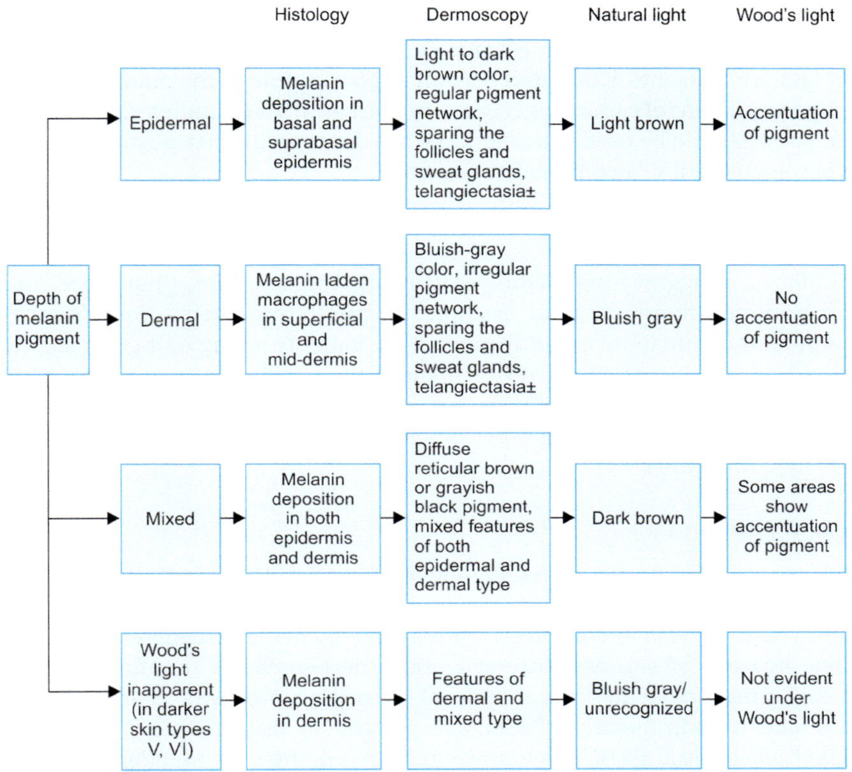

FLOWCHART 2: Classification of melasma depending on depth of pigmentation.

DIFFERENTIAL DIAGNOSIS

The disorders resembling melasma include solar lentigo with other forms of freckles and lentigines, acquired dermal macular hyperpigmentation, drug-induced and postinflammatory hyperpigmentation, Hori's nevus and nevus of Ota, actinic lichen planus, frictional melanosis, facial acanthosis nigricans, exogenous ochronosis, and poikiloderma of Civatte.

TREATMENT OF MELASMA IN PREGNANCY

The treatment of pigmentary changes during pregnancy is unsatisfactory and preventive strategies for hyperpigmentation during pregnancy are restricted.

The treatment of melasma is typically delayed until after delivery for several reasons:

- Most women experience a noticeable improvement in melasma after delivery, making therapy unnecessary;
- The hormonal cause for melasma persists during pregnancy, making it more resistant to treatment;
- The mainstay of treatment for melasma is contraindicated during pregnancy.

The most often recommended treatments for melasma during pregnancy include the use of broad-spectrum sunscreens, topical corticosteroids, and depigmenting agents. Cosmetics play an important role in the management as a temporary means of camouflage. Procedural treatments including chemical peels and lasers should be used with caution since they might cause postinflammatory hyperpigmentation, aggravating melasma.

General Management

Avoidance of aggravating factors—cosmetics, UV exposure, phototoxic drugs, and hormone therapy are all examples of phototoxic agents, so it is recommended to eliminate or avoid these factors. Patients taking oral contraceptives should be aware that effective treatment of their melasma may be impossible as long as the oral contraceptive is used. It is recommended that patients avoid irritation, trauma, or rubbing especially if they are prone to easy scarring (scars may hyperpigment).

Sunscreens

Melanocytes in melasma are readily activated by UVB, UVA, and visible radiation. Major lifestyle adjustments are required to maintain favorable treatment outcomes and prevent recurrences. Sunbathing is strictly forbidden since even a few minutes of sun exposure can undo the benefits of months of therapy. During pregnancy, the cornerstone of managing melasma is intensive and sustained photoprotection. Patients are urged to use opaque sunscreens to reduce all visible and UV light to prevent further pigment production.

Photoprotection comprises wearing wide-brimmed hats, sunglasses, photoprotective clothing, and sunscreen with sun protection factor (SPF) ≥30, reapplying every 2 hours when outdoors, and limiting sun exposure, especially during the daytime.

Role of Camouflage

Melasma lesions over the face may have psychological effects on patients. Cosmetic camouflage may be used to complement other treatments. Several ways are available to camouflage different skin tones. However, masking hypopigmented or depigmented lesions, such as vitiligo, is easier than concealing hyperpigmented lesions.

Various drugs have been used in treatment of melasma as summarized below **(Table 1)**.

BLEACHING AGENTS

Skin bleaching or lightening is using chemical compounds to lighten the skin tone or produce even complexion. Bleaching chemicals are classified into three types—phenolic compounds, nonphenolic compounds, and combinations. Bleaching agents have been used during pregnancy with varying but generally

TABLE 1: Summary of drugs used in melasma.

Agents	FDA pregnancy category	Mechanism of action	Comments
Hydroquinone	C	It inhibits the enzyme tyrosinase and also minimizes melanocyte destruction and distribution. Used in combination with retinoids or corticosteroids	More studies should be conducted to ascertain the effects on the fetus. No toxicity was reported to the fetus when applied in concentrations of up to 300 mg/kg
Arbutin	–	It inhibits tyrosinase activity, exerts a depigmenting effect, and reduces pigmentation	Due to its low systemic absorption and lower toxicity than HQ, it is assumed to be safe for use in pregnancy without any reported toxicity, irritation, or hypersensitivity reactions
Topical retinoids	C	It reduces pigmentation by preventing cell turnover and keratinocyte pigmentation. Superficial peeling occurs via reduced keratinization	Retinoids are not recommended due to potential teratogenic effects on the central nervous system, heart, and ears, and should be avoided during pregnancy, particularly in the first trimester
Azelaic acid	B	It is a dicarboxylic acid, derived from the yeast Malassezia furfur, and is vigorously used to treat melasma by inhibiting tyrosinase	Animal studies show no fertility, teratogenicity, or embryotoxicity risks during pregnancy, but should only be used for strict indications on small skin surfaces, and not in the first trimester
Alpha hydroxy acids (AHAs)	B	It improves hyperpigmentation and texture of skin by reducing stratum corneum thickness, stimulating cell growth and collagen formation	AHAs with a concentration of ≤10% and pH ≤3.5 are safe for use during pregnancy
Kojic acid	–	By chelating copper and ions, it inhibits tyrosinase, imparting it depigmenting and antiaging properties	Although it can induce contact allergies and sensitivities, it has not been demonstrated to be teratogenic
Topical steroids	C	Mechanism is unknown and typically ascribed to their direct antimetabolic influence on melanogenesis and change of melanocyte function	Mild-to-moderate potency topical steroids are considered safe for mothers and fetuses, while very potent steroids during pregnancy may raise the chance of low-birthweight babies

negative effects. Phenolic compounds are considered harmful because they can cause dyschromias, contact dermatitis, and severe skin irritation.

Hydroquinone (HQ) is a hydroxyphenolic compound, which inhibits the enzyme tyrosinase, which converts DOPA to melanin. Its mode of action also includes inhibiting DNA and RNA production, as well as minimizing melanocyte breakdown and distribution. HQ has been used commonly in the treatment of hyperpigmentation; however, pregnant women should exercise caution. It is US FDA pregnancy category C.

Arbutin (grape extract) is a naturally occurring plant substance and the beta-D-glucopyranoside derivative of HQ, that has been very efficient in reducing preexisting melasma by inhibiting tyrosinase. Compared to HQ, arbutin is less toxic and has dose-dependent activity. Typically used at concentrations of 2–3%. Higher dosages require extra caution as it might cause hyperpigmentation.

Ascorbic acid (vitamin C) possesses antioxidant and photoprotective properties, that inhibit melanogenesis, reduce dopaquinone to DOPA and prevent free radicals' production and absorption of UVR. It has no adverse effects and can be used alone or in conjunction with other demelanizing agents. Topical ascorbic acid has been demonstrated to improve melasma and hyperpigmentation and is particularly safe to use during pregnancy since it can aid in preventing preeclampsia. The percutaneous absorption of vitamin C can be enhanced by the use of iontophoresis.

Kojic acid, a naturally existing hydrophilic fungal product generated from certain *Aspergillus, Penicillium,* and *Acetobacter* species is used to treat pregnancy-induced melasma. It prevents the synthesis of free tyrosinase and is also an effective antioxidant. Kojic acid is often used in concentrations of 2–4%, alone or in conjunction with HQ, tretinoin, or a corticosteroid. Kojic acid has several benefits over traditional bleaching compounds; by being gentler on the skin and its antioxidizing characteristics help the product retain its efficacy.

Azelaic acid is a naturally occurring dicarboxylic acid obtained from the fungus *Pityrosporum ovale* and is present in wheat, rye, and barley. It inhibits tyrosinase, which leads to excellent outcomes in the treatment of melasma and postinflammatory hyperpigmentation. Its mechanisms of action include inhibiting the production of DNA and mitochondrial enzymes, therefore causing direct cytotoxic effects on the melanocyte. It is nontoxic and can be safely used during lactation and pregnancy. The FDA had previously classified azelaic acid as category B, but no well-controlled and sufficient studies have been undertaken in pregnant women. Considering this, azelaic acid should be used only in limited regions, ideally not during the first trimester, to avoid any possible harm to the baby.

Retinoic acid (RA) is a synthetic derivative of vitamin A. The mechanism of action of topical retinoids is yet unknown, however, they disrupt several steps in the melanization pathway. Tretinoin promotes rapid pigment loss via epidermopoiesis, increases epidermal turnover, and shortens the period of contact between keratinocytes and melanocytes. Retinoic acid inhibits UVB-induced pigmentation by lowering tyrosinase activity. The acid has post-transcriptional effects on tyrosinase and tyrosinase-related protein. Generating a desquamation (peeling), through the reduction of keratinization. Both systemic and topical retinoids are contraindicated during pregnancy. However, topical retinoids are considered safe during lactation, as only trace amounts are secreted in breast milk.

Topical steroids: The use of mild-to-moderate potency topical steroids during pregnancy is deemed safe since several studies have shown no increased risk to the mother or fetus from these drugs. Topical corticosteroids are seldom used alone for treating melasma due to their cutaneous side effects such as acneiform eruptions, skin atrophy, telangiectasias, hypertrichosis over the face, perioral dermatitis, and rosacea. Their direct antimetabolic effect on melanogenesis, inhibition of the synthesis of inflammatory mediators such as prostaglandins and leukotrienes, and/or modification of melanocyte function without being melanotoxic are some of the theories put forth to explain their skin-lightening effect, although the exact mechanism is still unknown. Topical use of a potent or super potent corticosteroid alone has shown promising results in the treatment of melasma. In triple combination therapy for melasma, corticosteroids including dexamethasone, hydrocortisone, fluocinolone acetonide, fluticasone, and mometasone furoate are still favored. Although fluticasone is less atrophogenic than other topical steroids, the latter is generally not recommended as monotherapy. Nevertheless, they are helpful when used with caution when pigmented cosmetic dermatitis is suspected or to lessen irritation from other topical treatments.

Nicotinamide: The amid form of vitamin B3 is called niacinamide, or nicotinamide. It has been demonstrated that topical nicotinamide, which inhibits the transfer of melanosomes from melanocytes to keratinocytes, is beneficial in treating hyperpigmentation and melasma. There are no documented side effects of nicotinamide in fetuses, even though it can accumulate in fetal blood and cross the placenta. Although there is uncertainty regarding the impact of high doses of nicotinamide and extended systemic use, topical nicotinamide seems to be a safe treatment option for pregnancy-related hyperpigmentation.

LYT2 serum in pregnancy-induced melasma: LYT2 serum is a novel and effective substitute for hydroquinone-based regimens for melasma during pregnancy. LYT2 is a topical pigment-correcting serum free of hydroquinone and retinol. Skin physiological metrics, including Melasma Area and Severity Index (MASI), brightness, global improvement, investigator-rated overall hyperpigmentation scale, and quality of life showed statistically significant decreases from baseline values. A noticeable decrease in hyperpigmentation compared to the baseline was also found.

Cysteamine: It is a thiol compound that is used as a depigmenting agent. It depletes dopaquinone and increases intracellular glutathione levels, thus decreasing the rate of melanin synthesis. It is a category C drug.

Turmeric: Turmeric contains curcumin and is a common spice used in many cultures and helps lighten skin by mediating oxidative damage and reducing cutaneous inflammation. The application of turmeric topically is deemed safe during pregnancy; several studies have shown the systemic use of turmeric via the probable role of curcumin in managing pregnancy complications, such as fetal intrauterine growth restriction, preeclampsia, and gestational diabetes.

SYSTEMIC THERAPIES

Tranexamic Acid

Tranexamic acid (TA), a lysine analog, is trans-4-(aminomethyl) cyclohexane carboxylic acid, which has been used as an antifibrinolytic drug for >30 years. It suppresses ultraviolet-induced plasmin activity in keratinocytes by restricting the attachment of plasminogen to the keratinocytes. Tranexamic acid can be used either topically, by intradermal microinjection or orally in melasma treatment. It is used orally in a dosage of 250 mg two times a day. However, it is contraindicated during pregnancy and lactation.

Chemical Peels

Alpha-hydroxy acids (AHAs) are a class of organic acids widely found in fruits and vegetables [tartaric acid, lactic acid (LA), glycolic acid (GA), citric, and malic acid] which when applied topically reduce the thickness of the stratum corneum by promoting the synthesis of collagen and cell proliferation, thus improving both the texture and hyperpigmentation of the skin. During pregnancy, there are no risks associated with AHAs that have a concentration of ≤10% and a pH of ≤3.5.

When treating the epidermal type of melasma, superficial peeling agents are helpful and can be used in conjunction with other melasma treatments. Considering the patient's skin type, needs, and sensitivity, the peel solution is chosen. In severe refractory cases of melasma, medium-depth peels may be an alternate therapy; however, in certain circumstances, this treatment may exacerbate the hyperpigmented lesion. Nonetheless, melasma's response to chemical peeling is erratic and might get worse due to postinflammatory hyperpigmentation. Therefore, chemical peeling is generally not advised for those with dark skin.

Glycolic Acid

Glycolic acid is an alpha-hydroxy acid naturally found in sugar cane juice. 10% GA peels mixed with 2% HQ were more effective than GA peels alone. Glycolic acid is an amino acid obtained from animals and plants that is safe to use during pregnancy and effectively improves hyperpigmentation.

Lactic Acid

Skin type IV patients with epidermal type of melasma could benefit from LA.

Lasers and Light Devices

There is no research on the usage of lasers during pregnancy. Laser therapy is another option for treating pregnancy-related hyperpigmentation and melasma. In general, laser therapy has been judged safe for both the infant and mother, however, the effectiveness varies depending on the particular laser, how it is used, and both operator and patient characteristics.

Various lasers that have been used for melasma include the following:

- *Red light:* Q switched alexandrite (755 nm), Q switched ruby (694 nm),
- *Green light:* Frequency-doubled QS Nd: YAG (532 nm), flashlamp-pumped pulsed dye laser (510 nm),
- *Near-infrared:* Q switched neodymium—yttrium aluminium garnet—1064 nm.

The rationale behind treating melasma with the more recent antiangiogenic lasers (copper bromide laser) and pulsed dye laser is that melanocytes and the cutaneous vasculature interact to cause melasma. Patients with severe telangiectasia and melasma can benefit from these laser therapies.

Intense pulsed light—a broadband light source that may target several cutaneous structures, such as vasculature and deeper pigmentation. Pulse-in-pulse (PIP) mode, which allows for numerous fractionated subpulses inside a single pulse width, is a novel form of IPL that holds promise as a safe therapy for melasma.

KEY POINTS

- Melasma is an acquired, generally symmetrical, blotchy hyperpigmentation that arises on sun-exposed areas such as the face and neck.
- Melasma can arise before or during pregnancy, with typical presentation during the second half of gestation or many years after delivery.
- The risk factors of melasma in pregnancy include UV radiation exposure, hormonal factors (OC pills, HRT, and pregnancy), genetic susceptibility, and medications.
- The treatment of melasma in pregnancy is restricted and limited due to safety concerns. The most often recommended treatment includes broad-spectrum sunscreens, topical steroids, depigmenting agents, and cosmetics.
- Melasma undergoes spontaneous resolution after delivery within 1 year but can persist in some patients with few pigmentary sequelae.

SUGGESTED READINGS

1. Espósito ACC, Cassiano DP, da Silva CN, Lima PB, Dias JAF, Hassun K, et al. Update on Melasma-Part I: Pathogenesis. Dermatol Ther (Heidelb). 2022;12(9):1967-88.
2. Lee AY. An updated review of melasma pathogenesis. Dermatologica Sinica. 2014;32: e233-9.
3. Sarkar R, Handog EB, Das A, Bansal A, Macarayo MJ, Keshavmurthy V, et al. Topical and Systemic Therapies in Melasma: A Systematic Review. Indian Dermatol Online J. 2023;14(6):769-81.
4. Cassiano DP, Espósito ACC, da Silva CN, Lima PB, Dias JAF, Hassun K, et al. Update on Melasma-Part II: Treatment. Dermatol Ther (Heidelb). 2022;12(9):1989-2012.

CHAPTER 7

Stretch Marks in Pregnancy

Mudita Gupta, Sanjeev Gupta

INTRODUCTION

Striae distensae, commonly known as stretch marks, are a form of dermal scarring that appears as linear bands or streaks on the skin. They develop as a result of rapid stretching of the skin, leading to the breakdown of collagen and elastin fibers in the dermis. This condition can occur in both males and females and is often associated with periods of rapid growth, significant weight changes, and certain medical conditions. Common causes include puberty, obesity, bodybuilding, and the use of systemic or topical corticosteroids.

Striae gravidarum (SG) are a specific type of striae distensae that develop during pregnancy. They are linear, atrophic scars that commonly appear on the abdomen, breasts, hips, buttocks, and thighs due to the rapid stretching of the skin as the body undergoes changes to accommodate the growing fetus. These stretchmarks can cause significant aesthetic and psychological impact on mother.

- Striae distensae are form of dermal scarring appearing as linear bands.
- Striae gravidarum (SG) is a specific type of striae distensae that develop during pregnancy.
- Striae gravidarum are located on abdomen, breasts, hips, buttocks, and thighs.
- Can cause significant aesthetic and psychological impact on mothers.

EPIDEMIOLOGY

Studies suggest that SG affects a significant proportion of pregnant women, with estimates ranging from 50 to 90%. Choi et al. observed that SG in second trimester developed in 55.9% primiparous and 63.1% of the multiparous mothers. Katta et al. observed overall SG in 99.1% of multipara and 89.2% of primiparas. Risk factors for development of SG may be various genetic (family history of striae), ethnical (less in Asians), demographic (younger females), obstetric causes (larger fetal size, multiparity, multigravida, polyhydramnios, elevated levels of estrogen, relaxin, and corticosteroids), greater prepregnancy body mass index, poor nutrition and lifestyle factors such as smoking, etc.

- Striae gravidarum (SG) prevalence estimates ranging from 50 to 90%.
- *Various risk factors are:*
  - Genetic predisposition
  - Ethnicity
  - Demographic factors
  - Obstetric factors
  - Overdistended abdomen
  - Increased hormones
  - Prepregnancy
    - Increased BMI
    - Smoking
    - Nutritional deficiency

PATHOGENESIS

Collagen type 1 provides strength, support, and resilience to the skin. These collagen fibers are present as bundles. Elastic fibers form a network and are responsible for elasticity of skin. Pathogenesis of the disease remains unclear. Why SG develops in specific areas in body, why it is not present in all pregnant females and why severity is more in some, are few questions which need to be addressed. It may be an interplay between various factors **(Box 1)**.

Mechanical Factors

The mechanical stretching of the skin is a significant factor in the development of striae gravidarum. During pregnancy, the rapid expansion of the abdomen and other areas can lead to the rupture of the dermal elastic fibers and collagen bundles. This mechanical stress exceeds the skin's capacity to stretch, leading to the tearing apart of the dermal fibers.

Hormonal Factors

Hormonal changes during pregnancy play a crucial role in the pathogenesis of striae gravidarum. Increased levels of hormones such as estrogen, relaxin, and corticosteroids can affect the skin's structure and function:

- *Estrogen*: SG skin has more estrogen receptors. Estrogen is known to influence the integrity of collagen, elastic fibers and decrease migration and proliferation of fibroblasts in the dermis. These weakened fibers, make them more susceptible to tearing under mechanical stress.

BOX 1 Pathogenetic factors in striae gravidarum.

- Mechanical—overdistension
- Hormonal—increased estrogen, relaxin, and adrenocotropic
- Genetic—family history
- Molecular—structural alteration in dermal products

- *Relaxin*: This hormone increases during pregnancy and helps relax the connective tissue in preparation for childbirth. However, it also contributes to the weakening of collagen fibers, making the skin more prone to developing striae. In addition, it increases the production of sulfate-free mucopolysaccharides. These mucopolysaccharides absorb water relaxing the interfibrous cohesive forces, leading to a cleavage or fraying of the collagen fibers.
- *Corticosteroids*: Increased corticosteroid levels can lead to the atrophy of the dermal layer and decrease collagen synthesis, which weakens the skin's structure and increases the likelihood of stretch marks.

Genetic Factors

Genetic predisposition is another significant factor in the development of SG. Studies have shown that women with a family history of stretch marks or pre-pregnancy stretch marks are more likely to develop them during pregnancy. Specific genetic markers and polymorphisms have been associated with the susceptibility to developing striae:

- *Collagen synthesis genes:* Variations in genes responsible for collagen synthesis, such as *COL1A1* and *COL3A1*, can influence the strength and resilience of the skin, making it more prone to tearing and scarring.
- *Elastin genes:* Polymorphisms in elastin-related genes can affect the elasticity and recoil properties of the skin, contributing to the development of striae.

Molecular Pathways

At the molecular level, the pathogenesis of striae gravidarum involves alterations in the extracellular matrix (ECM) and the inflammatory response:

- *Extracellular matrix (ECM) remodeling:* The degradation of collagen and elastic fibers is a key feature in the development of striae. Matrix metalloproteinases (MMPs), which are enzymes that degrade ECM components, are upregulated in striae-affected skin. This leads to the breakdown of collagen and elastin, weakening the dermal structure.
- *Inflammatory response:* The initial stage of striae development involves an inflammatory response characterized by the infiltration of immune cells and the release of cytokines and growth factors. This inflammation contributes to ECM remodeling and the formation of striae.
- *Formation of tropoelastin-rich fibrils*
- *Altered collagen fibers arrangement*—do not form bundles, instead show branching and the accompanying blood vessels get intertwine.

CLINICAL PRESENTATION

The development of SG occurs in distinct stages, each characterized by specific clinical and histological features. SG begin as dark red or purplish red linear elevations [due to inflammation and vascularity and are termed as stria rubra (SR)]. At this stage SG may be pruritic or may cause discomfort. These striae may mature into white or silver colored linear streaks with wrinkled surface to

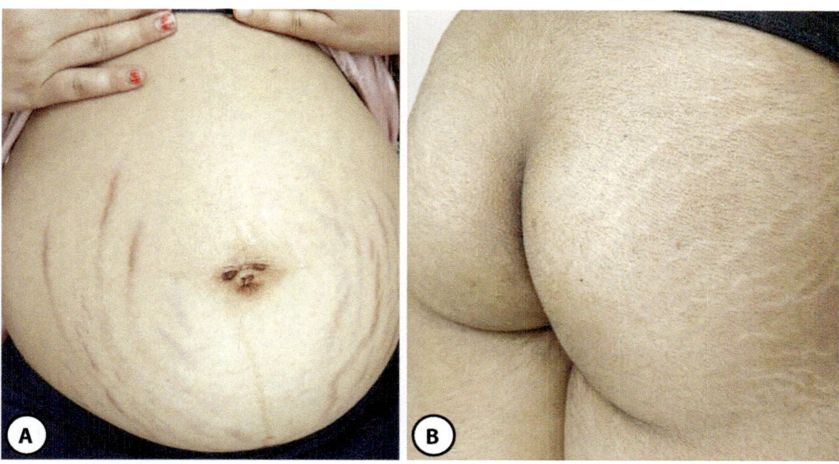

FIGS. 1A AND B: (A) Striae rubra on abdomen; (B) Striae on buttocks.

become converted into stria alba (SA) (**Figs. 1A and B**). Conversion of SR to SA takes around 6–10 months. SA then persists and becomes more prominent with age due to further loss of elastic fibers. In patients with darker skin type SA may appear as black (stria nigra) or blue (stria cerulae). Classically SG appears along skin tension lines on abdomen, breasts, medial upper arms, hips, lower back, buttocks, and thighs.

As clinical features are quite characteristic no specific investigations are required. Histologically, SG shows thinned out epidermis with loss of rete ridges. In SR there is lympho-histiocytic infiltrate in the dermis. In the center of early striae there is reduction in normal collagen, elastin, and fibrillin while periphery shows thick and tortuous elastic fibers. Collagen bundles unlike normal dermis fail to form bundles. Elastolysis presents as disorganized thin elastic fibers. There may be mast cell degranulation with macrophage activation. In SA no inflammatory cells are seen and thin collagen bundles arranged parallel to skin surface are seen.

Clinical features

- Linear streaks initially red/purple—striae rubrum
- Later silvery white—striae alba
- In dark skinned—black streaks (striae nigra) and bluish gray (striae cerulae)

Psychological impact of striae gravidarum may be immense on mother. Historical descriptions also show that stretch marks have always been a source of distress for pregnant women. In sixteenth century BC poet Ovid alluded to women who would self-abort due to fear of striae. Recent research suggests that severe SG increases the risk of perineal tears during delivery.

TREATMENT

While no treatment can completely eliminate stretch marks, several options have been shown to be effective to varying degrees hence pretreatment assessment

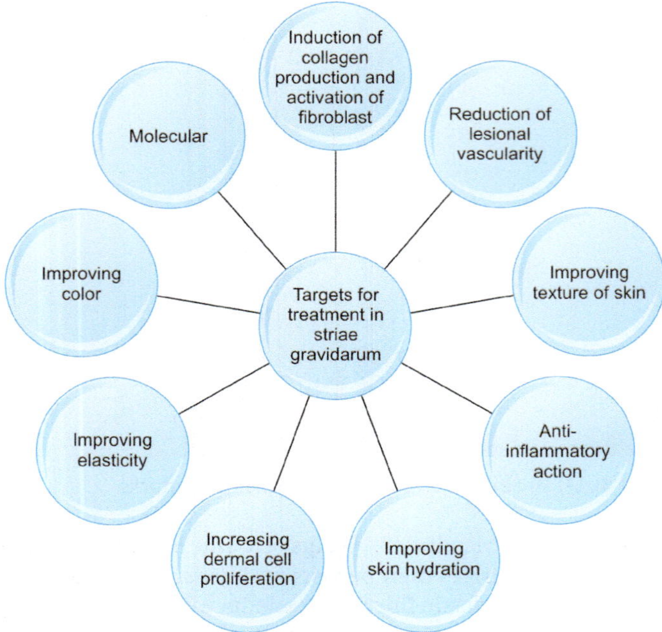

FIG. 2: Targets for treatment in striae gravidarum.

of patient is essential. Patient should have realistic expectations, should realize the cost of therapy and that a prolonged follow-up and treatment is required. In patients with darker skin types interventional therapies should be avoided. Occupation of patient and type of clothing of patient should also be assessed. Also, if SG is hampering patient's quality of life a more energetic approach is required. The various targets for treatment are as shown in **Figure 2**. These treatments can be categorized into topical therapies, procedural interventions, and emerging treatments.

Preventive therapies: Application of *Centella asiatica*, hyaluronic acid have been reported to be of preventive value.

Topical Therapies

Tretinoin (Retinoid Creams)

Tretinoin, a derivative of vitamin A, has been shown to improve the appearance of early stretch marks, by promoting collagen production and skin renewal. While 0.1% or 0.05% cream after 6 months of treatment reduce severity of SG lower concentrations were not found to be beneficial. If no improvement occurs within 6 months then tretinoin should be stopped. Topical tretinoin was not found to be effective in SA. However, it is not recommended during pregnancy and breastfeeding due to potential teratogenic effects. Also, at this concentration it may cause irritation. Tretinoin may be combined with 20% glycolic acid or trichloroacetic acid (TCA) peels which can penetrate into dermis.

Punica Granatum Seed Oil and Croton Lechleri Resin Extract

It causes increased derma thickness, elasticity and hydration.

Hyaluronic Acid

Hyaluronic acid-based creams can help hydrate the skin and improve its elasticity, thereby reducing the appearance of stretch marks. It is safe to use during pregnancy and breastfeeding. It also stimulates fibroblast activity and increases resistance to mechanical forces.

Centella Asiatica Extract

Centella asiatica popularly known as Indian pennywort, Gotu Kola in India. It is a member of Apiaceae family. Asiaticoside, madecassoside, and their respective aglycones asiatic acid and madecassic acid are the active ingredients of this plant. Fibroblasts from SG have increased expression of connective-tissue growth factor (CTGF). The exact mechanism of action of *Centella* is not known. Topical formulations containing *Centella asiatica* can be effective in treating both early and mature stretch marks. Enhanced fibroblast migration, maturation, and restoration of the orientation of collagen bundles without enhancing the quantity of collagen, elastic fiber networks formation. CTGF which is upregulated in SG is reduced by this compound and also extracellular matrix degradation gets rectified and micro-circulation is stimulated. Women who had a history of *striae distensae* at puberty stated that *Centella asiatica* treatment was 100% effective in preventing SG.

Silicone Gel and Sheets

Silicone products help maintain skin hydration and have been used successfully to reduce the appearance of scars and stretch marks. They are safe for use during and after pregnancy.

Topical Pirfenidone

It has immune modulatory effects and promotes collagenase and fibroblast activity.

Efficacy of these topical treatments though may be partially effective in stria rubra are not of much benefit in SA.

- Several topical treatments like punica granatum seed oil, croton lechleri resin extract, hyaluronic acid, centella asiatica extract, silicone gel, and pirfenidone may improve skin health and potentially reduce the appearance of stretch marks.

Procedural Interventions

Laser Therapy

Lasers target various chromophores such as water, hemoglobin, and melanin **(Table 1)**.

- *Ablative lasers* have wavelength >1,000 nm. These lasers get absorbed by water and cause vaporization and tissue destruction. Fractional ablative

TABLE 1: Laser and light therapies in striae gravidarum.

Lasers	Light and radiofrequency	Other interventional therapies
• Lasers • Ablative • Carbon dioxide • Erbium Yag • Fractional • Non ablative • Nd:Yag 1064 • Erbium glass • Diode 1450 • Pulsed dye laser 585 • Cu bromide • Excimer 308	• Light based • Intense pulsed light • Phototherapy • Infrared • Radiofrequency • Ablative • Non ablative • Microneedle	• Platelet-rich plasma • Carboxy therapy • Galvanotherapy • Microneedling • Microdermabrasion • Microneedling • Chemical peeling • Botulinum toxin

lasers cause intermittent destruction with intervening normal epidermis. Ablative lasers work better for SA than SR. The lasers target different chromophores such as water, hemoglobin, and melanin and thus improve overall appearance of SD by increasing collagen production, decreasing vascularity (especially in SR) and by increasing melanin pigmentation. Various ablative lasers used are carbon dioxide ablative laser (10,600 nm), Erbium Yag (2940 nm) laser, and fractional laser. Fractional laser causes formation of intermittent channels by thermolysis with intervening normal epidermis which helps in healing. Ablative lasers are more painful and take longer time to recover.

- *Nonablative lasers*
  - *Neodymium-doped yttrium aluminum garnet (Nd:YAG) laser:* This laser targets hemoglobin, water and melanin.
  - *Erbium glass* (1540 nm) is usually used as fractional laser. It improves color, texture, and elasticity of SG.
  - *Diode (1450 nm)* improves collagen production.
  - *Pulsed dye laser (PDL):* Effective for treating striae rubrae, PDL targets blood vessels, reducing redness, and promoting collagen production.
  - Copper bromide laser (577 nm) selective for hemoglobin
  - Excimer (308 nm) improves pigmentation in SA.
- *Fractional laser therapy:*
  - Suitable for both early and mature stretch marks, fractional lasers create micro-injuries in the skin, stimulating collagen remodeling and improving skin texture and stimulating pigmentation. Ablative fractional laser with 10,600 nm fractional CO_2 lasers and nonablative 1,540 nm laser. Both types of lasers were reported to be equally efficacious but ablative laser had more downtime.

Light Therapy

- *Intense pulse light*—using a 590 nm filter.
- *Phototherapy:* It causes re-pigmentation.
- *Infrared light*: Thermal energy which is produced helps in collagen remodeling and new collagen formation.
    - Used primarily for striae albae promoting repigmentation

Radiofrequency Therapy

It uses radiofrequency energy to heat the dermis and subcutis, promoting collagen, fibroblast proliferation, and elastin production. It is a noninvasive method to improve skin firmness and reduce the appearance of stretch marks.

Microdermabrasion

This minimally invasive procedure exfoliates the skin, promoting cell turnover, and collagen production. It can improve skin texture and the appearance of stretch marks over multiple sessions.

Microneedling

It involves creating tiny punctures in the skin with fine needles, stimulating collagen production and improving skin texture. Microneedling can be combined with topical treatments for enhanced results. It results in reduced risk of dyspigmentation in darker skin types.

Platelet-rich Plasma

Platelet-rich plasma (PRP) therapy involves injecting concentrated platelets from the patient's own blood into the stretch marks. Platelets contain growth factors that can stimulate collagen production and skin repair.

Botulinum Toxin

Emerging research suggests that botulinum toxin (Botox) injections may improve the appearance of stretch marks by relaxing the skin and enhancing collagen production.

Carboxy therapy

In this procedure, carbon dioxide gas is injected subcutaneously in striae, at weekly interval for 3–12 sessions. Improved vascularity leads to release of oxygen which produces increased collagenase, elastin, and hyaluronic acid.

Galvanotherapy

In this procedure microcurrent is passed by microneedles into dermis causing collagen stimulation.

- Lasers and light, microneedling, platelet rich plasma, botulinum toxin, carboxytherapy, galvanotherapy may help in treatment of striae gravidarum.

Supportive Measures

- *Moisturizers and emollients:*
  - Regular use of moisturizers can help maintain skin hydration and elasticity, supporting overall skin health and complementing other treatments.
- *Sun protection:*
  - Using sunscreen on areas with stretch marks can prevent further skin damage and pigmentation changes, helping to maintain the effectiveness of other treatments.

SUGGESTED READINGS

1. Katta TP, Panthalla V, Bondugula HR, Gunda P. Keywords Pregnancy, Prurigo, Trimester, Dermatoses. Pregnancy Dermatoses. 2016:95244.
2. Choi H, Kim YS, Kim MS, Na CH, Shin BS. A survey of the awareness, prevalence, and characteristics of striae gravidarum in dermatologic outpatients of a university hospital. Korean J Dermatol. 2017;55(9):588-96.
3. Yu Y, Wu H, Yin H, Lu Q. Striae gravidarum and different modalities of therapy: a review and update. J Dermatol Treat. 2022;33(3):1243-51.
4. Mendes N, Alves PJ, Barros M, Rodrigues JM, Machado J. A Narrative Review of Current Striae Treatments. Healthcare. 2022;10:2565.
5. Salter SA, Kimball AB. Striae gravidarum. Clin Dermatol. 2006;24:97-100.
6. Farahnik B, Park K, Kroumpouzos G, Murase J. Striae gravidarum: Risk factors, prevention, and management. Int J Womens Dermatol. 20166;3(2):77-85.
7. Lokhande AJ, Mysore V. Striae Distensae Treatment Review and Update. Indian Dermatol Online J. 2019;10(4):380-95.
8. Osman H, Rubeiz N, Tamim H, Nassar AH. Risk factors for the development of striae gravidarum. Am J Obstet Gynecol. 2007;196(1):62.e1-5.

CHAPTER 8

Immunobullous Disorders

Aakansha Sharma, Mudita Gupta

INTRODUCTION

Immunobullous disorders are autoimmune diseases characterized by the formation of blisters on the skin and mucous membranes, caused by the immune system attacking various adhesion molecules within the skin. Immunobullous disorders can be categorized into subepidermal and intraepidermal bullous disorders **(Table 1)**.

The hormonal and immunological changes that occur during pregnancy can influence the course of these diseases, potentially leading to either exacerbations or remissions. Managing these conditions during pregnancy presents unique challenges, as it requires balancing the control of maternal symptoms with minimizing risks to the developing fetus. Autoimmune bullous disorders (AIBDs) are more prevalent in females, largely due to the role of sex hormones in regulating immune responses. While androgens and progesterone primarily act as immunosuppressants, estrogen and prolactin have overall immunoenhancing effects and may contribute to the pathogenesis of autoimmune diseases.

TABLE 1: Classification of immunobullous disorders.

Intraepidermal bullous disorders	Subepidermal bullous disorders
• Pemphigus vulgaris and its variants • Pemphigus foliaceus and its variants • Paraneoplastic pemphigus • IgA pemphigus • Drug-induced pemphigus Characterized by autoantibodies attacking desmosomal adhesion proteins, specifically desmoglein 1 and 3	• Bullous pemphigoid • Pemphigoid gestationis • Mucous membrane pemphigoid • Epidermolysis bullosa acquisita • Linear IgA bullous dermatosis • Anti-p200 pemphigoid Characterized by autoantibodies targeting components of the basement membrane zone, like BP180 and BP230

PEMPHIGUS VULGARIS

Etiological Aspects of Pemphigus Vulgaris seen in Pregnancy

Pemphigus vulgaris (PV) is an epidermal blistering disorder characterized by the formation of flaccid vesicles and bullae, with a notable female predominance. Moreover, it is associated with worse outcomes in women. The HLA alleles *DRB104:02 and DQB1*03:02 have been linked to severe PV, with DQB1*03:02 being more frequently observed in female patients. PV is a Th2-mediated disease, and the shift from a Th1 to a Th2 response, along with a higher population of T regulatory cells and an increase in mast cell numbers during pregnancy, may contribute to the predisposition to develop PV.

Typically, PV affects women between the ages of 40 and 60, but it is not uncommon in younger women of reproductive age, particularly among Asians. While earlier studies suggested an increased incidence of infertility in PV patients, more recent research has found no such association.

Effect on Disease Course

Pemphigus vulgaris may flare during the first two trimesters but tends to improve after the third trimester, often reactivating in the postpartum period. Improvement in third trimester may be attributed to increased levels of endogenous corticosteroids and the resulting immunosuppression. The relationship between pemphigus and pregnancy is complex, with multiple factors influence the outcome. The interplay of various pregnancy hormones, including estrogen, progesterone, prolactin, dehydroepiandrosterone (DHEA), cortisol, and norepinephrine, plays a critical role in determining the disease course. Some studies suggest that if a PV patient is in remission at the time of conception, the likelihood of developing the disease during pregnancy is reduced. However, others report that in approximately one-third of cases, the disease may present for the first time during pregnancy.

- Pemphigus vulgaris (PV) shows female preponderance.
- In Asians, females of active reproductive age group may be involved.
- PV does not affect fertility.
- Immunomodulation during pregnancy may be responsible for flare during pregnancy (first and second trimester) or de novo occurrence.
- Endogenous corticosteroid reduces PV activity in third trimester.

There are limited studies exploring the relationship between pemphigus and pregnancy. However, two case series reported flares in 53.8% and 61.9% of patients, an unchanged disease course in 28.8% and 28.6%, and improvement in approximately 9% of cases. Additionally, the morphology of lesions may change during pregnancy, with variations such as polycyclic lesions or lesions that are exclusively mucosal or cutaneous.

Maternal and Fetal Complications

Pemphigus vulgaris during pregnancy can lead to both maternal and fetal complications. Poor pregnancy outcomes may occur in approximately 10% of cases. The various complications observed are outlined in **Table 2**.

Neonatal Pemphigus

Neonatal pemphigus is a transient condition resulting from the transplacental transfer of maternal antibodies. It usually presents at birth but can be delayed up to 2 weeks. The condition typically resolves within 2–6 weeks due to the natural apoptosis of maternal antibodies. The expression of desmogleins in neonatal skin differs from that in maternal and adult skin, leading to varied clinical manifestations. In neonates, desmoglein 3 is expressed throughout the epidermis, while desmoglein 1 is absent. This difference results in more severe manifestations when neonates are exposed to antibodies against desmoglein 3, as there is no desmoglein 1 to compensate.

Adverse outcomes in neonates are closely linked to various factors; poor control of disease in mother, high maternal serum and umbilical cord antibody levels (≥1:160), and fetal/neonatal immaturity all pose significant risks. In some cases, even when the mother is in remission or has low antibody titers, neonates may still be sensitive to maternal autoantibodies.

Use of immunosuppressive therapy during pregnancy is aimed at reducing maternal serum antibody titers and, consequently, the transplacental passage of pathogenic IgG and maternal disease activity. However, the safety and efficacy of this approach during pregnancy are not yet fully established.

Managing PV during pregnancy presents significant challenges due to the rarity of this condition, the need for immunosuppressive therapies, and the potential side effects of the available medications. These challenges are further compounded by the mother's apprehension and stress, making an already difficult situation even more complex. Disease control becomes particularly challenging due to the hormonal changes of pregnancy and the associated complications, such as preeclampsia, gestational diabetes, intrauterine growth restriction, and preterm birth.

TABLE 2: Maternal and fetal effect of PV on pregnancy outcome.

Maternal complications	Fetal and neonatal complications
• Preeclampsia and eclampsia • Hyperglycemia • Corticosteroids may increase risk of infections, gestational diabetes, and hypertension • Disorders of neuroendocrine system	• Abortion • Stillbirth (1.4–27%) • Intrauterine growth retardation • Premature delivery • Neonatal pemphigus • Increased perinatal mortality

(PV: pemphigus vulgaris)

Hurdles in management of pemphigus vulgaris during pregnancy are:
- Rarity of disease
- Need for immunosuppressive therapies
- Side effects of medications
- Maternal apprehension and stress
- Hormonal changes and pregnancy complications

- *Medication safety*: It is essential to administer medications that are safe for use during pregnancy. The treatment plan should be carefully tailored, considering the severity of the maternal disease, the stage of pregnancy, and the risk-benefit profiles of different medications for both mother and fetus. Following a specific treatment algorithm is crucial for optimal management **(Flowchart 1)**.

Medication and Treatment Planning

- *Topical treatments*:
  - *Corticosteroids*: For mild disease, topical corticosteroids are recommended. However, their use is debated, as there are reports linking the use of potent or very potent topical corticosteroids (exceeding 300 grams throughout pregnancy) with low birth weight. Topical corticosteroids have not been associated with congenital malformations, premature births, or low Apgar scores, making them safe for maintenance therapy.
  - *Calcineurin inhibitors*: These have been used but are not considered highly effective. They may be used as adjuncts to treatment for small areas, with a recommended dose of <5 g/day for 2–3 weeks, or as needed.

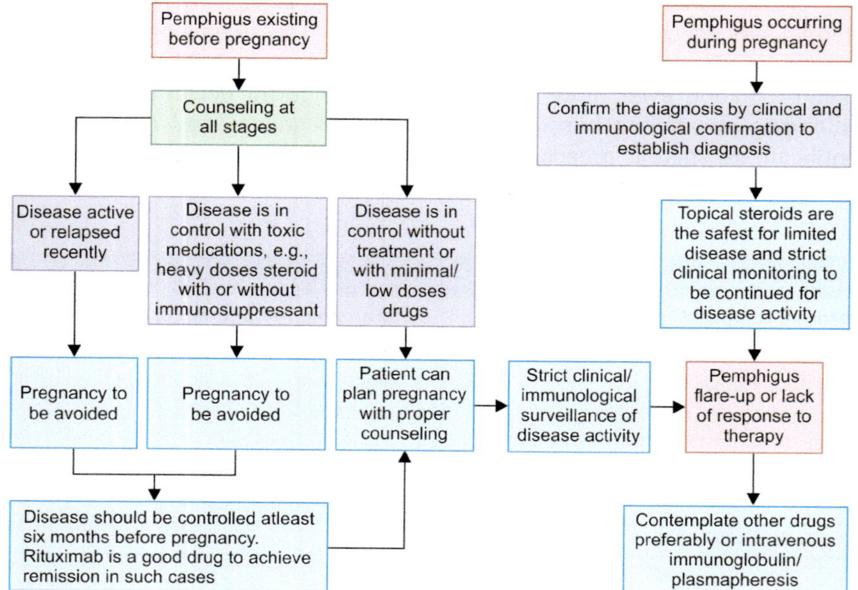

FLOWCHART 1: Algorithm for management of pemphigus vulgaris in pregnancy.

- *Systemic therapies*:
  - *Corticosteroids*: Systemic corticosteroids are the first-line therapy for AIBDs during pregnancy. A starting dose of 20 mg/day of prednisone is recommended. The fetus is less exposed to prednisolone due to the activity of 11-β-hydroxysteroid dehydrogenase-2 in the placenta, which reduces fetal exposure by approximately 90%. This protective effect is not shared by fluorinated steroids. If necessary, a steroid-sparing agent can be added as a second-line treatment, tailored to the patient's needs.
    Breastfeeding considerations: Systemic steroids are generally compatible with lactation, as only small amounts are transferred to breast milk. Prednisone has a half-life of 60 minutes, with its concentration peaking in breast milk around 2 hours after administration and rapidly eliminated thereafter. To minimize the infant's exposure, it is recommended that breastfeeding takes place at least 4 hours after a dose of prednisone.

> - Corticosteroids are the first-line treatment for auto-immune bullous diseases (AIBDs) during pregnancy.
> - Prednisone is often used, with minimal fetal exposure due to placental enzymes.
> - Breastfeeding is generally possible while on corticosteroids. Spacing feedings after medication can minimize infant exposure.

  - *Intravenous immunoglobulin (IVIg)*: Intravenous immunoglobulin is a therapeutic option for pemphigus during pregnancy, particularly when standard treatments, such as corticosteroids and immunosuppressive agents, are either insufficient or contraindicated.
    Mechanism of action: Intravenous immunoglobulin works by modulating the immune system, primarily through the following mechanisms:
    - *Neutralization of autoantibodies*: IVIg can neutralize pathogenic autoantibodies that are responsible for the blistering in pemphigus.
    - *Inhibition of autoantibody production*: It may reduce the production of these autoantibodies by modulating B-cell activity.
    - *Anti-inflammatory effects*: IVIg exerts anti-inflammatory effects that can help reduce disease activity and tissue damage.

    Indications in pregnancy:
    - *Refractory disease*: When pemphigus is not responding adequately to corticosteroids and other immunosuppressive therapies.
    - *Steroid-sparing agent*: IVIg can be used to reduce the dose of corticosteroids needed, minimizing potential side effects.
    - *Concerns about fetal safety*: IVIg is considered relatively safe for use during pregnancy and can be an alternative to more teratogenic medications.
      Safety: Intravenous immunoglobulin is generally considered safe during pregnancy, with no significant adverse effects reported on the fetus. It does not cross the placenta in large amounts, which limits fetal exposure.

    Administration and dosage:
    - *Dosing*: The typical IVIg dose ranges from 2 g/kg per cycle, administered over 2–5 days each month.

- *Frequency*: Treatment cycles may be repeated every 4–6 weeks or as required based on the clinical response.

> - IVIg is a valuable treatment option for pemphigus during pregnancy, especially when other therapies are ineffective or unsuitable.
> - IVIg works by neutralizing autoantibodies, inhibiting their production, and exerting anti-inflammatory effects.
> - IVIg can help reduce the need for high-dose corticosteroids, minimizing potential risks to both mother and fetus.

- *Biologics*:
  Rituximab (anti-CD20 monoclonal antibody):
  - *Mechanism of action*: Rituximab targets CD20-positive B cells, reducing the production of autoantibodies responsible for the blistering in PV.
  - *Use during pregnancy*: While rituximab has been used in some cases during pregnancy, it crosses the placenta after the first trimester, leading to fetal B-cell depletion. This could potentially affect the infant's immune system, particularly in the second and third trimesters.
    Recommendations: Rituximab is generally recommended to be discontinued before conception if possible, and pregnancy should be deferred for 1 year after treatment due to the long half-life and prolonged effect on B-cells.
    Tumor necrosis factor-α (TNF-α) inhibitors (e.g., infliximab and adalimumab):
  - Less commonly used in PV. These agents also cross the placenta, especially in the third trimester, and are generally avoided unless absolutely necessary.
    Precautions in neonates if mother has received biologics: Regarding biologics, it is advised that children exposed to these medications after the 22nd week of gestation should avoid live-attenuated vaccines (such as measles, mumps, oral polio, oral typhoid, varicella zoster, and yellow fever vaccines) during the first 6 months of life. This recommendation is based on the fact that IgG antibodies can cross the placenta and remain detectable in the infant's circulation for up to 6 months after birth, potentially leading to fetal immunosuppression and a heightened risk of severe, widespread infections following live vaccinations.

> - Rituximab is not advised during pregnancy conception needs to be planned atleast after 1 year wash out period.
> - If mother has received rituximab during pregnancy live vaccines in infancy need to be postponed.

- *Other adjuvant therapies*:
  Azathioprine (AZA):
  - *Safety in pregnancy*: Azathioprine is considered a safe steroid-sparing agent during pregnancy when used at a dosage not exceeding 2 mg/kg/day.

- *Breastfeeding considerations*: A significant portion of its main metabolite, 6-mercaptopurine, is excreted in breast milk within 4 hours after AZA intake. Although the amount ingested by the infant is extremely low, it is recommended to breastfeed at least 4 hours after AZA administration, similar to the guidelines for corticosteroid use.

Dapsone:
- *Safety in pregnancy*: Dapsone is considered safe for use during pregnancy.
- *Precautions*: It is crucial to measure glucose-6-phosphate dehydrogenase (G6PD) levels before initiating treatment, both in pregnant women and other patients. Strict blood monitoring is required after starting treatment due to the risk of maternal or neonatal anemia.

Colchicine:
- *Safety in pregnancy*: Colchicine is deemed safe during pregnancy and lactation, as supported by data from rheumatologic studies.

Mycophenolate mofetil (MMF):
- *Safety concerns*: MMF is highly teratogenic and is contraindicated during pregnancy and lactation due to significant risks, including first-trimester miscarriage and various congenital anomalies (e.g., microtia, external auditory canal atresia, cleft lip/palate, and cardiac, renal, ocular, and CNS anomalies). Therefore, MMF should be avoided in pregnant or breastfeeding women.

Mode of Delivery

Vaginal delivery remains the preferred mode of delivery even though trauma caused during vaginal delivery can result in extension and deterioration of mucosal lesions. In a cesarean section, patients who receive long-term steroid therapy will increase the risk and may complicate wound healing.

Counseling before Conception and Planning for Pregnancy

It is recommended to carefully plan pregnancy only after the disease has entered remission. Medications such as methotrexate, mycophenolate mofetil (MMF), and cyclophosphamide should be discontinued well before conception, with minimum discontinuation periods of 12 weeks, 6 weeks, and 4 weeks, respectively. For rituximab, pregnancy should be postponed for at least 1 year following the last dose, in accordance with standard guidelines. It is also crucial to advise expectant mothers not to stop their medication on their own upon discovering they are pregnant.

PEMPHIGUS FOLIACEUS

Pemphigus foliaceus (PF) is an autoimmune blistering disorder which presents with erosions, and rarely flaccid bullae on the skin, sparing the mucosa. The disease is less severe than PV, but more challenging to manage. It presents as scaly, moist, and oozy erosions, usually involving the seborrheic areas but may be widespread. Blisters are not obvious as the plane of cleavage is superficial and, therefore, the flaccid blisters rupture easily.

Pemphigus foliaceus has two forms—the classic and the endemic form which is known as *fogo selvagem (FS)*. The latter corresponds to the South American endemic form of the disease, which presents at an age of 20–40 years. There is no confirmation of gender predominance in PF or FS, but the endemic forms of PF observed in North Africa (Tunisia) show a characteristic female predominance, especially among young women (<20 years).

Course of Pemphigus Foliaceus in Pregnancy

As seen in PV, PF also follows a similar course with exacerbations during the first and second trimesters of pregnancy. PF also similarly improves in third trimester to flare again in postpartum period. Treatment is also same as in PV.

Fetal Effects

- No significant effect on the fetus.
- The association with neonatal PF is extremely rare, and may be related to exceptionally high antibody titers. As explained earlier, desmoglein 3 is expressed throughout the epidermis, including the subcorneal layers in neonatal skin. This stark difference between the adult and neonatal skin has been proven to be protective against disease-causing anti-desmoglein 1 antibodies.

> - *Pemphigus foliaceus*: Immunobullous disease characterized by moist erosions and rarely flaccid bullae in seborrheic distribution.
> - *Peak frequency*: 20–40 years, may present for the first time in pregnancy.
> - Pemphigus foliaceus has two forms—the classical disease and endemic PF (fogo selvagem).
> - Fetal growth and survival may be compromised.
> - *Neonatal PV*: Not observed with PF.

- There are case reports of PF, paraneoplastic pemphigus, and pemphigus herpetiformis being triggered during pregnancy, as well as the onset of de novo postpartum pemphigus vegetans.

BULLOUS PEMPHIGOID

Bullous pemphigoid is the most common blistering disorder. It is a subepidermal blistering disorder which commonly affects elderly people, but, younger patients may also be affected.

Disease progression is seen in **Figure 1**.

It is known that BP and pemphigoid gestationis behave similarly: both are characterized by subepidermal blisters which are formed by complement-binding antibodies of IgG class. Pemphigoid gestationis is also considered to be a

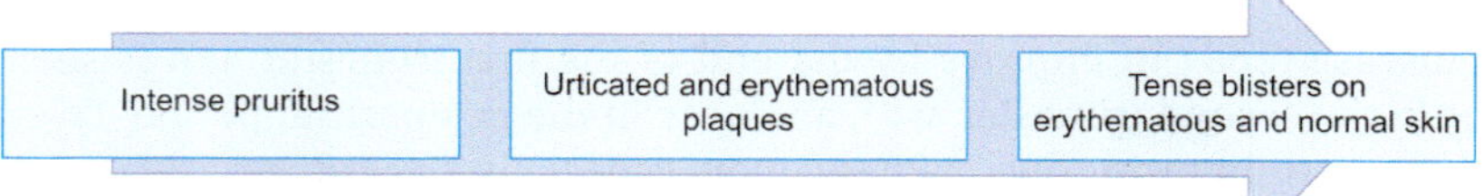

FIG. 1: Evolution of lesion in bullous pemphigoid.

TABLE 3: Difference between bullous pemphigoid and pemphigoid gestationis.

Bullous pemphigoid	Pemphigoid gestationis
• IgG4 (alternate pathway) in BP is the main pathway • Less restricted antigenic epitopes being found intracellularly: NC16A domain and the shed ectodomain • Seen in nonfertile age group with no documented association with pregnancy and hormones • Fetal risk is high	• IgG1 (classical pathway) in PG is the main pathway • Antigenic epitopes restricted to the NC16A domain • Associated with pregnancy, puerperium, trophoblastic tumors, hydatidiform mole and choriocarcinoma • Fetal risk is low

(BP: bullous pemphigoid; PG: pemphigoid gestationis)

variant of BP seen in pregnancy, hence, the nomenclature. Both the diseases have the same antigenic targets in the hemidesmosome, BPAG1 (230 kDa), and BPAG2 (180 kDa). However, certain differences have been observed between both the diseases **(Table 3)**.

Pemphigoid gestationis has been discussed under specific dermatosis chapter.

LINEAR IGA DERMATOSIS

Linear IgA bullous dermatosis (LABD) is an uncommon subepidermal autoimmune blistering disease characterized by the presence of IgA autoantibodies, which most commonly target the 120-kDa and 97-kDa shed ectodomains of type XVII collagen (COL17, BP180) located in the basement membrane zone (BMZ). The disease is characterized by subepidermal blisters, which are characteristically seen in a "string of pearls" appearance. Patients are categorized into two groups—one with prepubertal (childhood) onset and the other with a later onset (adult LAD). It is the most common autoimmune blistering disorder in infants and children.

Pregnancy and Linear IgA Dermatosis

Linear IgA dermatosis has been observed in young pregnant females. Its antigen is known to be expressed in the amniotic basement membrane and IgA deposition occurs in the area of the amniotic basement membrane of the affected mother's fetus.

Course in Pregnancy

The disease tends to improve by the end of the first trimester and is seen to recur in the second trimester, with a relapse in the postpartum period. Overall, LAD tends to improve during pregnancy, especially around the 10th week of pregnancy. One hypothesis to explain this is the glycosylation of IgA antibodies during pregnancy (leading to change in configuration), which further explains the remission, and Treg cells would also play a role. The disease is also known to reactivate years later, even after a prolonged period of remission, which is the usual course of the disease (as seen in children and adults). Case reports of LAD being associated with hydatidiform mole pregnancy have also been published.

Clinical Features

The disease presents with tense blisters, vesicles, and annular erythema with the blisters arranged in a classical "crown of jewels" formation. Skin lesions have the same morphology in adults as in children. However, in adults, the disease progression is gradual in comparison with children. Mucosal involvement is seen in 75–80% of patients. The disease is also known to be triggered by drugs, with lesions healing 4–8 weeks after drug discontinuation. The lesions heal with hyperpigmentation usually, but there may be milia formation. Scarring is not seen after the lesions heal.

EPIDERMOLYSIS BULLOSA ACQUISITA

Epidermolysis bullosa acquisita (EBA) is a rare, phenotypically different subtype of AIBD, predominant seen in females. The basic pathophysiology is the formation of autoantibodies against type VII collagen. In this disease, both mother and newborn may present with superficial and deep erosions on the face, chest, abdomen, and extremities. It is an acquired mechanobullous disorder which is chronic and refractory to treatment. The disease has a predominant acral involvement and heals with atrophic scarring, milia, hyper- and hypopigmentation. Rarely, the disease has been reported in pregnancy.

DERMATITIS HERPETIFORMIS

Dermatitis herpetiformis (DH) has been known for its close association with celiac disease which has been studied widely, with both conditions being mediated by IgA autoantibodies and targeting the transglutaminase autoantigen. DH is known to be modified by pregnancy in a variable way, with some patients improving and others exacerbated by the unsteady state of female hormones during pregnancy. Patients with untreated celiac disease, which is known to be associated with DH, have higher miscarriage rates, increased fetal growth restriction, and lower birth weights due to malabsorption. However, adverse pregnancy outcomes are possibly related to both—immune-mediated mechanisms and nutrient deficiency.

TABLE 4: Maternal and fetal effects in AIBD.

Condition	Maternal outcomes	Fetal outcomes
Pemphigus vulgaris (PV)	• Can flare during pregnancy • Improve in third trimester • Complications from long-term immunosuppressive therapy	• Possible risks of preterm birth and low birth weight, especially with active disease or immunosuppressive therapy • Rare neonatal pemphigus due to transplacental transfer of autoantibodies (typically mild and self-limited)
Pemphigus foliaceus	Similar course as pemphigus vulgaris	• Preterm birth and low birth weight • No neonatal pemphigus foliaceus
Bullous pemphigoid	• Rare in pregnancy but can present similar to PG; chronic and relapsing course • Flare-ups possible during pregnancy and postpartum	Low risk to fetus
Linear IgA bullous dermatosis (LABD)	Chronic, relapsing course, may or may not be affected by pregnancy	Generally low risk of adverse fetal outcomes
Epidermolysis bullosa acquisita (EBA)	• Chronic, relapsing condition that may persist or worsen during pregnancy • Blistering, skin fragility, and scarring can cause significant discomfort and risk of secondary infections	• Limited evidence of direct impact on fetal outcomes, but potential risk due to maternal disease activity • Rare cases of neonatal blisters due to passive transfer of maternal antibodies (usually mild)
Dermatitis herpetiformis (DH)	Generally has a mild course in pregnancy, with symptoms potentially improving due to immunological changes. Sometimes worsening symptoms may be seen	• Dapsone use requires monitoring for potential side effects (hemolytic anemia, methemoglobinemia), especially in the fetus • If associated with celiac disease then higher miscarriage rates, increased fetal growth restriction, and lower birth weights due to maternal malnutrition may be seen

(AIBD: autoimmune bullous disorder)

The maternal and fetal effects in autoimmune bullous disorders are mentioned in **Table 4**.

No cases of anti-p200 pemphigoid have been reported in pregnancy yet.

SUGGESTED READINGS

1. Patsatsi A, Marinovic B, Murrell D. Autoimmune bullous diseases during pregnancy: Solving common and uncommon issues. Int J Womens Dermatol. 2019;5(3):166-70.
2. Genovese G, Derlino F, Berti E, Marzano AV. Treatment of autoimmune bullous diseases during pregnancy and lactation: A review focusing on pemphigus and pemphigoid gestationis. Front Pharmacol. 2020;11:583354.

3. Ikkaku N, Tateishi C, Oda Y, Tsuruta D, Horikawa T. Linear immunoglobulin A bullous dermatosis developing during late pregnancy. J Dermatol. 2017;44(3):e44-5.
4. De D, Shah S, Mahajan R, Handa S. Pemphigus and Pregnancy. IDOJ. 2024;15:749-57.
5. Fagundes PPS, Santi CG, Maruta CW, Miyamoto D, Aoki V. Autoimmune bullous diseases in pregnancy: clinical and epidemiological characteristics and therapeutic approach. An Bras Dermatol. 2021;96(5):581-90.

CHAPTER 9

Urticaria in Pregnancy

Shivani Gauba Wadhwa, Sanjeev Gupta, Aditi Dabhra

INTRODUCTION

Urticaria is a common dermatological disorder. Since urticaria, especially chronic urticaria (CU), affects mostly the females in their reproductive age, pregnancy is an important aspect to consider in the context of urticaria. In addition to increased frequency, urticaria is more resistant in females. Hormonal and immunological changes happening in pregnancy modify the course of many skin diseases and urticaria is no exception.

Lifetime prevalence of acute urticaria is reported to be up to 20% in general population. Prevalence of CU on the other hand is reported to be 0.5% to up to 5% and women are affected twice as often as men. There are no published data regarding the prevalence of urticaria in pregnancy; however, because it occurs in young women, its prevalence is expected to be the same or even greater in pregnancy than in the general population.

Urticaria is often classified according to its duration and triggers **(Flowchart 1)**, but it is important to note that different types of urticaria may coexist in the same patient. Signature lesions of urticaria are wheals/hives which may coexist with angioedema. If hives/angioedema appears daily or almost daily for 6 weeks or more, urticaria is termed as CU and when these last lesser than 6 weeks, it is called as acute urticaria. Acute urticaria is more commonly associated with identifiable external triggers like food, drugs, infections, or insect bites. CU on the other hand either has physical triggers [symptomatic dermographism (stroking), cold, cholinergic, delayed pressure, solar, heat, aquagenic, contact urticaria, and vibratory angioedema] or there are no identifiable external triggers. The former is termed as chronic inducible urticaria and the latter chronic spontaneous urticaria (CSU) **(Flowchart 1)**.

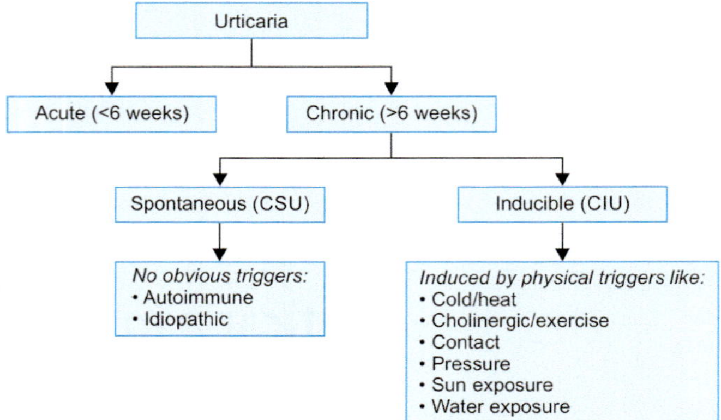

FLOWCHART 1: Classification of urticaria.

(CSU: chronic spontaneous urticaria; CIU: chronic inducible urticaria)

PATHOGENESIS OF URTICARIA

Chronic Spontaneous Urticaria

The pathogenesis of CSU involves interaction of autoimmunity, complement, coagulation, and inflammation. CSU can be further of two types depending on the autoantibody–autoimmune CSU and autoallergic CSU **(Flowchart 1)**.

Autoimmune CSU (also known as type IIb autoimmune urticaria) is mediated by IgG (IgG 1 and 3). These autoantibodies bind to FcεRI and IgE, i.e., IgG-anti-FcεRI and IgG-anti-IgE complex is formed which activates mast cells (MCs). Other immunoglobulins IgA, IgE, or Ig M may also occasionally have a role. Like other autoimmune diseases, JAK-STAT pathway and IL-17 may also be involved in this variant of CSU. This type is a resistant variant of CSU.

Autoallergic CSU (type I autoimmune urticaria) is the more common type and is mediated by IgE to autoallergens like thyroperoxidase, IL-24, dsDNA, etc. This type of CSU is usually less severe and better responsive to treatment.

Mechanism of Urticaria

Mast cells and release of preformed mediators play a central role in all types of urticaria. MRGPRX2 is activated by eosinophilic mediators and neuropeptides. This further activates MC. Various other cytokines, neuropeptides (substance P, etc.), and complement may activate MC.

Histamine is the main mediator which is released. Other important ones are leukotrienes, prostaglandins, and platelet-activating factor. There is also release of various cytokines [granulocyte-monocyte colony-stimulating factor (GMCSF), tumor necrosis factor-α (TNF-α), IL-3, -4, -5] and chemotaxis and migration of other inflammatory cells (basophils, eosinophils, neutrophils, and lymphocytes). The chemotaxis of inflammatory cells further activates MC. Histamine release through basophils is of doubtful significance in humans.

IMMUNOLOGICAL AND HORMONAL CHANGES IN PREGNANCY

Pregnancy is a unique physiological state with marked changes in hormonal and immunological milieu and their complex interplay. Several changes in hormones during pregnancy affect the immunological milieu, these changes are critical for the continuation of the pregnancy and prevent rejection of the "non self" fetus by the mother. Many of these changes influence the course of immune-mediated diseases including urticaria.

Immunological changes in pregnancy are not simply suppressive in nature but are dynamic and responsive based on the timing of pregnancy **(Table 1)**.

Several hormonal changes alter the immune response during pregnancy. Few important ones are as depicted in **Figure 1**.

Human chorionic gonadotropin (HCG) is a glycoprotein secreted by placenta that peaks during the first trimester then slowly declines till delivery. It also maintains the secretion of progesterone from the corpus luteum.

Progesterone is a steroid hormone that has a crucial role in maintaining the pregnancy, in early pregnancy, it is secreted by the ovarian corpus luteum and by almost 10–12 weeks of pregnancy, the placenta takes over. The progesterone levels continue to rise as the pregnancy progresses and drops after delivery.

Estrogens are also steroid hormones and are of three types, estradiol, estriol, and estrone. Among them, estradiol is the most potent and predominant type of

TABLE 1: Changes in immunological milieu on different trimesters of pregnancy.

Trimester	Immune status	Physiological function
First trimester	Proinflammatory	Helps implantation and placental growth
Second trimester	Anti-inflammatory	Helps growth of fetus
Third trimester	Proinflammatory	For labor/delivery preparation

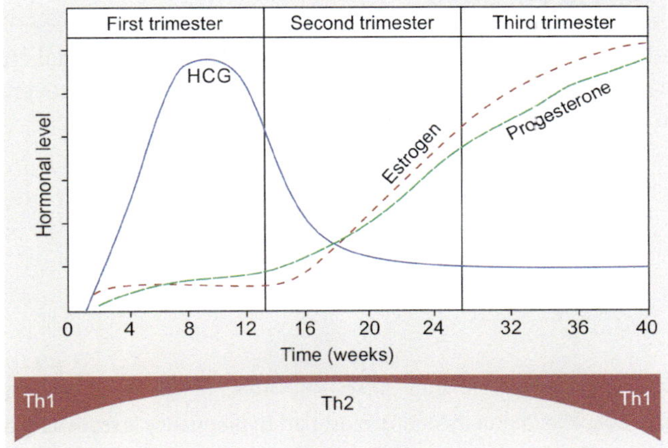

FIG. 1: Changes in hormone levels and adaptive immunity in pregnancy.

estrogen in females in the reproductive age; and is secreted by the ovaries. Estriol is the main type of estrogen seen in pregnant females, constituting about 90% of the estrogen in pregnancy. It is secreted by the placenta and its levels increase steadily over the trimesters and drop by the time of the delivery.

Estrogens, progesterone, and HCG are critical in maintaining the pregnancy as these promote gestational tolerance. These hormones also act as important immunomodulators in pregnancy as they influence many cells in the immune system. They act via specific receptors present on the MCs, T lymphocytes, B lymphocytes, eosinophils, macrophages, and dendritic cells (DCs) thus exert their effects on both innate and acquired immune system. They suppress the innate immunity by having an inhibitory effect on natural killer (NK) cells and by inducing more tolerogenic DCs. They favor Th2/Treg cytokine profile and have an inhibitory effect on Th1/Th17 response.

Cortisol levels start increasing by the end of the first trimester and are highest in third trimester. Though its source in pregnant women is adrenal cortex, placenta also contributes toward that by secreting the corticotropic hormone toward the end of third trimester which is also one of the important triggers for the initiation of labor. Cortisol exerts its significant anti-inflammatory effect by multiple pathways.

CYTOKINES IN PREGNANCY

Cytokines are polypeptides secreted by various immune cells that play an important role in cell-to-cell communication. Usually, there is a fine balance proinflammatory and anti-inflammatory cytokines. This balance shifts toward the proinflammatory side in early pregnancy and toward the end of the pregnancy to help in implantation and labor respectively. During the rest of the pregnancy, it is shifted toward the anti-inflammatory/tolerogenic side **(Figs. 2 and 3)**.

EFFECT OF PREGNANCY ON THE COURSE OF CHRONIC URTICARIA

The increased prevalence of CU in females suggests that hormonal changes may be one of the precipitating factor. Also, females usually have severer and less responsive to conventional treatment type of CU.

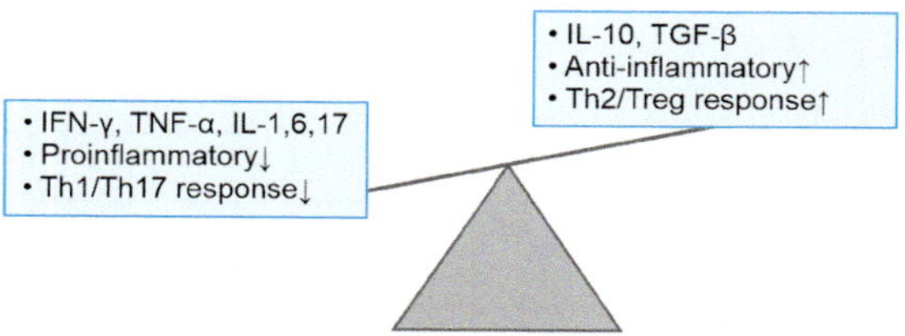

FIG. 2: Skewing of adaptive immunity during most part of pregnancy (except very early and very late pregnancy).

(IFN: interferon; IL: interleukin; TGF: transforming growth factor; TNF: tumor necrosis factor)

In a recent PREG-CU study, 288 patients of CU from 21 centers over 13 countries were evaluated. They participated by answering a questionnaire regarding the course of the disease during pregnancy. About 51% patients reported the improvement in disease whereas 29% patients reported worsening; 20% of patients reported that the disease was unchanged. CU exacerbations occurred mostly in the third trimester or in the first trimester because of the predominance of Th1 immune responses and proinflammatory signals during these times. The patients who improved during pregnancy, 50% of them experienced worsening in the postpartum period, whereas others reported no change **(Fig. 4)**.

There is no consistent pattern with regards to the course of CU in pregnancy, disease improves in some patients whereas flares in others. This could be attributed to the confounding influence of multiple hormones.

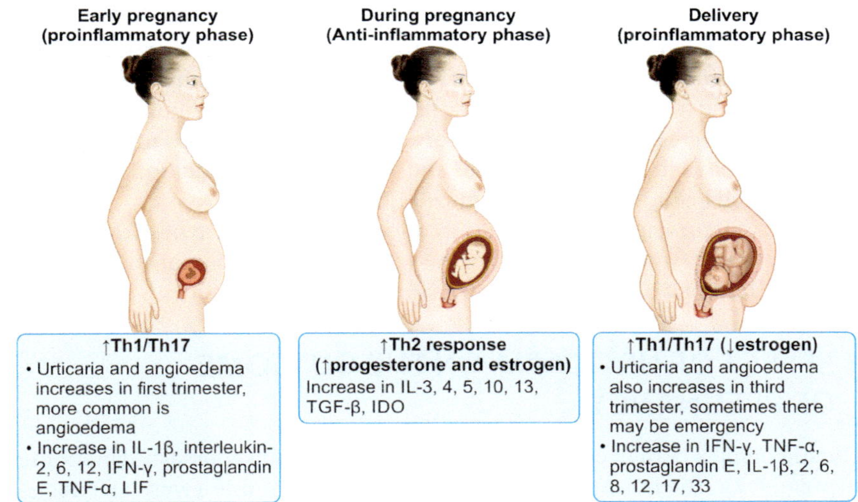

FIG. 3: Immunological shift during different phases of pregnancy.

(IFN: interferon; IL: interleukin; TGF: transforming growth factor; TNF: tumor necrosis factor)

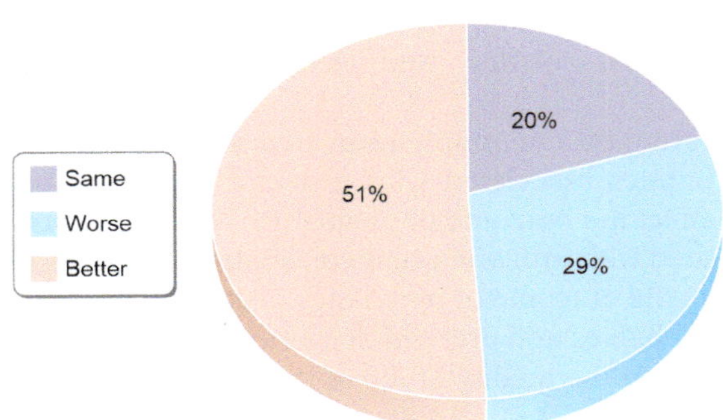

FIG. 4: PREG-CU study: The course of chronic urticaria in pregnancy.

Many chronic inflammatory diseases tend to change during pregnancy because of the changes in the immune response such as decrease in the Th1/Th17 type cytokines and increase in the Th2 type cytokines. In addition, there is also an increase in the Treg (T-regulatory) cytokines like IL-10 and TGF-β that suppress all T helper cell responses. Estrogens favor a Th2 response and enhance the release of histamine from the MC and basophils. Synthetic estrogen (present as pollutant/used in various foods) has been known to increase number as well as activate MC. Estrogen acts through ER-α (estrogen receptor) present on MC. Progesterone has an inhibitory effect.

Cortisol reduces the level of proinflammatory cytokines in the blood. It also reduces the number of T and B lymphocytes in some parts of the lymphoid system like spleen and lymph nodes thus reducing the antibodies production. These changes account for the improvement of many immunological type of urticaria during pregnancy. Dehydroepiandrosterone (DHEA), an androgenic hormone, levels have been found to be reduced in CU.

Prolactin which increases in third trimester may lead to increase in CU by increasing proinflammatory cytokines. Leptin, a hormone required to balance the pregnancy-induced hypermetabolic state, is secreted by placenta. This hormone activates MC increasing proinflammatory cytokines like TNF-α. In CU patients, there is decrease in IgE, eosinophils, and basophils in circulation of pregnant females which leads to decreased induced CU.

Various factors are hypothesized to affect CU; induced type CU, untreated prepregnancy CU, those with no previous history of angioedema, and less severe type of CU have more risk of aggravation during pregnancy.

EFFECT OF URTICARIA ON THE OUTCOME OF PREGNANCY

Urticaria being a benign condition is unlikely to affect the course and outcome of the pregnancy. The recent PREG-CU study reported that there were no effects on the outcome of pregnancies of the patients having CU, compared to the normal population. Both groups had a similar incidence of complications like preterm birth or neonatal medical conditions. This is irrespective of the prescribed treatments. Treatment was continued by 60% of the pregnant females enrolled in this study during pregnancy. Prescribed medications included standard as well as higher doses of first- and second-generation antihistamines and omalizumab.

Though urticaria and commonly used treatments do not affect pregnancy directly, comorbidities associated with urticaria and some of the treatments can potentially affect the outcome of pregnancy. Anxiety, depression, and sleep disorders associated with urticaria can increase stress levels in the mother which in turn may affect the outcome of pregnancy negatively, increasing the chances of low birth weight babies and preterm deliveries. Thus, it is critical to assess the impact of urticaria on the quality of life of the patient and manage the disease accordingly.

Also, the indiscriminate use of systemic treatments like glucocorticoids or cyclosporine can cause complications like hypertension, nephrotoxicity, gestational diabetes, preeclampsia, and macrosomia. This warrants judicious use of medications during pregnancy along with a close watch on the adverse effects.

CLINICAL FEATURES AND DIFFERENTIAL DIAGNOSES

The diagnosis of urticaria is generally straightforward. Classical lesions of urticaria are itchy, erythematous raised lesions that resolve within 24–48 hours, without leaving any postinflammatory changes. There are two pregnancy-specific dermatoses which need to be mentioned as differential diagnosis of urticaria, at least in their initial stages. These are pruritic urticarial papules and plaques of pregnancy (PUPPP) and pemphigoid gestationis (PG). Both can initially present with urticarial-like lesions, but as the disease evolves, other features of these dermatoses can be helpful to clinch the right diagnosis **(Boxes 1 and 2)**.

Urticarial lesions can also be seen in autoimmune progesterone and estrogen dermatitis. History of exposure to synthetic progesterone, prepregnancy cyclical changes, and intradermal testing can distinguish these conditions from CU.

BOX 1 Salient features of PUPPP.

Differential diagnosis—PUPPP:

- Seen usually in primigravida, in late third trimester
- Associated with extensive stretching of abdomen (e.g., obesity twin/triplet pregnancy)
- Starts as itchy urticarial papules/plaques on striae, spreads to limbs and trunk
- Palms, soles, and face are usually spared
- No evanescence seen, excoriations are frequent
- Responds well to topical steroids and emollients
- Resolves spontaneously after the delivery

(PUPPP: pruritic urticarial papules and plaques of pregnancy)

BOX 2 Salient features of pemphigoid gestationis.

Differential diagnosis—pemphigoid gestationis:

- Autoimmune vesiculobullous disease (Ag-BPAG2)
- Usually starts in 2nd/3rd trimester in periumbilical skin as itchy urticarial wheals, soon develops vesiculobullous lesions
- No evanescence of the lesions seen
- Skin biopsy confirms subepidermal bulla on H and E stain and C3 and IgG deposits at DEJ on immunofluorescence
- Recurrent and more severe in subsequent pregnancies

MANAGEMENT OF URTICARIA DURING PREGNANCY

In induced urticaria, proper history and stimulation tests can be done. In autoimmune CU, positive autologous serum skin test (ASST), basophil histamine release assay (BHRA), and immunoassay for specific IgG autoantibodies against FcεRIα/IgE can be done to confirm diagnosis.

Though urticaria is unlikely to affect the outcome of pregnancy but it can severely affect the quality of life of the patient. The disease activity assessment can be done using the standard scoring systems like weekly UAS 7 (urticaria activity score). The impact of the disease on the quality of life can be measured with DLQI (Dermatology Quality of Life Index); whereas, the success of the ongoing treatment is measured with scores like UCT (urticaria control test) score.

Patient should be counseled regarding the unpredictable nature and course of the disease and possible red flag signs. The importance of avoiding the possible triggers and regular follow-ups should be emphasized **(Box 3 and Flowchart 2)**.

The International guideline for the management of urticaria recommends starting treatment with standard doses of second-generation, nonsedative H1 antihistamines. In case of no response to standard doses, the dose can be increased gradually up to fourfold and if there is still no response, omalizumab may be added as the third step. Autoimmune CU is normally resistant to conventional antihistaminics and omalizumab and may require cyclosporine. The recommended treatment in omalizumab-resistant cases is cyclosporine-A **(Box 3)**.

Though these guidelines for the management of urticaria are like those for general population but they emphasize the lack of "evidence-based information" on the safety of these drugs during pregnancy. It is important that the patients should be well informed, and the risk-benefit ratio should be contemplated in each patient individually.

H1 Antihistamines

The H1 antihistamines are the cornerstone of urticaria pharmacotherapy. About 15% of pregnant women use antihistamines during their pregnancy for various indications and many of these are used in the first trimester. Unlike the older reports, recent studies have not found significant associations between the use of standard dose of various antihistamines and major congenital anomalies. The safety of the higher than standard dose of antihistamines has not been confirmed thus the higher doses should be used only after discussing potential risk and

BOX 3 Key aspects in the management of urticaria in pregnancy.

Management of urticaria in pregnancy:

- Assessment of disease activity and monitoring the response to treatment
- Control of triggering factors if any
- Pharmacotherapy
- Psychological support and counseling

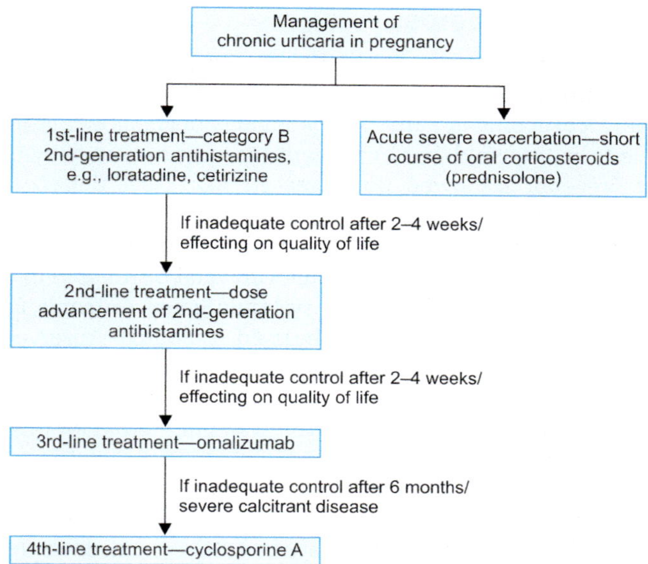

FLOWCHART 2: Guidelines for the management of chronic urticaria in pregnancy.

benefits with the patients. Many of first- and second-generation antihistamines are classified as category "B" in the FDA category system for pregnancy but loratadine and cetirizine are the antihistamines of choice based on the data on their safety.

Omalizumab

Omalizumab is a recombinant IgG1 anti-IgE monoclonal antibody which is recommended in the treatment of antihistamine-resistant CSU. In severe CU patients, that fail to respond to even higher than standard doses of antihistamines, omalizumab may be considered as a reasonable choice of treatment (FDA Category B).

Cyclosporine-A

Cyclosporine is generally recommended by the guidelines for CSU cases who do not respond to omalizumab treatment for at least 6 months. It has significant side effects, most prominent of which are nephrotoxicity and hypertension, because of which it needs significant monitoring. It could potentially cause pregnancy-related complications, e.g., preeclampsia and may have a negative effect on the outcome of pregnancy. Cyclosporine should be preserved only for very severe cases of CSU and should only be used, in case all other treatments have failed (FDA Category C).

Systemic Glucocorticoids

The use of systemic corticosteroids in the management of chronic spontaneous urticaria is recommended only for the acute exacerbations of the disease. The use of oral glucocorticoids in early pregnancy has been shown to increase the risk of oral clefts by threefold, but in a recent case-control study by US National Birth Defect Prevention showed no increased risk. Nevertheless, the use of systemic glucocorticoids in pregnancy may potentially cause adverse effects like preeclampsia and gestational diabetes leading to poor pregnancy outcomes (i.e., intrauterine growth retardation, intrauterine fetal death, and macrosomia). Therefore, as far as possible, the use of systemic glucocorticoids for urticaria should be avoided in pregnancy. If it must be used, it should be reserved for severe cases, at the lowest effective dose (≤20 mg/day of prednisone/prednisolone) and that too, only for 1–5 days.

Prednisone/prednisolone is the preferred systemic steroid for this indication owing to the following two reasons:

1. It has a short half-life of 2–3 hours and thus is cleared from the body quickly.
2. It is effectively metabolized in the placenta thus fetal plasma concentration is reported to be significantly lower (about 10%) compared to the maternal plasma concentration.

Commonly used drugs for urticaria during pregnancy are summarized in **Table 2**.

TABLE 2: Safety of commonly used drugs for urticaria in pregnancy.

Drugs	FDA pregnancy category#	Remarks
Chlorpheniramine (fg AH)*	B	
Diphenhydramine (fg AH)*	B	
Hydroxyzine (fg AH)*	C	
Cetirizine (sg AH)**	B	
Loratadine (sg AH)**	B	
Omalizumab	B	Use in severe disease refractory to antihistamines
Prednisolone/ methylprednisolone	B***	Use minimal possible dose (≤20 mg/day) for shortest possible duration; reserved only for acute exacerbations
Cyclosporine A	C	Reserved for very severe cases, refractory to all other treatments with close monitoring of adverse effects

*fg AH—first-generation antihistamines.
**sg AH—second-generation antihistamines.
***In the dose and duration mentioned, details in text.
#FDA category B—Animal studies show no risk and no adequate studies in pregnant women.
#FDA category C—Animal studies show adverse effect and no adequate studies in humans, but potential benefits may warrant use of the drug in pregnant women despite potential risks.

CONCLUSION

An array of hormonal and immunological changes seen in pregnancy affect the course of many dermatological diseases. Chronic spontaneous urticaria is more likely to improve rather than worsen during pregnancy. There are many safe treatment options available to control the disease. The optimum treatment should be chosen considering the risk-benefit ratio individually for each patient.

SUGGESTED READINGS

1. Pope EM, Laageide L, Beck LA. Management of Allergic Skin Disorders in Pregnancy. Immunol Allergy Clin North Am. 2023;43(1):117-32.
2. Kocatürk E, Podder I, Zenclussen AC, Kasperska Zajac A, Elieh-Ali-Komi D, Church MK, et al. Urticaria in Pregnancy and Lactation. Front Allergy. 2022;3:892673.
3. Khalili A, Sadeghi B. Chronic Urticaria in Pregnancy: Physiologic and Hormonal Background for an Immune Skin Disease. J South Asian Feder Obs Gynae. 2024;16(2):145-9.

CHAPTER 10

Pregnancy and Sexually Transmitted Diseases

10.1 Syphilis in Pregnancy

Rohit Batra, Aishwarya Dua

INTRODUCTION

Syphilis is a chronic, sexually transmitted infection (STI) caused by the bacterium *Treponema pallidum*, a spirochete characterized by its corkscrew shape. This bacterium is highly infectious and primarily spread through direct contact with syphilitic sores, known as chancres, which are typically found on the external genitals, vagina, anus, or in the rectum. Syphilis can also be transmitted from an infected mother to her baby during pregnancy, leading to congenital syphilis.

If untreated, syphilis progresses through several stages: primary syphilis, marked by a painless sore or chancre; secondary syphilis, characterized by skin rashes and flu-like symptoms; latent syphilis, which is asymptomatic but detectable by tests; and tertiary syphilis, which can cause severe damage to the heart, brain, nerves, and other organs.

Understanding syphilis in pregnancy is critically important due to its significant implications for both maternal and fetal health.

EPIDEMIOLOGY

The World Health Organization (WHO) estimates that 7 out of every 1,000 pregnant women worldwide have maternal syphilis infection. This has resulted in over 200,000 yearly neonatal fatalities and 1.5 million cases of infected babies recorded globally in 2023, with nearly two-thirds of all cases discovered in Africa.

TRANSMISSION OF SYPHILIS

Mother to child transmission of syphilis can occur if either an infected woman becomes pregnant or a pregnant woman becomes infected.

Modes of Transmission

- Transplacental transmission is most common
- During passage through birth canal by contact with genital lesion
- Breastfeeding if lesion on breast

Risk of Transmission of Syphilis from an Infected Mother to Her Child

Risk of antepartum fetal infection or congenital syphilis at delivery is related to the stage of syphilis infection during pregnancy:

- Primary/secondary syphilis: 70–100% risk
- Early latent syphilis: 40% risk
- Late latent syphilis: 10% risk

Also, risk of in utero transmission increases with increasing gestational age. Pregnant women can transmit syphilis infection to the fetus as early as 9 weeks, but usually transmission takes place between 16 and 28 weeks of pregnancy. However, the risk of fetal morbidity and mortality is higher with infections contracted in the first trimester compared to those in the second trimester. In contrast, infections during the third trimester are more likely to result in asymptomatic cases.

Laws of Syphilis Transmission in Pregnancy

- *Colles' law (also known as Baumis law)*: A child born to an apparently asymptomatic mother with no signs of disease and present with syphilis after few weeks would infect the healthy nursemaid but not its mother (since mother is immune), i.e., syphilitic infants can transmit the infection to nursemaid but not to their mother.
- *Profeta's law*: Healthy infant born to a syphilitic mother is immune to the disease. At birth, an infected infant may not develop signs and appear healthy, till it is some weeks old.
- *Kassowitz law (also known as Diday's law)*: Pregnancy outcome of an untreated syphilitic mother improves with successive pregnancies, i.e., the longer the interval between syphilis infection and conception, better is the pregnancy outcome. It is thought that transmission rates decrease from 70–100% to 10% respectively in primary and latent syphilis.

EFFECT OF SYPHILIS ON PREGNANCY

Maternal Outcome

Clinical manifestations and course of syphilis infection do not seem to be much altered by pregnancy.

- Primary syphilis infection—chancre at the infection site
- Secondary syphilis—skin rash, mucocutaneous lesions, and lymphadenopathy
- Tertiary syphilis—cardiac gummatous lesions, tabes dorsalis, and general paresis

BOX 1 Fetal outcomes in maternal syphilis.

- Child can escape infection
- Spontaneous abortion usually after 12–16 weeks
- Stillbirth/IUGR/perinatal death/nonimmune hydrops fetalis
- Born with features suggestive of congenital syphilis
- Born well but develops early congenital syphilis after few weeks
- 40% of untreated children may develop late congenital syphilis in later years

(IUGR: intrauterine growth restriction)

Fetal Effects

Syphilis can be transmitted from a pregnant woman to her fetus, a condition known as congenital syphilis, which can lead to severe outcomes as shown in **Box 1**. Risk of developing syphilis infection in utero to the fetus is on an average 40–50% in a pregnant female with untreated syphilis Thus, timely diagnosis and management of syphilis infection during pregnancy is important to prevent adverse outcomes.

Syphilitic stillbirth—death of fetus >500 g weight or >20 weeks gestational age where mother has untreated or inadequately treated syphilis.

Treponema pallidum can cross the placenta, particularly as the pregnancy progresses. The bacteria infect the placenta, leading to placentitis, characterized by inflammation and thickening of the placenta. The presence of spirochetes in the placenta can disrupt its normal function, compromising nutrient and oxygen exchange between the mother and the fetus.

Once the bacteria cross the placenta, they enter the fetal circulation, infecting various fetal tissues and organs. The fetal immune system is immature and has limited capacity to mount an effective response against *Treponema pallidum*. This allows the bacteria to proliferate and cause significant damage.

SCREENING FOR SYPHILIS IN MOTHER

Screening Tests

- *Nontreponemal tests*: These include the rapid plasma reagin (RPR) test and the venereal disease research laboratory (VDRL) test. They are often used for initial screening because they are inexpensive and easy to perform. However, they can produce false-positive results, which require confirmation.
- *Treponemal tests*: TPHA (treponema pallidum hemagglutination) or ELISA (enzyme-linked immunosorbent assay), etc. are used to confirm syphilis infection if a nontreponemal test is positive. They detect antibodies specific to *Treponema pallidum*.

Time of Screening

- *First prenatal visit*: Routine screening for syphilis is recommended during the first prenatal visit for all pregnant women.

- *Third trimester and at delivery*: In areas with high prevalence rates or for women at increased risk (i.e., those with current or past history of STI, repeated abortions, stillbirth, past history of delivery of premature baby and neonatal death; injecting drug users; women with more than one sexual partner and sex worker), repeat screening in the third trimester (28–32 weeks of gestation) and at delivery is recommended.
- Monitoring for treatment response after 3 and 6 months of treatment
- Partner of pregnant patient
- Neonate of a syphilitic mother

Biological False-positive Nontreponemal Test

Biological false-positive RPR/VDRL can occur during the pregnancy and, therefore, positive results should be confirmed with the specific a treponemal tests (FTA-ABS, TPHA, or ELISA).

Reasons for Biological False Positives in Pregnancy

- *Hormonal changes*: Pregnancy induces various hormonal and immunological changes in the body that can sometimes lead to the production of antibodies that react nonspecifically with the antigens used in the VDRL test.
- *Autoimmune disorders*: Conditions such as systemic lupus erythematosus (SLE) or other autoimmune disorders are associated with increased production of antibodies that can cause false-positive VDRL results.
- *Infections*: Other infections, such as viral infections (e.g., HIV and hepatitis), malaria, or certain bacterial infections, can lead to the production of antibodies that cross-react with the VDRL test reagents.
- *Recent immunizations*: Certain vaccines or recent immunizations can sometimes stimulate the immune system in a way that causes a transient BFP.
- *Chronic medical conditions*: Chronic liver disease, intravenous drug use, and other chronic conditions might also be associated with BFP results.

To confirm whether a positive VDRL result is a true syphilis infection, further testing with a more specific treponemal test is needed.

Maternal nontreponemal titer if >1:8 should be considered a marker of early syphilis infection and bacteremia. Unless appropriate treatment history is documented in the medical records and antibody titer has declined sequentially, seropositive pregnant female should be considered infected. Women without any treatment/inadequate treatment history should be staged and treated accordingly.

All women who have syphilis infection should be offered testing for HIV infection.

TREATMENT

Management of syphilis in pregnancy involves multidisciplinary approach involving obstetrician and pediatrician. Penicillin is the mainstay of treatment and administered according to the stage of disease in pregnancy. Partner of seroreactive pregnant women should also be treated to prevent reinfection.

Recommended Regimen

Primary, secondary, and early latent syphilis:

- Benzathine penicillin G 2.4 million units intramuscular in a single dose
- Single dose of benzathine penicillin G decreases the risk of transmission by 95% and 98% in secondary syphilis and early latent syphilis. It ends infectivity in 24–48 hours. If untreated, 50% mothers can transmit infection.

Late latent syphilis: Benzathine penicillin G 2.4 million units administered intramuscularly weekly for 3 weeks.

Tertiary syphilis with normal cerebrospinal fluid (CSF) examination: Benzathine penicillin G 2.4 million units administered intramuscularly weekly for 3 weeks.

Neurosyphilis and ocular syphilis: Aqueous crystalline penicillin G 3–4 million units per day IV every 4 hours or continuous infusion (total dose of 18–24 million units per day) for 10–14 days.

Treatment in Penicillin Allergic Pregnant Females

Penicillin G is the only effective therapy for preventing maternal transmission of syphilis to the fetus and there is no proven alternative treatment to penicillin. Therefore, any pregnant women who has history of penicillin allergy should be desensitized and treated with penicillin.

In case of any missed dose, pregnant women should repeat the full course of therapy.

Monitoring and Follow-up

- Women treated for syphilis during pregnancy should be monitored with repeat serologic testing (RPR or VDRL) to assess the response to treatment.
- Pregnant women should be followed up at 3, 6, 12, and 24 months after pregnancy and VDRL/ RPR should be performed at each of these follow-up visit.
- The VDRL/RPR test should be performed again in late pregnancy following treatment to rule out reinfection or treatment failure.
- Pregnant women, who have been previously treated for syphilis and have stable, serofast low antibody titer, do not require additional treatment. However, rising or persistently high antibody titers are markers of reinfection or treatment failure and thus treatment should be reconsidered.

Management of Sexual Partners

Sexual partners should also be evaluated, tested, and treated as necessary to prevent reinfection and transmission.

Risk of Jarisch–Herxheimer Reaction

Women being treated for syphilis during second half of pregnancy might undergo Jarisch–Herxheimer reaction. Patient has fever with headache, myalgia, and other symptoms which can occur within 24 hours of treatment initiation. This reaction can induce preterm labor or fetal distress, so pregnant women should be informed about this possibility and monitored accordingly.

Ultrasonography

When syphilis is diagnosed, an ultrasound should be carried out for fetal evaluation for congenital syphilis. Sonographic signs of fetal syphilis include hepatomegaly, hydrops, fetal anemia, ascites, or a thickened placenta and indicate a higher risk for fetal treatment failure.

CONGENITAL SYPHILIS

Signs and Symptoms of Congenital Syphilis

Congenital syphilis can be classified as:
- *Early congenital syphilis*: If features appear within first 2 years of life.
- *Late congenital syphilis*: If features appear after 2 years of birth.
- *Stigmata of congenital syphilis*: Sequelae of early or late congenital syphilis.

Early Congenital Syphilis

Neonate may be asymptomatic in 1st weeks of life in around 50% cases. Symptoms usually start to appear in the 1st month of life but clinical manifestations may get delayed until the second year of life.

It is a triad of:
- *Skin rash*: A widespread maculopapular rash, often involving the palms and soles. Bullous lesions over palms and soles known as pemphigus syphiliticus or bullous syphiliticus (40%) may be seen.
- *Snuffles*: Thick or bloody nasal discharge and ulceration on upper lip and nasal vestibule known as syphilitic snuffles. These mucocutaneous lesions have high load of treponemes and are highly infectious.
- *Hepatosplenomegaly*: It is the most frequent sign of early syphilis (33–100%). It may or may not be accompanied with increased liver enzymes, increased bilirubin levels, and increased prothrombin time.

Other features of early congenital syphilis include:
- Jaundice/anemia/thrombocytopenia
- *Bony involvement*: Osteochondritis and periostitis of long bones (most commonly legs). Inflammation of bone and cartilage, leading to pain and deformities (e.g., saber shins). Due to pain caused by bone involvement, infected child will not move the limb, this is known as parrot's pseudoparalysis. Loss of density on medial aspect of upper tibia is seen on X-ray known as Wimberger's sign or Cat bite sign. Bony changes on X-ray are seen in 75–100% cases.
- Moth-eaten alopecia involving scalp and eyebrows may occur.
- Generalized nontender lymphadenopathy can occur in 20–50% cases.

- The child develops old man look because of low-birth weight giving wrinkled appearance to skin (10–40%). Radiating furrows may develop around the mouth leading to rhagades formation.
- Other associated features include fever (16%), bleeding (10%), respiratory distress, and abdominal distension.
- *Neurosyphilis*: Involvement of the central nervous system can cause seizures, developmental delays, and other neurological issues.

Late Congenital Syphilis

It is not infectious and corresponds to tertiary (gummatous) syphilis in adults. cardiovascular system (CVS) is usually spared in late congenital syphilis.

Stigmata of Syphilis

Musculoskeletal manifestations:

- Frontal bossing (Olympian brow)—seen in 30–90% of symptomatic cases. It is the most common or classical stigmata of congenital syphilis
- Square skull with prominent suture lines—also known as hot cross bun cranium or natiform skull
- Saddle nose—due to destruction of the nasal cartilage
- Short maxilla
- Prominent mandible
- Perforation of hard palate
- Hutchinson teeth—peg shaped, notched and widely spaced upper central incisors
- Mulberry molars—multiple cusps
- Higoumenakis' sign—there is unilateral thickening of sternoclavicular joint mostly on patients dominant hand side
- Dubois sign—shortened 5th finger
- Saber shin—anterior tibial bowing
- Clutton joint—painless effusion of knees and elbows
- *Interstitial keratitis*: Most common late manifestation. Occurs in 20–50% of infected children. It is usually bilateral (>75% cases) and can develop either simultaneously or sequentially.
- *Sensorineural hearing loss*: Least common manifestation of Hutchinson's triad. It occurs due to osteochondritis of otic capsule and fibrous adhesions between stapedial foot plate and membranous labyrinth and cochlear degeneration.
- *Neurological symptoms*: Seizure, mental retardation, hydrocephalus, cranial nerve palsy, and paresis
- *Rhagades*—perioral furrowing

Hutchinson's triad of late congenital syphilis: It includes Hutchinson teeth, interstitial keratitis, and sensorineural hearing loss.

Diagnosis of Congenital Syphilis

Diagnosis of congenital syphilis can be either by indirect serological testing of the neonate or direct detection of whole organisms or their components.

- *Indirect serological tests*:
  - FTA-ABS IgM or 19s FTA-ABS IgM—serological test for the neonate, if mother has untreated syphilis. It has low sensitivity and specificity and thus not recommended. Positive specific anti-treponema pallidum IgM test is diagnostic of congenital syphilis since maternal IgM antibodies do not cross placenta. Other standard serological tests like TPPA or ELISA have low sensitivity in congenital syphilis and also if positive, it reflects passive transfer of IgG antibodies from mother to fetus. These IgG antibodies become undetectable after 12–18 months of age.
  - Infection in neonate is suggested if serum nontreponemal antibody titer (VDRL/RPR) is > 4 times than mother's serum antibody titer. This approach is more commonly followed due to easier availability and affordability.
- *Direct detection of treponema pallidum or its components*:
  - From nasal discharge, intraocular discharge, mucous patches, vesicobullous lesions, etc.—using PCR, dark ground microscopy, or direct fluorescent antibody test
  - Histopathological examination of placenta and umbilical cord. Classical pathological features of placental involvement are focal proliferative villitis with plasma cell infiltration, hypertrophic immature crowded villi, and endothelial and adventitious proliferation of villous vessels with obliteration
- All proven or highly probable cases of congenital syphilis should be evaluated for neurosyphilis. CSF examination with WBC count > 25/mm^3, protein levels > 150 mg/dL, and positive CSF VDRL are suggestive of neurosyphilis.

Case definition of congenital syphilis (as per NACO):

- *Confirmed case of congenital syphilis*:
  - *A stillbirth, live birth, or child aged <2 years with microbiological evidence of syphilis infection*

    Or

  - *A child within first 2 years of life with clinical evidence of syphilis and reactive syphilis serology irrespective of mother's serology.*
- *Suspected case of congenital syphilis*: *A stillborn or live born baby of syphilis seroreactive mother*

Recommended evaluation in a neonate in case of proven or highly probable congenital syphilis:

- CSF analysis for cell count, protein, and VDRL
- Complete blood count and platelet count
- Long bone radiographs
- Chest radiograph
- Liver function tests
- Ophthalmic examination

- Auditory brainstem response
- Neuroimaging

Treatment of Congenital Syphilis

Effective prevention and early detection of congenital syphilis requires routine serologic screening during pregnancy as mentioned above.

- *Scenario 1*: Proven or highly probable congenital syphilis, i.e., definite diagnosis of congenital syphilis
    - Aqueous crystalline penicillin G—100,000–150,000 units/kg/day, administered as 50,000 units/kg/dose IV every 12 hours during first 7 days of life and every 8 hours thereafter for a total of 10 days

      Or
    - Procaine penicillin G 50,000 units/kg/dose IM in a single dose for 10 days

The entire course should be restarted if >1 day of therapy is missed.

- *Scenario 2*: Possible congenital syphilis, i.e., no definitive evidence of syphilis in neonate but mother was not treated or inadequately treated or mother has received treatment <4 weeks before delivery.
    - Aqueous crystalline penicillin G—100,000–150,000 units/kg/day, administered as 50,000 units/kg/dose IV every 12 hours during first 7 days of life and every 8 hours thereafter for a total of 10 days

      Or
    - Procaine penicillin G 50,000 units/kg/dose IM in a single dose for 10 days
- *Scenario 3*: Congenital syphilis less likely, i.e., no evidence of syphilis in neonate and mother was adequately treated during pregnancy and treatment was administered >4 weeks before delivery.
    - Benzathine penicillin G 50,000 units/kg/dose IM in a single dose

      Or
    - Close follow-up of the child every 2–3 months for 6 months whose mother's VDRL/RPR titers decreased at least fourfold after appropriate therapy for early syphilis or remained stable for low titer for latent syphilis.
- *Scenario 4*: Congenital syphilis unlikely, i.e., no evidence of syphilis in neonate and mother was adequately treated before pregnancy.
    - No treatment is required

All neonates with reactive VDRL/RPR test should undergo careful follow-up examination and serological testing every 2–3 months until the test becomes nonreactive. With appropriate treatment, clinical features (hepatomegaly, X-ray changes) resolve within 3 months of birth and serological markers (IgM) disappear by 6 months. The infant should be followed up at 3, 6, 12, and 24 months with VDRL/RPR test at each follow-up visit.

In neonates who were considered less likely or unlikely to develop congenital syphilis and did not receive penicillin treatment, the VDRL/RPR titers should decline and be nonreactive by 6 months of age indicating that reactive test was caused by passive transfer of maternal IgG antibody. If VDRL/RPR titer persists by 6–12 months of age despite treatment, neonates should be reevaluated through CSF examination.

KEY POINTS

- All pregnant females should be screened for syphilis at first antenatal visit. Additional testing at 28 weeks' gestation and again at delivery should be carried out for high-risk females.
- Risk for antepartum fetal infection or congenital syphilis at delivery is related to the stage of syphilis during pregnancy. 70–100% risk in primary/secondary syphilis, 40% risk in early latent syphilis, and 10% risk in late latent syphilis.
- Risk of transmission increases with increasing gestational age. Though risk of fetal morbidity/mortality occurs more in first trimester followed by second trimester infection and then third trimester infection which is more often asymptomatic.
- Penicillin is the mainstay of treatment and administered according to the stage of disease in pregnancy. Any pregnant women who have history of penicillin allergy should be desensitized and treated with penicillin.
- Infected neonates should also be treated with penicillin and followed up routinely.

SUGGESTED READINGS

1. National AIDS Control Organisation. (2014). Elimination of parent to child transmission of syphilis. NACO RTI/STI Guidelines. [online] Available from https://naco.gov.in/sites/default/files/National%20RTI%20STI%20technical%20guidelines%20Sep2014_0.pdf. [Last accessed January, 2025].
2. Workowski KA, Bolan GA. (2015). Syphilis during pregnancy. CDC, sexually transmitted diseases treatment guidelines. [online] Available from https://www.cdc.gov/mmwr/preview/mmwrhtml/rr6403a1.htm. [Last accessed January, 2025].
3. Saliny M, Joy B, Sridharan R. Laws and signs of congenital syphilis. J Skin Sex Transm Dis. 2020;2(1):62-4.
4. Kumar B, Gupta S. Syphilis in pregnancy. Sexually Transmitted Infections, 2nd edition. Gurugram: Elsevier India; 2011.

10.2 Herpes in Pregnancy

Rohit Batra, Aishwarya Dua

INTRODUCTION

Herpes genitalis is a very common sexually transmitted infection primarily caused by herpes simplex virus (HSV). HSV is an enveloped double-stranded DNA virus which belongs to the human Herpesviridae family. There are two subtypes, HSV-1 and HSV-2, which share up to 40% sequence homology of their genome structure. It is the most common infectious cause of genital ulceration worldwide. Women in reproductive age group can contract and transmit infection to the newborn causing severe neonatal infection which can be fatal or lead to long-term disabilities in the newborn. Thus, management of herpes infection in pregnancy is important to prevent transmission to the neonate.

PREVALENCE OF MATERNAL AND NEONATAL HERPES SIMPLEX VIRUS

Approximately 500 million people globally are estimated to be infected with HSV-2, which is the predominant cause of genital herpes. The overall global prevalence of genital herpes in pregnant women mirrors that of the general population. It is estimated that around 10–20% of pregnant women worldwide are infected with HSV-2, but this number can vary by region. A significant proportion of HSV infections in pregnant women are asymptomatic or have mild, unrecognized symptoms. Up to 80–90% of individuals with HSV-2 are unaware of their infection, leading to undiagnosed cases in pregnancy. Globally, the annual incidence of neonatal herpes is about 14,000 cases.

PATHOGENESIS

The word herpes is derived from Greek word "herpein" which means "to creep".

Herpes genitalis, primarily caused by HSV types 1 and 2, begins with the virus entering the body through mucosal surfaces or skin breaks, often via sexual contact. Once inside, HSV infects epithelial cells, leading to viral replication. It replicates in the nucleus and produces intranuclear inclusion bodies (Cowdry type A). Formation of painful vesicles or ulcers occurs in the genital area. The virus then travels to the sensory neurons, establishing latency in the nerve cell bodies located in regional ganglia. Reactivation of the virus can be triggered by factors such as stress, immunosuppression, or hormonal changes, leading to the production of new viral particles that travel back to the skin, causing recurrent lesions or asymptomatic shedding. The host's immune system, including both cell-mediated and humoral responses, plays a critical role in controlling the infection and limiting its spread, though it cannot eliminate the virus completely.

The HSV-2 is primarily responsible for genital herpes infection (two-thirds cases) and HSV-1 for predominantly orolabial herpes. However, incidence of HSV-1 infection causing genital herpes in rising is probably due to changing viral pathogenicity and increasing orogenital sex.

- Genital herpes can be caused by both HSV-1 and -2. Though HSV-2 more commonly causes genital infection
- Virus remains dormant in regional ganglia
- Reactivation occurs in periods of stress

TRANSMISSION

Sexual Transmission

It occurs through oral as well as genital sexual contact. Transmission from infected male to female partner occurs more commonly than infected female to male partner. Males more commonly have asymptomatic infection and thus may be responsible for higher male to female transmission of infection.

Mother to Child Transmission

Neonatal herpes, though rare, is a serious viral infection with a high morbidity and mortality caused by HSV-1 or HSV-2 as either of the viral type can cause genital herpes infection in the mother.

- Most of the neonatal herpes (85%) cases occur as a result of direct contact with infected maternal genital secretions at the time of birth. Mother may be having active lesions or asymptomatic viral shedding. The risk is highest (30–50%) when a pregnant women acquires infection for the first time (primary genital herpes) in the third trimester especially within 6 weeks of delivery, as viral shedding might persist and protective maternal antibodies have not been developed by the time the baby is likely to be born. Prenatal histories of recurrent genital herpes or who acquire infection during first half of pregnancy are associated with a low risk (<1%) of neonatal herpes.
- Postnatal infection (10%) as a result of exposure to orolabial herpes infection may also in few cases. Postnatally acquired HSV infection can be especially severe in newborns born to women without prior HSV infection.
- Congenital herpes infection occurs by in utero transfer of infection and is extremely rare (5%). This usually occurs when the mother has a primary HSV infection during pregnancy, especially if it happens in the first or second trimester. Congenital herpes can cause severe fetal complications, including intrauterine growth restriction, preterm labor, spontaneous abortion, and congenital malformations affecting the skin, eyes, and brain. Intrauterine infection that results from maternal primary HSV infection and viremia during pregnancy is HSV infection of placenta and causes infarcts, necrotizing, calcifying funisitis, plasma cell deciduitis, and lymphoplasmacytic villitis. Fetal damage manifests as hydrops fetalis and intrauterine death. Intrauterine infection can occur through vertical transmission or ascending infection (prolonged rupture of membranes in mothers with active HSV infection).
- Ascending infection in contrast to vertical transmission has milder fetal effects.

Transmission of herpes virus from mother to the child can occur during:
- *Intrapartum*: Most common. Highest risk of neonatal herpes especially in primary episode
- *Postnatal*: Contact with maternal secretions
- *Antenatal*: Causes congenital herpes (may lead to stillbirths and abortion). Ascending infection only mildly affects the neonate

CLASSIFICATION OF HERPES GENITALIS

- *Primary*: Infection developing for the first time. It is of two types:
  i. *True primary*: Infection in a person who has never got infection earlier, i.e., in a seronegative female
  ii. *Nonprimary*: Infection in a female who has had infection by a different strain earlier
- *Recurrent herpes*

CLINICAL FEATURES

Primary Genital Herpes in Pregnancy

First episode of genital herpes occurring first time during pregnancy presents with prodrome (headache, fever, lethargy, myalgia, backache, and photophobia) for 6–8 days. Itching, paresthesia, erythema, and pain at the local site (labia) precede the visible lesions by 1–2 days.

Multiple, small, grouped, and painful vesicles appear on erythematous base over the labia, and break to form superficial ulcers with polycyclic margin in next 2–4 days. New crops of lesions can appear in the 2nd week. Ulcers re-epithelize in 3-week time. It may be associated with cervicitis in 88% cases. Other associated symptoms include dysuria, discharge, urethritis, etc. Ulceration is usually accompanied with bilateral inguinal lymphadenopathy. Lymph nodes are tender, firm, and nonfluctuant. Asymptomatic viral shedding occurs for about 12 days after complete clinical recovery.

Maternal clinical features of herpes genitalis:
- Grouped vesicular painful lesions on external genitalia
- Cervicitis
- Dysuria
- Urethritis
- Asymptomatic

Risk of transmission of HSV infection from mother to the newborn is high (30–50%) when primary genital herpes infection occurs during second half of pregnancy especially within 6 weeks of delivery due to asymptomatic viral shedding into the maternal secretions.

Risk factors for mother to child transmission:
- Type of maternal HSV infection (primary > recurrent)
- Maternal HSV antibody status
- Duration of ruptured membranes
- Use of fetal scalp monitors
- Mode of delivery (cesarean less chances versus vaginal)

Recurrent Genital Herpes

Women with history of recurrent genital herpes can develop secondary episodes during pregnancy. Recurrent episodes are usually short lasting and less severe in comparison to primary episode. Patient may have minimal or absent prodromal symptoms, limited vesicles associated with mild itching, burning, or redness. Symptoms usually last 5–7 days and viral shedding occurs for about 4 days post clinical recovery.

Neonatal Herpes

Classification

- Isolated skin, eye, and mucous membrane (SEM) (approximately 35–45%)
- Combined involvement of SEM

- Central nervous system (CNS) involvement
- Disseminated

Disseminated herpes occurs in preterm infants and most exclusively as a result of primary herpes genitalis infection in mother. Neonatal herpes caused by HSV-1 is more frequent than that by HSV-2; however, the latter has a higher morbidity. HSV-1 is more likely to be associated with SEM disease, while HSV-2 is associated more often with CNS disease and with a poorer outcome.

Neonates with localized infection represent nearly 30% of neonatal herpes infection and have best prognosis with appropriate antiviral treatment, while disseminated disease carries the worst prognosis with around 30% mortality and 17% long-term neurological sequelae.

Diagnosis of neonatal herpes is often delayed as quite often mother is asymptomatic or may not recall history of herpes lesions. Also, the incubation period is of around 21 days, so a healthy child is taken home. Early features of neonatal herpes are quite vague like irritability, lethargy, poor feeding, etc.

Skin, eye, and mucous membrane disease: It usually manifests in the first 2 weeks of life but may be delayed up to first 6 weeks of life.

- *Cutaneous features:* Grouped vesicular lesions on an erythematous base. These lesions are seen at the presenting part of the body, or at sites of localized trauma, such as scalp monitor sites or in disseminated disease anywhere on the body.
- *Ocular features*: Increased lacrimation, conjunctival erythema, excessive crying due to eye pain, periorbital skin vesicles, etc. HSV keratoconjunctivitis may progress to corneal scarring, cataracts, and chorioretinitis ultimately leading to blindness.
- *Mucosal features*: Ulceration may be seen on mouth, palate, and tongue.

Central nervous system disease: Approximately one-third of neonatal HSV disease involves the CNS. Retrograde spread from the nasopharynx and olfactory nerves to the brain or through hematogenous spread in neonates with disseminated disease may lead to involvement of CNS. These features may resemble bacterial meningitis.

Disseminated disease: Approximately, 25–30% of neonatal HSV disease is the disseminated form, which is sepsis-like presentation, involving multiple organs (lungs, liver, hematological, renal, cardiac, adrenal, etc.). Neonates with disseminated HSV often present in the 1st week of life with nonspecific signs and symptoms of neonatal sepsis (temperature dysregulation, apnea, irritability, lethargy, respiratory distress, abdominal distension, hepatomegaly, and ascites).

DIAGNOSIS

All the pregnant females should be asked about history of genital herpes. Routine screening of genital herpes (serological testing) is not recommended during pregnancy. However, if partner has history of genital herpes, serological testing for HSV-1/-2 can be carried out for the patient. Seronegative pregnant women should be counseled to avoid unprotected intercourse in third trimester to avoid contracting herpes infection and in turn avoid neonatal transmission.

Herpes genitalis is a clinical diagnosis. In case of confusion, tests for direct viral detection and serological testing can be done.

Direct Viral Detection

- *Tzanck smear*: Can be prepared by deroofing a fresh vesicle and staining using freshly prepared Giemsa stain. Giemsa stain contains methylene blue, eosinate, azure A and B. Presence of enlarged multinucleated keratinocytes is pathognomonic of herpes infection. It has 80% sensitivity.
- *HSV polymerase chain reaction (PCR)*: It is the test of choice in symptomatic patients. Swab taken from fresh vesicle has a sensitivity of >90%.
- *Culture*: Can be done for viral isolation in MRC-5, Vero, or Hep-2 cell lines. Antiviral susceptibility testing can be done along with viral isolation. Culture is not specific and is not considered gold standard.
- *Other methods*: Enzyme immunoassay (EIA), electron microscopy, and immunofluorescence testing.

Serological Testing

Antibodies against HSV-1 and HSV-2 can be detected in the serum immunofluorescence or EIA. IgM antibodies can be detected within 1 week of infection, though it is not type specific. IgG antibodies can only be detected after 2 weeks of infection and are type specific. Seroconversion or rise of antibody titer can be used to differentiate primary episode from recurrent infection **(Table 1)**.

It is not recommended routinely in asymptomatic patients, but can be carried out in certain groups:

- Asymptomatic pregnant female where history of genital herpes is present in the partner so that seronegative women can be advised sexual abstinence in the last trimester to avoid contracting infection.
- To differentiate between primary genital herpes and recurrent herpes infection so as to guide counseling and management.

TABLE 1: Interpretation of serological testing.

	IgM (acute phase)		IgG (convalescent phase)		
HSV type	**HSV-1**	**HSV-2**	**HSV-1**	**HSV-2**	**Inference**
HSV-1	–	–	+	–	Primary HSV-1
HSV-2	–	–	–	+	Primary HSV-2
HSV-1	–	+	+	+	Primary HSV-1 in previously HSV-2 infected individuals
HSV-2	+	–	+	+	Primary HSV-2 in previously HSV-1 infected individuals
HSV-1	+	±	+	±	Recurrent HSV-1
HSV-2	±	+	±	+	Recurrent HSV-2

(HSV: herpes simplex virus; IgG: immunoglobulin G; IgM: immunoglobulin M)

- In case of clinical dilemma (atypical genital disease), where direct detection of virus is negative.
- In partner of patient with genital herpes infection where source of infection and its transmission is a concern and also to counsel the strategies to reduce risk of transmission to the serodiscordant couple.

All neonates suspected of HSV infection should be screened for any visible signs of infection and samples from skin, conjunctival mucosa, nasopharynx, oral cavity, and rectum should be collected and sent for HSV-PCR and culture within 24 hours of birth. In case of positive test results, CSF testing should be carried out.

TREATMENT

Pregnant women who have partners with known history or suspicion of genital herpes infection should be counseled to avoid vaginal intercourse during the third trimester. In addition to this, pregnant women, who do not have known history of orolabial herpes, should avoid receptive oral sex in third trimester with partners known to have orolabial herpes.

Pregnant women with first episode genital herpes:

- First or second trimester (until 27+6 weeks of gestation):
  - Tablet acyclovir 400 mg three times daily for 7 days. Intravenous acyclovir should be administered to pregnant women with severe disseminated.
  - Acyclovir is considered safe during all stages of pregnancy and lactation. There is no increased association of birth defects with acyclovir. It helps to reduce the duration and severity of symptoms as well as decrease the viral shedding. Valacyclovir also has similar results; however, it should be avoided in pregnancy due to lack of data.
  - Normal vaginal delivery at term should be anticipated (after ruling out other obstetric indications for cesarean section).
  - Daily suppressive dose of acyclovir 400 mg thrice a day starting from 36 weeks of gestation can be given to reduce asymptomatic viral shedding.
- *Third trimester (from 28 weeks of gestation)*:
  - Tablet acyclovir 400 mg three times daily for 7 days. Intravenous acyclovir should be administered to pregnant women with severe disseminated.
  - Treatment should be continued with daily suppressive acyclovir 400 mg thrice a day until delivery.
  - Cesarean section is recommended mode of delivery in those women developing first episode of genital herpes in the third trimester, especially those who develop symptoms within 6 weeks of expected delivery.

Pregnant women with recurrent genital herpes:

- Risk of transmission of herpes infection from mother to neonate with prenatal histories of recurrent herpes is low.
- If no symptoms of genital herpes at the onset of labor can deliver vaginally.
- In symptomatic mothers at time of labor, cesarean mode of delivery should be preferred to reduce risk of neonatal HSV transmission.

- Suppressive therapy with tablet acyclovir 400 mg thrice a day starting at 36 weeks of gestation helps in reducing the frequency of recurrences near expected delivery and thus in turn reducing the frequency of cesarean section.

Neonatal herpes: Intravenous acyclovir 20 mg/kg/dose every 8 hours should be started for 10–14 days for skin and mucosal involvement. Therapy is continued for 21 days in case of CNS involvement or disseminated disease.

SUGGESTED READINGS

1. Royal College of Obstetricians and Gynaecologists. Management of Genital Herpes in Pregnancy. [online] Available from https://www.rcog.org.uk/guidance/browse-all-guidance/other-guidelines-and-reports/management-of-genital-herpes-in-pregnancy/. [Last accessed January, 2025].
2. Straface G, Selmin A, Zanardo V, De Santis M, Ercoli A, Scambia G. Herpes simplex virus infection in pregnancy. Infect Dis Obstet Gynecol. 2012;2012:385697.
3. Centers for Disease Control and Prevention. (2015). Herpes in pregnancy. CDC: Sexually Transmitted Disease Treatment Guidelines. [online] Available from https://www.cdc.gov/mmwr/pdf/rr/rr6403.pdf. [Last accessed January, 2025].
4. American Academy of Pediatrics. Herpes simplex. In: Kimberlin DW, Banerjee R, Barnett ED, Lynfield R, Sawyer MH (Eds). Red Book: 2024-2027 Report of the Committee on Infectious Diseases, 33rd edition. Itasca, IL: American Academy of Pediatrics; 2024. p. 467.
5. Hyde SR, Giacoia GP. Congenital herpes infection: placental and umbilical cord findings. Obstet Gynecol. 1993;81:852.
6. Vasileiadis GT, Roukema HW, Romano W, Walton JC, Gagnon R. Intrauterine herpes simplex infection. Am J Perinatol. 2003;20:55.
7. Kimberlin DW. Neonatal herpes simplex infection. Clin Microbiol Rev. 2004;17:1.

10.3 Anogenital Warts

Rohit Batra, Aishwarya Dua

INTRODUCTION

Anogenital warts, also known as condylomata acuminata, are a common sexually transmitted infection (STI) clinically manifesting as benign growths or lesions. It is caused by *human papillomavirus (HPV)* a double-stranded DNA (dsDNA) virus from the *Papillomaviridae* family. In 90% of cases, the low-risk HPV strains 6 and 11 are implicated.

In the general population, the estimated prevalence of anogenital warts is about 1%. The annual incidence rate of anogenital warts is estimated to be between 160 and 200 cases per 100,000 persons. Since it most commonly affects sexually active age group, thus there are chances that it can occur during the pregnancy. It is estimated that 1–5% of pregnant women may develop anogenital warts. Management of anogenital warts during pregnancy is a little challenging because of limited number of safe treatment options. Transmission of HPV 6 and 11 infection from mother to the newborn, though less likely, can lead to respiratory papillomatosis in neonates and infants.

In these cases, the fetus could be infected through microabrasions in the membranes or through the placenta, from its tissue or the cord blood.

PATHOGENESIS

Human papillomavirus is a dsDNA virus and can be categorized as low risk (6, 11, etc.) and high risk (16, 18, 31, 33, 45, 52, 58, etc.) genotypically based on their malignant potential. Generally, these are HPV 6 and 11 strains which cause condyloma acuminata. While high-risk HPV strains cause intraepithelial neoplasia and carcinoma of cervix, penis, and anus.

Human papillomavirus infects the basal epithelial cells of the skin or mucosa, typically gaining entry through microabrasions or breaks in the skin resulting from sexual activity. Viral DNA integrates into that of host cell and keeps on replicating to the surface of skin. HPV-infected epithelial cells undergo hyperplasia and hyperkeratosis, leading to the thickening of the epithelium and the formation of visible warts. The warts can cluster and form a cauliflower-like appearance, which is characteristic of condylomata acuminata.

Human papillomavirus employs several mechanisms to evade the host immune system, allowing it to persist in the epithelial cells. These mechanisms include limited expression of viral proteins in the basal layers, lack of cell lysis (which reduces inflammation and immune detection), and downregulation of immune signaling molecules like interferons. Cell-mediated immune responses try to eliminate these virus infected cells. Changed immunological responses during pregnancy, e.g., Th1 to Th2 immunity, increased human β-defensin-1 and reduced protective α-defensins, alteration of pattern recognition proteins and toll-like receptors, and natural killer cell activity are responsible for altered behavior of human body to HPV infection.

Human papillomavirus infection is transmitted during vaginal, anal, or oral sexual contact. Only some of those who have contracted viral infection manifest clinically. HPV 6 and 11 infect the basal epithelial cells and remain latent in majority of patients. It may take months or years to develop genital warts in patients who have contracted HPV infection. During pregnancy, these latent viruses may get activated. Chances of transmission of HPV from an infected individual to his/her sexual partner are about 60%. There is no consistent conclusion whether pregnancy increases incidence of acquiring HPV infection, while few studies support this idea, others refute it. In a study by Pandey et al., HPV was found in vaginal secretions in 39.4% pregnant females in their first trimester.

Human papillomavirus can be transmitted to the sexual partner even in absence of visible signs of warts. Since virus remains latent in the basal keratinocytes, it is difficult to eradicate HPV infection even after treatment and there is always a risk of recurrence especially within first 3 months.

- Anogenital warts are caused by low-risk HPV (6 and 11)
- HPV replicates in basal layer of skin and mucosa
- HPV evades the maternal immune system
- Cell-mediated immunity helps in destruction of virus-infected cells
- Anogenital warts have a transmission rate of 60%
- Increased risk of HPV infection during pregnancy is debatable

MODES OF TRANSMISSION

As the incubation period of HPV (3 weeks to 8 months) is long, so determining the transmission route is difficult.

- *Perinatal*: During delivery, contact with HPV-infected cells can get deposited on any abrasion on the neonate. Conjunctival, buccal, pharyngeal, and genital swabs of the neonates have been sampled and same strain of HPV as that of mother has been detected. Medeiros et al. reported a transmission probability of 6.5%. Though HPV was detected in higher percentage of neonates at birth but after 5 weeks no HPV was seen. Thus is the advantage of elective cesarean section. But as the virus is not seen in a child after 5 weeks so certain studies deny this indication for not allowing vaginal delivery.
- Ascending infection from cervical warts especially HPV 16 can lead to involvement of trophoblast. HPV-infected trophoblasts decrease in numbers and lose their ability to adhere to endometrial cells. Thus, prepregnancy vaccines are advisable to reduce abortions and infertility.
- Hematogenous spread is very low.
- Anogenital warts in father around the period of conception may transmit HPV to oocyte through sperms and semen. Also, this could be a cause for infertility in men. Mothers can also be a source of periconceptual transmission.

Nonsexual horizontal transmission:

- Heteroinoculation
- Fomites

- Perinatal transmission is the most common mode of fetal HPV
- Lack of persistent growth of HPV in the neonate refutes the need for elective cesarean delivery

CLINICAL FEATURES

Condyloma acuminata presents as multiple, asymptomatic finger-like projections with irregular surface affecting the labia minora and majora, introitus, posterior fourchette, perineum, and perianal region.

During pregnancy, lesions may proliferate rapidly, become friable, and individual lesions may even coalesce to form larger lesions and in severe cases can fill the vaginal outlet and cause obstruction of the birth canal. Though less likely, HPV infection can transmit vertically to the neonate causing respiratory papillomatosis during vaginal delivery. Also, response to treatment could be incomplete during pregnancy.

Alteration in clinical course of anogenital warts in pregnancy:

- Warts become larger in size and friable
- Bleeding from wart surface may be seen
- Can cause obstruction of birth canal
- Very rarely may cause respiratory papillomatosis in the newborn
- May cause psychological impact on the mother
- Some studies have reported poor pregnancy outcome and pregnancy complication
- Clearance of HPV during pregnancy is delayed in first two trimesters while it increases postpartum

A rare, locally invasive HPV 6 and 11 associated lesion is known as Buschke-Lowenstein tumor. It is a giant tumor characterized by downward growth into the dermal structures. It does not metastasize usually; however, there is a risk of transmission to squamous cell carcinoma in immunocompromised patients.

MATERNAL SIDE EFFECTS

Spontaneous abortion, preterm birth, preeclampsia, and premature rupture of membranes are reported to be adverse effects of HPV infection during pregnancy. The ways in which HPV infection may impact pregnancy outcomes are thought to include changes in cervical competence, alterations to the vaginal microbiota, infections of the placenta or amniotic fluid, effects from cervical procedures done to treat HPV during pregnancy, and infections transmitted through semen.

FETAL EFFECTS

Effect of maternal HPV infection has less adverse effects on the fetus. The various changes which have been reported are:

- Intrauterine growth restriction, fetal death
- Juvenile recurrent respiratory papillomatosis (JRRP), though is rare but has high morbidity and is seen in neonates born by vaginal delivery. Genetic susceptibility is seen in those with HLA-DQB1*0201, DQB1*0202, and DRB1*0301. Hoarseness of voice is the most common presentation. They my present with choking, weak cry, and failure to thrive. Patient usually presents in 2–6 years age group.
- Other manifestations of HPV infection are conjunctival papilloma and probably retinoblastoma.

> - HPV infection rarely causes maternal and fetal adverse effects
> - *Maternal effects*: Preeclampsia, premature rupture of membrane, abortion, and preterm labor
> - *Fetal effects*: Fetal death, intrauterine growth retardation, and juvenile recurrent respiratory papillomatosis

MANAGEMENT

- Safe sexual practices using condom should be advised to the couple presenting at the antenatal clinic. Since genital warts are transmitted sexually, pregnant female should be offered testing for other STIs also. Patient should be advised to avoid sexual activity with a new partner till the warts are removed.
- Physical examination of the partner can be done to detect genital warts and should be offered treatment.
- Mother should be counseled regarding the low risk of HPV infection transmission to their offspring (respiratory papillomatosis).
- Patients may experience great psychosocial impact after learning about the diagnosis and thus should be counseled about their concerns. Treating

medical professional should educate the patient about the HPV virus types and that the strains causing genital warts and cervical cancer are different. Female should be educated about tests for screening of cervical cancer (pap smear and HPV test). The couple should be counseled that HPV infection does not affect woman's fertility.
- Pregnant women with anogenital warts, at the time of birth, should deliver vaginally unless there is pelvic outlet obstruction due to warts or if normal vaginal delivery would lead to excessive blood loss. Cesarean section should not be performed to prevent respiratory papillomatosis in newborn as the risk of neonatal transmission is less.

Safer and efficacious treatment options for management of warts during pregnancy include:
- *Cryotherapy*: Using liquid nitrogen is the treatment of choice. It helps in controlled and targeted destruction of warts by freezing the tissue. The ice field should extend up to 1–2 mm of normal surrounding tissue. Freeze time starts once the ice has formed over the entire affected area and should not be >2 minutes. This is followed by thawing, i.e., the lesion is slowly allowed to come back to normal temperature. It can be repeated every 2 weeks till the lesions have completely resolved. Cryoprobe should not be used for vaginal warts because of risk of vaginal perforation and fistula formation. Although it is safe, patient may experience local side effects like pain, swelling, erythema, and exudation.
- *Chemical cauterization using trichloroacetic acid (80–90%)*: It destroys the warts by chemical coagulation of proteins. It can be repeated weekly till the warts are gone. It is safe in pregnant females as it does not get absorbed into skin and mucous membranes. Trichloroacetic acid has low viscosity and can damage adjacent tissues if not applied carefully.
- *Electrocautery/radiofrequency ablation*: Use of electrical energy or heat energy to destroy the lesions
- Surgical excision

Safe modalities of treatment of anogenital warts during pregnancy are:
- Cryotherapy
- Chemical cauterization with trichloroacetic acid
- Radiofrequency ablation
- Surgical excision

Use of podophyllin, podophyllotoxin, and sinecatechins should not be used in pregnancy. Podophyllin and podophyllotoxin have antimitotic action and contain mutagens like quercetin and kaempferol, thus leading to increased (theoretical) risk of teratogenicity. Imiquimod acts by immunomodulation (stimulates TLR-7/8) and induces transcription of genes for interferon-α (IFN-α) and tumor necrosis factor-α (TNF-α). Though imiquimod poses less risk and has been used in pregnancy in few studies, but it is better to avoid its use during pregnancy.

PREVENTION OF ANOGENITAL WARTS

Human papillomavirus vaccine: Gardasil vaccine (tetravalent and nonavalent) can be used to prevent genital warts in both males and females and, at the same time, provides protection against HPV-associated cancers (cervical, penile, and anal).

- Gardasil-4 provides protection against HPV 6, 11, 16, and 18 strains.
- Gardasil-9 provides protection against HPV 6, 11, 16, 18, 31, 33, 45, 52, and 58 strains.

Human papillomavirus vaccines are made up of noninfectious, virus-like particles (VLPs) and can prevent genital warts in those who have not yet been exposed to those HPV strains. However, it cannot treat the existing HPV infection or genital warts.

According to Advisory Committee on Immunization (ACIP), HPV vaccine should be routinely recommended to all boys and girls at 11–12 years of age (can be started at 9 years of age). Catch up vaccine is recommended for all persons up to 26 years of age. For adults aged 27–45 years, clinical decision making is recommended depending on the behavioral risk factors (e.g., HIV infected, MSM, and immunocompromised states). Vaccine can be administered regardless of anogenital warts, abnormal pap smear test, or HPV-associated precancer lesions.

Dosing schedule:

- *<15 years of age*: Two doses (0 and 6–12 month)
- *≥15 years of age*: Three doses of HPV (0, 1–2 month, and 6 month)

Dose: 0.5 mL intramuscular injection (preferably deltoid muscle).

Human papillomavirus vaccine provides 90% protection against anogenital warts lasting for about 5 years. Gardasil-4 protects against 66% of cervical cancer, while gardasil-9 provides additional 15% protection against cervical cancer as it targets five additional cancer causing HPV types.

Human papillomavirus vaccine is not recommended during pregnancy. If the female conceives after initiating vaccination series, remaining doses can be continued after delivery. If the vaccine is mistakenly administered during pregnancy, no further intervention is required.

KEY POINTS

- Management of anogenital warts during pregnancy is a little challenging because of limited number of safe treatment options.
- Transmission of HPV 6 and 11 infection from mother to the newborn, though less likely, can lead to respiratory papillomatosis in neonates and infants. During pregnancy, lesions may proliferate rapidly, become friable, and individual lesions may even coalesce to form larger lesions.
- Pregnant women with anogenital warts, at the time of birth, should deliver vaginally unless there is pelvic outlet obstruction due to warts or if normal vaginal delivery would lead to excessive blood loss.
- Cryotherapy, trichloroacetic acid, electrocautery/radiofrequency ablation, and surgical excision are considered safe during pregnancy.
- Gardasil vaccine (tetravalent and nonavalent) can be used to prevent genital warts in both males and females.

SUGGESTED READINGS

1. Workowski KA, Bolan GA. (2015). Anogenital warts in pregnancy. CDC: Sexually Transmitted Diseases Treatment Guidelines. [online] Available from https://www.cdc.gov/mmwr/preview/mmwrhtml/rr6403a1.htm. [Last accessed January, 2025].
2. Sugai S, Nishijima K, Enomoto T. Management of Condyloma Acuminata in Pregnancy: A Review. Sex Transm Dis. 2021;48(6):403-9.
3. Khayargoli P, Niyibizi J, Mayrand M, Audibert F, Monnier P, Brassard P, et al. Human Papillomavirus Transmission and Persistence in Pregnant Women and Neonates. JAMA Pediatr. 2023;177(7):684-92.
4. Ardekani A, Taherifard E, Mollalo A, Hemadi E, Roshanshad A, Fereidooni R, et al. Human Papillomavirus Infection during Pregnancy and Childhood: A Comprehensive Review. Microorganisms. 2022;10:1932.
5. Bruno MT, Caruso S, Scalia G, Costanzo M, Di Pasqua S, Boemi S, et al. Papillomavirus Infection as Potential Cause of Miscarriage in the Early Gestational Age: A Prospective Study. Diagnostics. 2023;13:1659.

10.4 Human Immunodeficiency Virus in Pregnancy

Rohit Batra, Aishwarya Dua

INTRODUCTION

Human immunodeficiency virus (HIV) belongs to Retroviridae family. Human infection is caused either by HIV-1 or HIV-2. Infection with HIV-1 is more prevalent and has higher virulence and infectivity.

Human immunodeficiency virus is a global health challenge, and its management in pregnancy is crucial for both maternal and fetal health. Without appropriate treatment, HIV can be transmitted from mother to child during pregnancy, childbirth, or breastfeeding. With timely interventions, however, the risk of mother-to-child transmission (MTCT) can be significantly reduced. This chapter outlines the impact of HIV on pregnancy, maternal and fetal outcomes, management strategies, and the prevention of MTCT.

EPIDEMIOLOGY

Globally, around 1.3 million women living with HIV become pregnant each year, and without intervention, the rate of MTCT ranges from 15 to 45%. Out of a total of 38 million people living with HIV/AIDS (PLHA), 1.5 million are children <15 years of age. Among these, 90% children have acquired disease through MTCT. According to reports, India has third highest number of PLHA. Overall prevalence of HIV infection in India in adults (15–49 years) is 0.22% and in pregnant women is 0.35%. Each year, approximately 22,000 new cases are reported in children accounting for 6.5% of the new HIV infections.

STRUCTURE OF HUMAN IMMUNODEFICIENCY VIRUS

Genome of HIV-1 contains the following genes:
- *Gag* gene—encodes for p24 (viral capsid) and p17 (matric protein)
- *Pol* gene—encodes for viral enzymes reverse transcriptase, integrase, and protease
- *Env* gene—encodes for viral envelope gp120 and gp41 proteins
- *Tat, rev, nef, vif, vpr, and vpu*—help in transcription and post-transcription of various structural proteins

PATHOGENESIS

Human immunodeficiency virus infects CD4-positive T cells and macrophages by interaction of gp120 envelope glycoprotein with CD4 receptor and chemokine coreceptor CXCR4 or CCR5. This induces formation of gp120-gp41 complex which facilitates fusion of the virus with host cell. Viral DNA is formed by reverse transcription and transported to host cell nucleus. Viral integrase enzyme catalyzes integration of viral DNA with host DNA leading to formation of provirus. The provirus may not produce new copies of HIV and remain latent for years. When it replicates, it uses RNA polymerase II to create viral RNA copies followed by formation of viral mRNA encoding viral proteins. Viral RNA is subsequently packaged into virions and mature virions are released from the plasma membrane with the help of protease enzyme.

Various antiretroviral therapy (ART) drugs according to the target of action are as follows:
- *Reverse transcriptase inhibitors*:
  - Nucleoside reverse transcriptase inhibitors (NRTI)—zidovudine, lamivudine, stavudine, abacavir, and emtricitabine
  - Non-nucleoside reverse transcriptase inhibitors (NNRTI)—nevirapine and efavirenz
  - Nucleotide reverse transcriptase inhibitors (NtRTI)—tenofovir
- Protease inhibitors—ritonavir, saquinavir, and lopinavir
- Integrase inhibitors—raltegravir and dolutegravir
- Fusion inhibitors—enfuvirtide
- Entry inhibitors (CCR5 antagonist)—maraviroc

MODE OF TRANSMISSION

Vertical transmission of HIV from mother to child can occur through:
- In utero
- Peripartum
- Breastfeeding

There are various maternal risk factors and intrapartum factors which increase MTCT **(Table 1)**. HIV-2 is less virulent, slowly multiplying, and is less commonly transmitted to the fetus.

TABLE 1: Maternal risk factors which increase mother-to-child transmission of HIV.

Maternal risk actors	Intrapartum factors
• Genotype of virus (HIV-1) • High viral load • Decreased CD4 count • P24 antigenemia • Advanced AIDS • Preterm delivery • Chorioamnionitis • Micronutrient deficiency • Rupture of membranes • >4 hours before delivery, concurrent sexually transmitted infections (STIs)	• Artificial rupture of membranes • Repeated vaginal examination • Prolonged labor • Delayed clamping of cord • Invasive fetal monitoring and delivery tools, e.g., scalp monitors, suction delivery, forceps delivery • Episiotomy

(HIV: human immunodeficiency virus)

BOX 1 Risk factors for MTCT during breastfeeding.

Risk factors of transmission of HIV through breastfeed:
- High viral load
- Longer duration of breastfeed especially in untreated mother
- Mixed feeding
- Mastitis or cracked nipples
- Infant's health

(HIV: human immunodeficiency virus; MTCT: mother-to-child transmission)

Risk of transmission of HIV from untreated breastfeeding mother to the child is as high as 30–45% compared to as low as 2% from breastfeeding mother on ART. Thus, National AIDS Control Organization (NACO) suggests lifelong ART for all pregnant and lactating females with HIV regardless of clinical stage and CD4 count. In a resource-poor parents, breastfeeding is encouraged. Mixed feeding during infancy predisposes the newborn to contract HIV infection and thus should be avoided. Mastitis and cracked nipples due to increased inflammatory cells and contact with blood may increase risk of transmission of HIV to baby. If the child has inflamed oral or gastrointestinal mucosa or oral thrush transmission is increased. There are various factors which increase transmission to newborn via breast milk **(Box 1)**.

CLINICAL FEATURES

Clinical course of HIV does not seem to alter much due to pregnancy. Clinical stages of HIV infection depending on the stage of the disease are as follows:

Stage 1:
- Asymptomatic
- Persistent generalized lymphadenopathy

Stage 2:
- Moderate unexplained weight loss (<10%)
- Herpes zoster
- Recurrent oral ulceration
- Papular pruritic eruption
- Fungal nail infection
- Seborrheic dermatitis

Stage 3:
- Unexplained severe weight loss (>10%)
- Unexplained chronic diarrhea (>1 month)
- Unexplained persistent fever (>1 month)
- Persistent oral candidiasis
- Oral hairy leukoplakia
- Pulmonary tuberculosis
- Acute necrotizing ulcerative stomatitis, gingivitis, or periodontitis
- Unexplained anemia (<8 g/dL), neutropenia, and/or chronic thrombocytopenia

Stage 4:
- Pneumocystis pneumonia
- Chronic herpes simplex infection
- Esophageal candidiasis
- Kaposi sarcoma
- Disseminated nontuberculous mycobacterial infection (NTM)
- Progressive multifocal leukoencephalopathy (PMLE)
- Disseminated mycosis
- Atypical disseminated leishmaniasis

Acquired immunodeficiency syndrome (AIDS) is defined as "occurrence of life-threatening opportunistic infections, malignancies, neurological diseases, and other specific illnesses in patients with HIV infection and CD4 count <200 cells/mm^3." Tuberculosis and candida albicans infection usually develop at CD4 counts 200–500 cells/mm^3. Pneumocystis pneumonia occurs at CD4 count <200 cells/mm^3 and cytomegalovirus (CMV) infection at counts below 100 cell/mm^3.

EFFECT OF HUMAN IMMUNODEFICIENCY VIRUS ON PREGNANCY

Though pregnancy does not alter the course of HIV much but HIV can have a variety of effects on pregnancy, influencing both maternal health and the health of the developing fetus as shown in **Figure 1**. Pregnant patient is more susceptible to opportunistic infections. Malaria occurring in HIV-positive pregnant female may be even fatal. There is high risk of nutritional deficiencies and anemia. ART may cause certain adverse effects such as nausea, vomiting, liver and renal compromise which a pregnant patient may find difficult to tolerate. Protease inhibitors may increase risk of preterm labor and drugs like efavirenz may increase risk of congenital malformations.

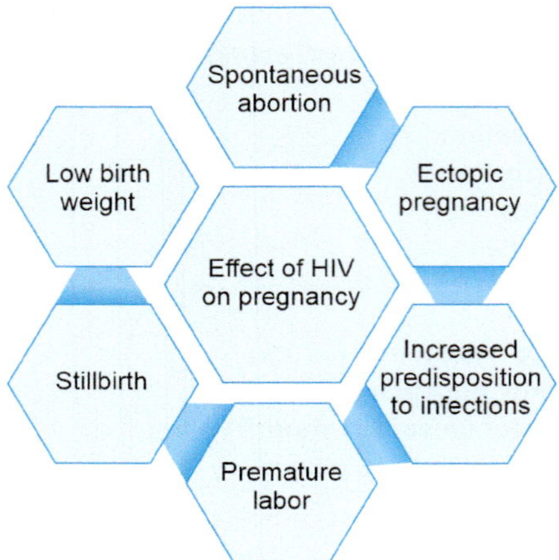

FIG. 1: Effect of HIV on pregnancy outcome.
(HIV: human immunodeficiency virus)

PREVENTION OF PARENT-TO-CHILD TRANSMISSION OF HUMAN IMMUNODEFICIENCY VIRUS

The goal of prevention of parent-to-child transmission (PPTCT) services in India is to work toward elimination of pediatric HIV and improve maternal, newborn, and child health and survival in the context of HIV infection.

Prevention of parent-to-child transmission program adopts a four-pronged strategy:

Prong 1: Primary prevention of HIV infection in general population
Prong 2: Prevent unintended pregnancies in HIV positive females
Prong 3: Prevention of MTCT by timely diagnosis and starting ART in HIV-positive pregnant females
Prong 4: Care, support, and treatment to HIV-positive mother and HIV-exposed infant

Some of the services under PPTCT include:
- Routine HIV counseling and testing to all pregnant women with "opt out" option
- Lifelong ART to all HIV-infected pregnant and lactating females
- Promotion of institutional deliveries
- Provision of detection and management of associated conditions (e.g., opportunistic infections)
- Psychological support and nutritional counseling
- Antiretroviral prophylaxis for infants
- Follow-up of HIV-exposed infants
- Community follow-up and outreach

Interventions during pregnancy to prevent transmission of HIV infection to the newborn aim at primary prevention of HIV in pregnant females, counseling, and educating pregnant women about HIV, promoting regular antenatal visits, prevention of accidental pregnancies in HIV-positive females, and following safe obstetric practices.

DIAGNOSIS

Routine HIV screening during pregnancy:

- First prenatal visit
- Opt-out screening (HIV testing is automatically included unless the patient specifically declines)
- Repeat testing in the third trimester (in high-risk/high-prevalence areas) at 28–36 weeks

Same testing kits and procedure are used as in general population.

Human immunodeficiency virus testing should be offered to all females at first antenatal visit. Any pregnant women detected HIV positive for the first time during routine antenatal should be linked to ART center immediately, where CD4 count is done and ART is initiated regardless of the CD4 count. If a pregnant woman is already aware of her positive HIV status and is on ART, same ART regimen should be continued. Viral load testing should be done at 32–36 weeks' gestation to assess for risk of transmission to the baby. Sexual partner of the pregnant female should also be evaluated for HIV infection. Testing for other sexually transmitted infections (STIs) like venereal disease research laboratory (VDRL), hepatitis B/C, and physical examination for genital warts, genital molluscum, etc. should be done.

Importance of Preconception Counseling

- *Reducing the risk of HIV transmission*: Preconception counseling helps to ensure the HIV-positive person is on effective ART before conception.
- *To the partner*: For HIV-discordant couples (where one partner is HIV-positive and the other is not), counseling helps them understand ways to prevent transmission during conception.

Optimizing Maternal Health

- Helps to encourage patient for regular ART and encourages individuals to achieve viral suppression before pregnancy
- Screening and treating AIDS-associated coinfections and conditions
- Nutritional and mental health support
- Tailor a safe ART plan that supports both maternal health and fetal development
- *Fertility options*: For couples where one or both partners are HIV-positive, counseling provides information on various fertility options to help them conceive safely. This might include timed intercourse, assisted reproductive technology, or sperm washing.

Postnatal Care Planning

- *Newborn care*: Counseling allows for discussions on newborn care, including the importance of early HIV testing and the prevention of postnatal transmission through breastfeeding (in some cases, formula feeding may be recommended depending on the resources available and the viral load).
- *Maternal health post-pregnancy*: Planning for continued ART use postpartum ensures both the mother's long-term health and reduces the risk of future transmission.

Mode of Delivery

- Plasma viral load <1,000 copies/mL—normal vaginal delivery
- Plasma viral load >1,000 copies/mL—beyond 34 weeks' gestation (e.g., not taking ART, presenting late in pregnancy, ART resistance), cesarean delivery at 38 weeks, prior to labor onset and rupture of membranes can be considered

TREATMENT

Any pregnant female who is tested HIV positive during pregnancy should be started on lifelong ART (same as all adults) irrespective of the CD4 count and stage of the disease. Fixed drug combination (FDC) of tenofovir 300 mg + lamivudine 300 mg + dolutegravir 50 mg daily once a day.

Dolutegravir is a new antiretroviral drug added in the regimen for faster viral load suppression, lesser toxicity, decrease risk of sexual transmission of HIV, greater maternal viral suppression, fewer maternal deaths, and fewer MTCT. However, there is very small potential (theoretical) risk of neural tube defects with first trimester exposure, thus women should be allowed to make an informed choice.

Females (reproductive age group) who do not wish to use dolutegravir:

- Fixed drug combination of tenofovir 300 mg + lamivudine 300 mg + efavirenz 600 mg daily once a day
- Any HIV-positive female on ART who becomes pregnant should continue with the same ART regimen as prepregnancy. ART should be continued even during labor, postpartum period, and lactation.
- During labor, all the triggering factors as described in **Table 1** should be avoided. Unless there is any obstetric contraindication, the baby may be delivered vaginally.

Breastfeeding practices: Exclusive breastfeeding should be promoted for first 6 months. Breastfeeding can be continued for up to 12–24 months with introduction of complementary feeds at 6 months of age. Mixed feeding in the early months is not recommended as it leads to inflammation of the child's gut, and hence, increases the chance of infection from breast milk.

Difference in risk of transmission of HIV infection from mother (on ART) to the child with and without breastfeeding is 2% and 1% respectively, thus making exclusive breastfeeding a preferred choice, as exclusive replacement feeding adds to the cost of treatment, and hygiene and availability become an issue.

Neonatal Prophylaxis and Monitoring for Infants (Table 2)

All infants born to HIV positive mothers should be given prophylaxis. Infants born to mother with suppressed viral load (<1,000 copies/mL) done at 32–36 weeks' gestation are considered low-risk infants and should receive single-dose prophylaxis with syrup nevirapine for at least 6 weeks **(Table 2)**.

If mother has history of taking NNRTI in past or there is HIV-2 coinfection, syrup zidovudine is given for prophylaxis in place of nevirapine.

Infants born to mother not on ART or who have been put on ART within 6 weeks of delivery and where mother has high viral load (>1,000 copies/mL) at 32–36 weeks or viral load has not been done are considered high-risk infants and should receive dual drug prophylaxis with syrup nevirapine and syrup zidovudine for 6 weeks in case of exclusive replacement feeding and till 12 weeks of age in case of exclusive breastfeeding.

Dosage of prophylactic drugs: Zidovudine (AZT) 4 mg/kg every 12 hours.

Nevirapine dosing is based on age:
- *Birth to 1 week*: Nevirapine 12 mg/kg once daily
- *1–2 weeks*: Nevirapine 12 mg/kg twice daily
- *2 weeks and older*: Nevirapine 12 mg/kg three times daily

All HIV-exposed infants should receive cotrimoxazole at 6 weeks of age. During infancy, observe for signs and symptoms of HIV infection at follow-up visits and standard immunization schedule should be followed.

TABLE 2: Infant prophylaxis and monitoring born to HIV-positive mother.

Step	Criteria	Action	Duration
Determine infant prophylaxis	• Maternal viral load undetectable (<1,000 copies/mL) • Maternal viral load undetectable (<1,000 copies/mL) with history of HIV-2 coinfection or mother has taken NNRTI • Maternal viral load >1,000 copies/mL	• Syrup nevirapine • Add zidovudine • Nevirapine + zidovudine	• 4–6 weeks • 4–6 weeks • 6–12 weeks
HIV testing of infant	• First test (birth) • Second (4–6 weeks) • Third (4–6 months) • At 18 months • Positive HIV test result	• Perform HIV DNA PCR or RNA • Repeat HIV DNA • Repeat HIV DNA • HIV antibody test • Confirm HIV test	

(HIV: human immunodeficiency virus; NNRTI: non-nucleoside reverse transcriptase inhibitor; PCR: polymerase chain reaction)

TABLE 3: Age- and weight-wise treatment of children living with HIV.	
Weight and age of child	**Recommended treatment**
<20 kg; <6 years	Abacavir + Lamivudine + Lopinavir
20–30 kg; 6–10 years	Abacavir + Lamivudine + Dolutegravir 50 mg
>30 kg; >10 years	Tenofovir + Lamivudine 300 + Dolutegravir 50 mg
(HIV: human immunodeficiency virus)	

A HIV-exposed newborn should be given antiretroviral prophylaxis and tested for HIV at 6 weeks by HIV DNA polymerase chain reaction (PCR) using dried blood spot (DBS) sample. If HIV is detected, collect and send another DBS sample of the baby for confirmatory HIV PCR test. On confirmation of HIV infection, baby is referred to ART center for starting treatment.

If HIV is not detected, repeat HIV testing using serological test at 6 months or 6 weeks after last breast milk feeding (whichever is earlier). Final antibody test is done at 18 months.

Treatment of Human Immunodeficiency Virus-positive Neonate

According to NACO 2021, age- and weight-wise treatment of children living with HIV is given in **Table 3**.

KEY POINTS

- Vertical transmission of HIV infection from mother to child can occur in utero, in peripartum period, and during lactation.
- HIV testing should be offered to all females at first antenatal visit.
- Lifelong ART should be given to all pregnant and breastfeeding women infected with HIV regardless of CD4 count or clinical stage.
- Exclusive breastfeeding for first 6 months is recommended for HIV-infected mothers.
- All neonates born to HIV-positive mothers should be given nevirapine prophylaxis for at least 6 weeks.

SUGGESTED READINGS

1. NACO. (2021). National guidelines for HIV care and treatment, 2021. [online] Available from https://naco.gov.in/sites/default/files/National_Guidelines_for_HIV_Care_and_Treatment_2021.pdf. [Last accessed January, 2025].
2. World Health Organization. WHO guidelines on HIV prevention, testing, treatment. [online] Available from https://www.who.int/publications/i/item/9789240031593. [Last accessed January, 2025].
3. Chilaka VN, Konje JC. HIV in pregnancy – An update. Eur J Obstet Gynecol Reprod Biol. 2021;256:484-91.

10.5 Gonorrhea

Rohit Batra, Aishwarya Dua

INTRODUCTION

Gonococcal infection is the second most prevalent bacterial sexually transmitted disease (STD) globally and is a major public health concern worldwide. It is caused by obligate human pathogen *Neisseria gonorrhoeae*.

Gonorrhea infection is associated with several complications in women, for example, cervicitis, urethritis, salpingitis, pelvic inflammatory disease (PID), ectopic pregnancy, and infertility.

Pregnant women and their newborn are all at the greater risk of infection sequelae, thus making timely diagnosis and management important. If it is not timely diagnosed and treated, it may have severe health, social, and economic implications caused by adverse pregnancy outcomes on mother, fetus, and newborn.

ETIOLOGY

Gonorrhea is caused by the bacterium *Neisseria gonorrhoeae*, a gram-negative diplococcus that infects the mucous membranes of the genital tract, rectum, pharynx, and conjunctiva.

EPIDEMIOLOGY

Global prevalence of gonorrhea among pregnant women is estimated to be 1.85%. According to WHO, prevalence of gonorrhea in pregnant women is up to twofold higher than that of general population of women. The incidence of gonorrhea in pregnancy is higher in populations with limited access to prenatal care, lower socioeconomic status, and those with a history of multiple sexual partners or inconsistent condom use. Also, patients may not seek medical care in absence of symptoms.

- Gonorrhea is a sexually transmitted infection caused by *Neisseria gonorrhoeae*
- Pregnant females are more likely to get the infection

PATHOGENESIS

Neisseria gonorrhoeae is a gram-negative, nonmotile, intracellular diplococci displaying high variability both genetically and phenotypically. The extensive genetic exchange within the species using transformation and conjugation helps it in adapting to the host immune response and developing antibiotic resistance. The pathogenetic mechanism of *N. gonorrhoeae* causing disease is as detailed below and shown in **Figure 1**.

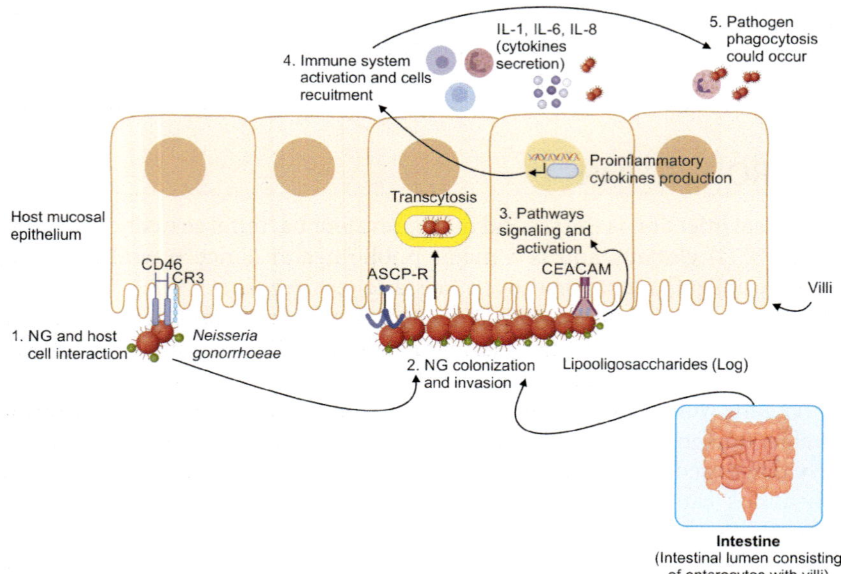

FIG. 1: The adhesion, invasion, and pathogenesis of *N. gonorrhoeae*.
(IL: interleukin; NG: *Neisseria gonorrhoeae*)
Courtesy: Gauri Thakural and Aanya Bedi, MMIMSR, Mullana, Haryana, India.

Adherence to and Invasion of Mucosal Surfaces

Neisseria gonorrhoeae has predilection for nonciliated columnar epithelium. The bacteria adhere to the mucosal cells by pili and outer membrane proteins (Opa protein). Then it is pinocytosed into the epithelial cells where it multiplies and becomes resistant to immune response. The lipid A moiety of the LOS (lipooligosaccharide) in the cell wall has endotoxin activity. Epithelial damage is mediated by enzymes like phospholipase and peptidase.

In pregnant women, the primary site of infection is the cervix. The cervical epithelium is more susceptible to infection due to hormonal changes in pregnancy that increase blood flow and mucus production. These changes create a favorable environment for bacterial adherence and colonization.

Avoidance of Host Immune Response

Neisseria gonorrhoeae has several mechanisms to evade the host's immune system, allowing it to persist and cause infection.

- *Antigenic variation*: The bacteria can alter surface proteins (such as pili and Opa proteins) to evade immune recognition.
- *Phase variation*: It can turn certain genes on and off, which helps avoid detection by antibodies.
- *Complement resistance*: *N. gonorrhoeae* produces proteins that interfere with the complement system, which is part of the innate immune response responsible for clearing pathogens.

Inflammatory Response

The invasion of *N. gonorrhoeae* triggers an intense local inflammatory response. The bacteria induce the production of proinflammatory cytokines (e.g., IL-1, IL-6, IL-8, and TNF-α) by infected epithelial cells and immune cells. This inflammatory response leads to the recruitment of neutrophils into the site of infection (lumen of urethra/cervix), which is responsible for the characteristic purulent discharge.

Pathogenesis of gonorrhea:
- Bacteria adhere to cervical/urethral mucosa
- Invades host cells
- Evades the host immune responses
- Recruits inflammatory cells—purulent discharge

MODE OF TRANSMISSION

Risk of transmission of gonorrhea from an infected male to female after single exposure is 50–90% and from an infected female to male is 20%.

Mother to child transmission rate of untreated gonorrhea infection during passage from birth canal is approximately 30%.

Also, gonorrhea is associated with higher risk of HIV transmission from mother to fetus.

SIGNS AND SYMPTOMS

- Gonococcal infections are commonly asymptomatic (50–80%) among women until complications have occurred.
- Endocervicitis—presents as profuse yellow to yellowish-green purulent vaginal discharge, dysuria, dyspareunia, and postcoital bleeding. On per speculum examination, severe edema and erythema of the cervix can be appreciated along with copious discharge at the external cervical os.
- Urethritis, skenitis, and bartholinitis can also occur.
- In first trimester, there is increased risk of ascending infection leading to PID and salpingitis.
- The PID and salpingitis result in scarring of the fallopian tubes leading to infertility and ectopic pregnancy.
- After first trimester, choroid membrane gets attached to the decidua and obliterates the uterine cavity. Thus, post this period, the risk of PID decreases and risk of chorioamnionitis, premature rupture of membranes, low-birth weight, preterm birth, and septic abortion increases. Pregnant women with untreated, asymptomatic sexually transmitted infections (STIs) are 3.3 times more likely to experience preterm delivery compared to those who receive treatment. Also, mother becomes more susceptible to postpartum endometritis and puerperal sepsis.
- Disseminated gonococcal infection (DGI) resulting from hematogenous spread of infection is reported to be more common during pregnancy. DGI can manifest as septic arthritis, dermatitis, endocarditis, meningitis, etc.

Complications of gonococcal infection:
- *General*: Cervicitis, urethritis, bartholinitis, skenitis, pelvic inflammatory disease, salpingitis, and disseminated gonococcal infection
- *Pregnancy related*: Ectopic pregnancy, chorioamnionitis, premature rupture of membrane, preterm labor, and septic abortion
- *Fetal/neonatal*: Low-birth weight, ophthalmia neonatorum, neonatal sepsis, and localized gonococcal abscess

GONOCOCCAL INFECTIONS AMONG NEONATE

In addition to low-birth weight, preterm baby, other complications due to gonococcal infection in neonates occur due to perinatal exposure to mother's infected birth canal. Symptoms manifest 2–5 days after birth ranging from less severe rhinitis, urethritis, vaginitis, to severe manifestations as ophthalmia neonatorum and sepsis. Thus, screening and treatment of women during pregnancy is important to prevent gonococcal infection among neonates.

Ophthalmia neonatorum manifests as mucopurulent to purulent discharge pouring out when eyelids are separated with intensely inflamed, bright red, and swollen conjunctiva with marked chemosis. If untreated, it can lead to corneal ulceration, iris prolapse, synechiae formation, anterior staphyloma, and even panophthalmitis. Approximately, 3% neonates with untreated gonococcal infection can suffer from blindness and up to 20% can have corneal damage. Ideally ophthalmia neonatorum prophylaxis should be given to all neonates soon after birth regardless of the mode of delivery. Erythromycin 0.5% ophthalmic ointment in each eye at birth in single application is given.

Newborns who do not receive ophthalmia prophylaxis and whose mother has not received any antenatal care or has a history of STDs or drug abuse are at increased risk for ophthalmia neonatorum.

Infants who have ophthalmia neonatorum should be evaluated for signs of DGI presenting as sepsis, arthritis, or meningitis.

Localized gonococcal infection of scalp (scalp abscess) may also occur, resulting from fetal monitoring through scalp electrodes.

DIAGNOSIS

Diagnosis of gonorrhea:
- Screening
- *Gram staining*: Gram-negative intercellular diplococci
- *Culture*: In nonspecific chocolate agar medium or selective media such as the modified Thayer–Martin medium
- Nucleic acid amplification test

Ideally, antenatal screening should be done at the first visit or in the first trimester as gonococcal infections are mostly asymptomatic in women. In high-risk females (e.g., those females with other STIs during pregnancy or those who have a new sex partner, more than one sex partner, a sex partner with concurrent partners, or a

TABLE 1: Recommended diagnostic test for different specimens in gonorrhea.

Specimen	Culture	NAAT
Endocervical swab	+	+
Urine	–	+
Vaginal swab	+	+
Rectal swab	+	+
Oropharyngeal swab	+	+
Conjunctival swab	+	+

Note:
- Though NAATs are more sensitive than culture for testing rectal, pharyngeal, and conjunctival swabs, NAATs are not FDA approved for these samples.
- Culture is not recommended for testing urine sample because of low sensitivity.
- Gram-negative intracellular diplococci on Gram stain in urethral specimen from male are useful for diagnosing gonococcal infection. However, urethral swabs from women are not recommended for testing because of low sensitivity.

(NAAT: nucleic acid amplification test)

sex partner who has an STI or is exchanging sex for drugs or money), screening should be repeated in third trimester to prevent postnatal complications in mother and gonococcal infection in the neonate. Culture and nucleic acid amplification test (NAAT) are available for the detection of genitourinary infection with *N. gonorrhoeae.* Culture requires endocervical swab specimen and NAAT allows for endocervical swabs, vaginal swabs, and urine sample. Culture is also available for rectal, oropharyngeal, and conjunctival gonococcal infection and is the only diagnostic method that allows testing **(Table 1)**. But NAAT is not FDA approved for use with these specimens.

Tests for other STI/RTI should also be advised—rapid plasma reagin (RPR) and HIV testing.

Identification of intracellular gram-negative diplococci within the polymorphonuclear leukocytes (PMNs) on Gram stain of conjunctival discharge is strongly suggestive of gonococcal ophthalmia. Detection of DGI in neonates requires cultures of blood, joint aspirate, and cerebrospinal fluid (CSF).

TREATMENT

Dual antibiotic therapy is recommended for treating gonococcal infection as combination therapy helps to improve the efficacy of treatment and slower the emergence and spread of antibiotic resistance against cephalosporins. In addition, persons infected with *N. gonorrhoeae* are frequently coinfected with *Chlamydia trachomatis*, further supporting the use of dual therapy to target both the infections.

According to CDC 2020, pregnant women infected with *N. gonorrhoeae* should be treated with:

- Ceftriaxone 500 mg in a single intramuscular injection and azithromycin 1 g orally as a single dose.

- Tablet cefixime 800 mg single oral dose should only be considered an alternative cephalosporin regimen because it does not provide as high and sustained bactericidal blood levels as 500 mg dose of ceftriaxone.
- In case of cephalosporin allergy, spectinomycin 2 g IM single dose is considered safe in pregnancy.

Female should be called for follow-up of patient after 7 days. To avoid reinfection, patient should be advised abstinence from unprotected intercourse till 7 days after treatment and resolution of symptoms and until partner is not adequately treated.

Education and counseling of patient regarding prevention of infection during the course of pregnancy and the adverse pregnancy outcomes is important.

All sex partners in last 60 days or most recent sex partner (i.e., if patient's last potential sexual exposure was >60 days before onset of symptoms) should also be referred for testing, evaluation, and presumptive dual treatment with oral tablet cefixime 800 mg single dose and tablet azithromycin 1 g single dose.

Recommended treatment regimen for DGI:

- Ceftriaxone 1 g intramuscular or intravenous every 24 hours for 2–3 days followed by oral tablet cefixime 800 mg once a day for a total course of 7 days and tablet azithromycin 1 g oral single dose on day 1.

  However, gonococcal meningitis and endocarditis require parenteral therapy for 10–14 days and at least 4 weeks, respectively.

Treatment of gonococcal infection among neonates:

- *Ophthalmia neonatorum*: Injection ceftriaxone 25–50 mg/kg (not >125 mg) intravenous or intramuscular single dose.

Presumptive treatment is indicated for:

- High-risk neonates who have increased WBCs but not gram-negative intracellular diplococci in conjunctival exudate.
- Neonates born to mother who have gonococcal infection

  Topical treatment is unnecessary and inadequate if systemic treatment is administered.

  Mother of infected child should be tested and presumptively treated for gonorrhea.
- Disseminated gonococcal infection and scalp abscess in neonate

  Injection ceftriaxone 25–50 mg/kg/day intravenous or intramuscular single dose daily for 7 days.

  In case of gonococcal meningitis, therapy should be continued for a longer duration of 10–14 days.

MANAGEMENT OF SEXUAL PARTNERS

To prevent reinfection, all sexual partners of infected pregnant women should be tested and treated for gonorrhea. Sexual activity should be avoided until treatment has been completed by both the patient and their partner(s).

CONCLUSION

Gonococcal infection in pregnancy is a serious health issue that can result in adverse outcomes for both mother and baby if left untreated. WHO has set a global goal for 2030 to 90% reduction in gonorrhea incidence compared to 2018 levels. Early screening, timely treatment, and effective partner management are essential to preventing complications such as preterm labor, neonatal infections, and long-term reproductive issues. Proper prenatal care and public health interventions are crucial for reducing the burden of gonorrhea in pregnant women and improving maternal and neonatal outcomes.

KEY POINTS

- Mother to child transmission rate of untreated gonorrhea infection during passage from birth canal is approximately 30%.
- There is increased risk of PID and salpingitis in first trimester. PID and salpingitis can result in scarring of the fallopian tubes leading to infertility and ectopic pregnancy.
- After first trimester, risk of chorioamnionitis, premature rupture of membranes, low-birth weight, preterm birth, and septic abortion increases. Also, mother becomes more susceptible to postpartum endometritis and puerperal sepsis.
- Neonates may develop ophthalmia neonatorum, localized scalp abscess, or sepsis due to perinatal exposure to mother's infected birth canal.
- Thus, screening and treatment of women during pregnancy is important to prevent gonococcal infection among neonates.

SUGGESTED READINGS

1. Workowski KA, Bolan GA. (2015). Syphilis during pregnancy. CDC: Sexually Transmitted Diseases Treatment Guidelines, 2015. [online] Available from https://www.cdc.gov/mmwr/preview/mmwrhtml/rr6403a1.htm. [Last accessed January, 2025]
2. Cavenee MR, Farris JR, Spalding TR, Barnes DL, Castaneda YS, Wendel GD Jr. Treatment of gonorrhea in pregnancy. Obstet Gynecol. 1993;81(1):33-8.
3. Nguyen D. Gonorrhea in pregnancy and in the newborn. Am Fam Physician. 1984;29(1):185-9.
4. Olaleye AO, Babah OA, Osuagwu CS, Ogunsola FT, Afolabi BB. Sexually transmitted infections in pregnancy – An update on *Chlamydia trachomatis* and *Neisseria gonorrhoeae*. Eur J Obstet Gynecol Reprod Biol. 2020;255:1-12.

10.6 Miscellaneous Sexually Transmitted Diseases

Rohit Batra, Aishwarya Dua

INTRODUCTION

Sexually transmitted infection (STI)/reproductive tract infection (RTI) is an important cause of maternal and perinatal morbidity and mortality. It can lead to severe life-threatening complications such as pelvic inflammatory disease (PID), ectopic pregnancy, and poor pregnancy outcomes such as spontaneous abortion, stillbirth, low-birth weight, preterm birth, and congenital infections.

PELVIC INFLAMMATORY DISEASE

Pelvic inflammatory disease refers to the inflammation of the upper reproductive tract, which includes the uterus, fallopian tubes, and ovaries. This condition encompasses various issues such as endometritis, salpingitis, tubo-ovarian abscess, and pelvic peritonitis. It is typically an ascending infection, spreading from the lower genital tract. The majority of cases of PID are related to an STI.

Pelvic inflammatory disease is a significant concern, especially among young, fertile women, although it is relatively uncommon during pregnancy.

Pathogenesis

It is believed that a healthy conceptus acts as a protective barrier against the development of PID by preventing the upward movement of bacteria from the cervix into the endometrial cavity and the fallopian tubes. Nevertheless, the uterine cavity does not completely seal off until approximately 12 weeks of gestation.

Pelvic inflammatory disease often arises from an infection that ascends from the lower genital tract, frequently linked to STIs like *Neisseria gonorrhoeae* and *Chlamydia trachomatis*. Other microorganisms, including *Mycoplasma genitalium, Mycoplasma hominis, Ureaplasma urealyticum,* those associated with bacterial vaginosis (*Peptostreptococcus* species, *Bacteroides* species), and certain respiratory (*Haemophilus influenzae, Streptococcus pneumoniae,* and *Staphylococcus aureus*) and enteric pathogens (*Escherichia coli, Bacteroides fragilis,* and group B *Streptococci*), may also play a role.

Several alternate mechanisms of infection have been proposed for the initiation of PID in pregnancy.

- *Infection at time of fertilization*: With the infecting organism might travel with and be introduced by the sperm. It is possible that the infection develops since the initial sexual encounter.
- *Infection after fertilization before decidua fusion*: Cervical infection could ascend to the fallopian tubes before the occlusion of the uterine cavity by fusion of the decidua and chorion.
- Spread through lymphatic or vascular routes from the cervix or vagina
- Reactivation of preexisting PID, i.e., acute exacerbation of chronic PID
- *Instrumentation*: Infections secondary to medical procedures or illegal abortion attempts
- Contiguous spread from adjacent organs (i.e., appendix)

Clinical Features

Symptoms of PID in the pregnant patient include:

- Pain in lower abdomen
- Loss of appetite, nausea, and vomiting

- Low-grade fever
- Copious and purulent vaginal discharge
- Dyspareunia
- Physical examination varies from mild abdominopelvic tenderness to frank peritonitis. Purulent cervicitis may be present especially in gonococcal disease presenting as cervical motion tenderness.
- Peripheral blood count shows leukocytosis with left shift.

It is essential to consider other potential causes of abdominal pain, such as appendicitis and ectopic pregnancy. Because of multiple potential causes of pelvic pain during pregnancy, PID is often overlooked in favor of more common causes.

Differential diagnosis of acute abdominal pain in pregnancy:
- Appendicitis
- Torsion of ovarian cyst/adnexal tumor
- Threatened/incomplete abortion
- Ectopic pregnancy
- Placental abruption
- Bowel obstruction/infarction
- Pancreatitis
- Renal stone
- Degeneration of leiomyoma

If left untreated, PID can lead to severe complications, including a high incidence of fetal loss (around 50%) and the risk of septic abortion and long-term sequelae like permanent tubal scarring, infertility, ectopic pregnancy, etc.

The spontaneous septic abortion rate is significant. Prompt diagnosis and management may reduce the rate of fetal loss and prevent inflammatory sequelae.

Since PID has no characteristic clinical or laboratory findings, and is rare during pregnancy, it is understandable why the diagnosis is missed in most cases, and the patient is treated as an abdominal emergency.

Diagnosis

Diagnosing PID can be difficult due to its vague symptoms and its uncommon occurrence during pregnancy.

Ultrasound pelvis should be done to rule out other causes of lower abdominal pain and to check for fetal well-being. Swabs from cervical discharge should be collected and sent for nucleic acid amplification test (NAAT) for detecting gonorrhea and chlamydia infection. Gram stain from vaginal secretion shows abundant numbers of PMNLs. Erythrocyte sedimentation rate and C-reactive protein (CRP) might be elevated.

All pregnant females diagnosed with PID should be tested for HIV.

Treatment

Pelvic inflammatory disease is treated with antibiotics to cover the primary pathogens, including *Neisseria gonorrhoeae* and *Chlamydia trachomatis*. Approximately, 10–15% of women with endocervical *N. gonorrhoeae* or *C. trachomatis* will go on to develop PID. Any pregnant female with PID should be hospitalized and treated with parenteral antibiotic treatment.

VAGINAL DISCHARGE

Normal thin, clear, or milky white vaginal discharge with mild odor, also known as leukorrhea, is one of the earliest signs of pregnancy. It progressively increases in amount throughout the pregnancy whereas abnormal or pathological vaginal discharge (PVD) is foul smelling and varies in color from dirty white to yellowish green. PVD commonly occurs due to vaginal infections such as bacterial vaginosis, trichomonas vaginalis, and vulvovaginal candidiasis.

Bacterial Vaginosis

It is a common vaginal infection resulting from imbalance and replacement of lactobacillus (accounts for 90% of normal vaginal flora) in vagina with increased number of anaerobic bacteria, i.e., *Gardnerella vaginalis, Mycoplasma hominis, Ureaplasma, Mobiluncus, Prevotella, Fusobacterium,* etc.

It presents as homogenous, copious, grayish white vaginal discharge with unpleasant fishy odor. Vaginal pH is >4.5 and Gram's stain from vaginal discharge shows clue cells (epithelial cell coated with bacteria obscuring the cell border), reduced lactobacilli, and polymorphonuclear cells.

It can lead to adverse pregnancy outcomes such as premature rupture of membranes, chorioamnionitis, premature delivery, low-birth weight, and puerperal sepsis.

Vaginal Candidiasis

Vaginal candidiasis is caused by the overgrowth of candida species. *Candida* species are part of normal vaginal flora present in the lower genital tract in healthy and asymptomatic women. *Candida albicans* is the most common type of vaginal *Candida* species followed by *Candida glabrata*. It presents as curdy white vaginal discharge associated with inflamed vaginal mucosa with edema and fissuring, vulval pruritus, and external dysuria.

Pregnant women are more likely to have symptomatic vaginal candidiasis attributing to increased estrogen levels, increased vaginal glycogen production, and immunologic alteration. It has been described in chapter on vulvovaginal candidiasis.

Trichomoniasis

It is caused by pear-shaped protozoa *Trichomonas vaginalis*. Infection is usually asymptomatic in 70–80% individuals. In females, it presents with copious, frothy, malodorous, yellow green colored discharge per vaginum associated with pruritus, dyspareunia, and dysuria. It causes cervicitis with punctate hemorrhage on cervical mucosa giving strawberry cervix appearance. Wet mount preparation from vaginal discharge shows pear-shaped protozoa with twitching/jerky motility.

Untreated or delayed treatment of trichomonas infection can lead to premature rupture of membranes, low-birth weight, and preterm labor. Infection might ascend and lead to PID.

Treatment

Per speculum examination should be done to rule out cervicitis and pregnancy complications like abortion and premature rupture of membranes. Wet mount microscopy, 10% KOH preparation, and Gram stain of the vaginal smear should be prepared. Oral fluconazole is contraindicated in pregnancy. Treat with clotrimazole vaginal pessary/cream for vaginal candidiasis. Tablet metronidazole 400 mg twice a day for 7 days is given for bacterial vaginosis and trichomonas vaginalis.

CHLAMYDIA

Chlamydia trachomatis is a gram-negative obligate intracellular bacterium which preferentially infects squamocolumnar epithelial cells. Majority of infected women are asymptomatic and thus serve as reservoir of infection.

It causes cervicitis presenting as mucoid or mucopurulent discharge per vaginum, dyspareunia, postcoital bleeding, cervical mucosal congestion, and cervical motion tenderness.

Chlamydia infection is not uncommon during pregnancy and thus increases risk of chorioamnionitis and postpartum sepsis.

If untreated during pregnancy, chlamydia infection can lead to conjunctivitis in the newborn due to infected birth canal.

Treatment: Tablet azithromycin 1 g oral single dose or tablet erythromycin base 500 mg orally four times a day for 7 days

CHANCROID

It is caused by *Haemophilus ducreyi* infection. It is a gram-negative, nonspore forming, and facultative anaerobic bacterium. It has a short incubation period of 3–7 days and leads to formation of solitary or multiple tender, nonindurated ulcers with undermined edges and yellow dirty gray slough over the base. It is associated with unilateral inguinal bubo in 30–60% cases bubo may rupture to form sinus.

No negative outcomes of chancroid on pregnancy have been reported. However, due to increased vascularity during pregnancy, ulcers may increase in size.

Treatment: Tablet azithromycin 1 g oral single dose or tablet erythromycin base 500 mg orally four times a day for 7 days

Summary of various fetomaternal effects in different STIs is given in **Table 1**.

TABLE 1: Overview of STIs in pregnancy.

STI/RTI	Interaction between STI/RTI and pregnancy
Gonorrhea	• Prematurity • Premature rupture of membranes • Disseminated gonococcal infection is more commonly reported in infected pregnant females
Chlamydia	• Chorioamnionitis • Postpartum sepsis • Conjunctivitis in newborn
Syphilis	• Abortion • Prematurity • Intrauterine growth retardation • Stillbirth • Congenital syphilis
Chancroid	Ulcers may be more enlarged and vascular
HSV infection	• Longer duration of symptoms and viral shedding. Primary infection may be more severe and dissemination of lesions • Abortion • Intrauterine growth retardation • Premature delivery • Congenital HSV • Neonatal herpes
HPV infection	• Size and number of warts may increase • Rarely associated with laryngeal papillomatosis
Bacterial vaginosis	• Chorioamnionitis • Premature rupture of membranes • Low-birth weight • Premature delivery • Puerperal sepsis
Candidiasis	• Increased frequency of infection • More severe symptoms
Trichomoniasis	• Premature rupture of membranes • Preterm labor • Low-birth weight

(HPV: human papillomavirus; HSV: herpes simplex virus; RTI: reproductive tract infection; STI: sexually transmitted infection)

SUGGESTED READINGS

1. Acquavella AP, Rubin A, D'Angelo LJ. The coincident diagnosis of pelvic inflammatory disease and pregnancy: are they compatible? J Pediatr Adolesc Gynecol. 1996;9(3):129-32.
2. Blanchard AC, Pastorek JG 2nd, Weeks T. Pelvic inflammatory disease during pregnancy. South Med J. 1987;80(11):1363-5.
3. National AIDS Control Organisation. (2007). RTIs/STIs among special populations. National Guidelines on Prevention, Management and Control of Reproductive Tract Infections including Sexually Transmitted Infections. [online] Available form https://naco.gov.in/sites/default/files/14%2C%20National_Guidelines_on_PMC_of_RTI_Including_STI.pdf. [Last accessed January, 2025].

CHAPTER 11

Infections and Pregnancy

11.1 Leprosy and Pregnancy

Sandhya Chauhan, Mudita Gupta

INTRODUCTION

- Leprosy has minimal effects on pregnancy.
- Pregnancy worsens leprosy/lepra reactions due to alteration of cell-mediated immunity.
- Psychological issues may be associated with both pregnancy and leprosy.
- Standard multidrug therapy (MDT) is safe in pregnancy and lactation.
- Dapsone-associated hemolysis may aggravate physiological anemia of pregnancy.
- Lepromatous leprosy in pregnancy can affect fetus, neonates, and infants.

Globally, leprosy affects 10–12 million people with one-third of them being women. Many of these females are in the reproductive age group and some of them become pregnant or lactating mothers or have close contact with infants and growing children. While the direct effects of leprosy on pregnancy are minimal, pregnancy can significantly alter the course of leprosy and trigger lepra reactions (LRs). Pregnancy is a state of relative immunosuppression, with a shift from Th1 to Th2 immunity, which can worsen leprosy, particularly in the third trimester. The regain of cell-mediated immunity (CMI) after childbirth can exacerbate reversal reactions (RRs). Type 2 lepra reactions (T2LRs) can manifest throughout pregnancy and the postpartum period due to intercurrent infections, stress, and an increased bacillary load in the third trimester.

Both pregnancy and leprosy are associated with psychological issues, such as anxiety, depression, and other mood disorders, with depressive disorders being the most common in both conditions. Leprosy patients also face unique psychosocial challenges, including divorce, economic difficulties, and displacement from their families. The stigma and deformities associated with leprosy further increase the prevalence of psychiatric comorbidities, ranging from 6 to 70% in various studies.

Antileprosy treatment is considered safe during pregnancy, although minor side effects such as dapsone-induced hemolytic anemia can worsen the physiological anemia commonly seen in pregnancy. Maternal anemia can impair placental and fetal development due to inadequate blood supply. Additionally, maternal leprosy increases the risk of transmitting the disease to newborns, given their immature immune systems and close familial contact. Pregnant women with leprosy should be closely monitored for worsening symptoms, LRs, anemia, and uterine growth to assess fetal development.

HISTORY

Psychiatric morbidity was found to be positively correlated with physical disability and marital status. The antileprosy treatment is safe in pregnancy but minor adverse events like dapsone-induced hemolytic anemia may aggravate the physiological anemia of pregnancy. Maternal anemia may impair placental and fetal development because of poor blood supply. Maternal leprosy also increases the incidence of leprosy transmission to neonates due to immature immunity and close intrafamilial contact. Pregnant women with leprosy should be closely monitored for progression of disease leprosy, LRs, anemia, and uterine growth.

In the past, individuals with leprosy were ostracized from society. They were prohibited from getting married, divorces were allowed legally, and remarriages of healthy partners were practiced. Mothers with leprosy were separated from their husbands, society, and their children. The most dreadful history of burying a leprous mother with her baby exists in the literature. However, the discovery of dapsone and the implementation of multidrug therapy (MDT) have significantly improved the situation. Today, leprosy is no longer considered a major public health problem.

EPIDEMIOLOGY

Leprosy was declared eliminated in 2005, but cases are still prevalent in certain endemic regions. The global data of 2022 revealed 174,087 new leprosy cases of which 67,657 (39%) were females. India contributed to the global burden by 53.6% by reporting 75,394 new leprosy cases in 2022. The relatively lower incidence is seen in females and is attributed to underreporting or underdiagnosis of leprosy. Limited mobility, illiteracy, financial dependence, stigma, and discrimination toward leprosy are sociocultural factors responsible for underreporting in females.

EFFECTS OF LEPROSY ON MENSTRUAL CYCLE AND FERTILITY

- Menstrual irregularities have been reported in females with leprosy.
- Leprosy causes infertility and sterility in males.
- Failure to conception in females may be related to male hypogonadism.
- Ovarian failure in multibacillary (MB) leprosy needs to be explored.
- Autoantibodies against ovarian tissue are a postulated theory for infertility.

Recent studies are very limited but literature from pre-MDT era has reported significant menstrual irregularities and primary infertility in 10–54% of female patients. Recently in 2014, Khanna et al. found substantial ovarian dysfunction in multibacillary (MB) leprosy cases evidenced by significantly elevated hormones [follicle-stimulating hormone (FSH), luteinizing hormone (LH), and prolactin] and menstrual irregularities in MB leprosy patients. Infertility in leprosy-affected couples is more related to male hypogonadism because testicular atrophy is seen in 10–50% (90% lepromatous cases) of leprosy patients.

The induction of autoimmune phenomena in leprosy may be associated with ovarian dysfunction resulting in irregular cycles and infertility. The sera of MB leprosy patients may show positivity for various autoantibodies like antinuclear antibody (ANA), antineutrophil cytoplasmic antibody (ANCA), antiphospholipid, antithyroid, RA factors, etc. Consequently, it is postulated that autoantibodies targeting ovarian tissue may result in ovarian failure and infertility in females with leprosy.

EFFECTS OF LEPROSY ON PREGNANCY, CHILDBIRTH, AND LACTATION

- Pregnancy-related complications are not affected by leprosy.
- A biological false-positive venereal disease research laboratory (VDRL) test for syphilis may be seen.
- Dapsone-induced hemolysis may aggravate physiological anemia of pregnancy.
- Intrapartum transmission of leprosy is nil so both normal vaginal delivery and cesarean sections are safe.
- *Mycobacterium leprae* as well as antileprosy drugs is secreted in breast milk.
- Exclusive breastfeeding is recommended.

Sixty years ago, Ryrie observed that pregnancy has profound effects on leprosy while vice versa is not true. Pregnancy-related complications like antepartum hemorrhage, postpartum hemorrhage, pregnancy-associated diabetes, and hypertension remain unaffected in leprosy patients. The occurrence of a biological false-positive venereal disease research laboratory (VDRL) test for syphilis has been reported in pregnant patients with coexisting leprosy. Some patients are mistakenly treated for syphilis due to skin lesions and a positive VDRL test until leprosy is diagnosed. In patients with lepromatous leprosy, anemia of chronic disease and dapsone-induced hemolysis may aggravate physiological anemia of pregnancy. Maternal anemia may impair placental and fetal development because of poor blood supply.

Leprosy does not have any relation with intrapartum/labor-related complications like delayed or precipitated labor or postpartum bleeds. Birth asphyxia and low APGAR scores have been reported in neonates of lepromatous mothers. Intrapartum transmission of leprosy to neonates is negligible so a normal vaginal delivery as well as cesarean section (if obstetric indication is there) is safe.

In a pre-MDT era when dapsone resistance was prevalent, leprosy has been reported in infants on breastfeeding. Acid-fast bacilli-like particles were also demonstrated in the breast milk of lepromatous mothers not on MDT. There is still uncertainty about the viability of orally ingested *M. leprae* to cause leprosy. If a lactating mother is on MDT or has completed MDT, the chances of mother-to-child transmission of leprosy (airborne or close contact or through gastrointestinal route) through breast milk are negligible. Experts recommend that mothers should be encouraged to take MDT and continue breastfeeding. Antileprosy drugs are secreted in breast milk and protect infants from leprosy. Breastfeeding is always safer than alternative feeding in leprosy-endemic regions, due to the risk of malnutrition, and ill hygienic water and food resources.

EFFECTS OF LEPROSY ON PLACENTA, FETUS, NEONATES, AND INFANTS

Placental Changes

In the post-MDT era, studies on placental morphology and bacteriology in leprosy patients are lacking. Pre-MDT literature has documented inflammation, granuloma formation, and vascular involvement lepromatous lesions and *M. leprae* has been detected in 38% placenta of lepromatous mothers. Some studies have reported that small placental size and intrauterine growth retardation are seen in lepromatous cases. *M. leprae* detection in placental tissue suggests the possibility of vertical leprosy transmission from the placenta to the fetus.

- Lepromatous placentitis is seen in animals and few studies on humans.
- Small placental size is seen in lepromatous leprosy patients.
- Prematurity, fetal loss, intrauterine growth retardation, and low-birth weight are reported fetoneonatal complications of lepromatous leprosy.
- Congenital leprosy is unreported but vertical transmission may be possible from lepromatous mothers.
- Newborns of mothers on MDT can present with exfoliative dermatitis secondary to dapsone and brownish skin discoloration due to clofazimine.
- Infants of lepromatous mothers may have a higher incidence of respiratory problems, severe childhood infections, and a higher infant mortality rate.

Fetal Adverse Effects

As early as 1897, neonates born to lepromatous mothers were observed to experience abortions, fetal distress, prematurity, stillbirths, and a high susceptibility to intercurrent and respiratory infections. It was noted that 59% of lepromatous women had subnormal estriol levels, which contributed to impaired placental-fetal function, resulting in smaller placental size, prematurity, and low-birth weight-related consequences. Significantly higher neonatal and infant mortalities were reported due to fetal distress and respiratory problems in babies born to borderline lepromatous (BL) and lepromatous (LL) mothers.

Leprosy Transmission to Neonates and Infants

The lepromatous patients discharge plenty of bacilli (through the mouth, nasal blows, or ulcerated skin) which can survive in the environment for 9 days or longer as per housing conditions. It is believed that nasal droplets and direct contact with skin are the main routes for leprosy transmission in neonates/ infants. In a review of 91 infants, the mother was the most common source of infection followed by the father, relatives, or other unknown sources.

The development of leprosy at the age of 3 weeks suggests intrauterine or transplacental transmission of leprosy. Breastfeeding or the gastrointestinal route has never been established in leprosy transmission despite the demonstration of *M. leprae* in breast milk of lepromatous mothers. Congenital leprosy has not been reported but cases have been described in neonatal (the youngest case 3-week-old neonate) and infantile period. Earliest in 2014, Nakajo reported leprosy in a 2.5-month-old girl and since then many cases have been reported. A literature review from the United States has described infantile leprosy in 91 cases.

A significant bacillemia, intact acid-fast bacilli in the placenta plus cord blood, and rising titers of specific IgA and IgM antibodies have been documented in infants born to lepromatous mothers. This indicates that these babies have been stimulated by *M. leprae* or its antigen during intrauterine life and suggests a possibility of vertical transmission of leprosy.

Psychological Issues

The hormonal changes (estrogens and progesterone) in pregnancy can exacerbate various psychological issues like depression, anxiety, and other mood disorders. Low confidence, loss of interest, altered temperament, altered hunger, feelings of weakness, etc. are common problems seen in normal pregnancy. Pregnancy-related psychological issues may be aggravated by coexisting leprosy. Depression is the most common mental health problem seen in both leprosy (8–71%) and pregnancy (15–65%) ranging in severity from dysthymia to suicidal ideation. Leprosy-induced stigma and deformities increase the prevalence of psychiatric comorbidities to significantly higher levels (6–70% in different studies). Additionally, leprosy patients face psychosocial issues like divorce, conflicts in marital relationships, economic problems, displacement from families, etc.

Leprosy-associated psychosocial problems are neglected but persist during and even after the completion of treatment. Concomitant leprosy in pregnancy may impair the psychological health of mothers but clinical studies are needed to establish the exact relationship.

EFFECTS OF PREGNANCY ON LEPROSY AND LEPRA REACTIONS (TABLE 1)

In pregnancy, susceptibility to infections is increased due to suppressed CMI and predominance of humoral immunity. Pregnancy-associated hormones (progesterone, cortisol, and norepinephrine) transform maternal CMI immunity from the Th1 toward the Th2 arm to accept the foreign fetus. Th2 cytokines like IL-10 are immunosuppressive and anti-inflammatory (fetus supportive) so they are elevated in pregnancy. Th1 cytokines including IL-12 and IFN-γ (fetal destructive) are suppressed in pregnancy and raised in the postpartum period. Infective conditions like leprosy or tuberculosis get aggravated during pregnancy while autoimmune and inflammatory diseases (e.g., LRs) get remitted. The scenario gets reversed after a postpartum period during lactation.

The paucibacillary tuberculoid form of leprosy develops when CMI is high in the presence of high levels of IFN-γ and low IL-10 (postpartum period). MB (lepromatous cases) leprosy occurs during pregnancy when CMI is depressed and the bacterial load is high. In the postpartum period, Th2 shifts back to Th1 immune response and triggers RRs by the release of proinflammatory cytokines like IL-12 and IFN-γ (Th1 mediators).

EFFECTS OF PREGNANCY ON LEPROSY

New Cases, Exacerbation, Relapse, and Reactivation of Leprosy

In pregnancy and puerperium, the altered secretions of steroids, and altered immunological and metabolic profile affect the course of leprosy. It has been recorded that new onset, exacerbation, reactivation or relapse of leprosy

TABLE 1: Effects of pregnancy on leprosy and lepra reactions.

Leprosy	T1LR	T2LR
There is a worsening of leprosy in pregnancy and early puerperium due to a decrease in CMI • Incubating leprosy shows overt signs • Established leprosy and nerve deficits downgrade • Cured leprosy may relapse	• Upgrading reactions develop during puerperium due to rapid regain of deficient CMI • Downgrading reactions occur in pregnancy particularly in 3rd trimester due to decreased CMI	• Particularly seen in 3rd trimester and puerperium due to infections and physical stress respectively • T2LR can occur throughout the pregnancy because of mental stress and intercurrent infections

(CMI: cell-mediated immunity; T1LR: type 1 lepra reaction; T2LR: type 2 lepra reaction)

occurs in 46% of cases either during pregnancy or within the first 12 months of lactation.

New Cases

Pregnancy is a state of immune suppression, mineral depletion, and metabolic derangements. Depressed CMI in pregnancy results in the multiplication of dormant bacilli and manifests incubating leprosy **(Fig. 1)**. In about 20–30% (10–35% in some studies) of females, the signs of leprosy appear for the first time during pregnancy and in >50% during puerperium.

Disease Activity in Pregnancy

In untreated cases, pregnancy-induced immunosuppression downgrades preexisting leprosy toward the lepromatous pole. Recent studies are lacking but literature from the dapsone era has described worsening of leprosy in 48–78% of pregnancies. The worsening has been noted from the second half of pregnancy till the first 3 months of puerperium. The highest number of cases (56% and 27.2%) have been observed in the third trimester of pregnancy which corresponds to peak hormonal levels and lowest CMI. Deterioration of leprosy in pregnancy is a compounded effect of suppressed CMI and avoidance of antileprosy drugs (fear of harmful effects of MDT on the growing fetus). The appearance of lesions of the lower pole, new or aggravated nerve function impairment, and worsening of BI and MI are the features described in downgrading leprosy in pregnancy.

Relapse and Reactivation

The relapses and reactivation of leprosy in pregnancy have been reported in the third trimester of pregnancy during the pre-MDT era. The multiplication of persisters' bacilli due to suppressed CMI contributes to relapses and reactivation of leprosy in pregnancy. The exacerbation/reactivation of leprosy has been reported in 38% of TT and BT, 44% of BL, and 63% of LL cases. A relapse rate of 36% has been described in pregnant women during dapsone monotherapy.

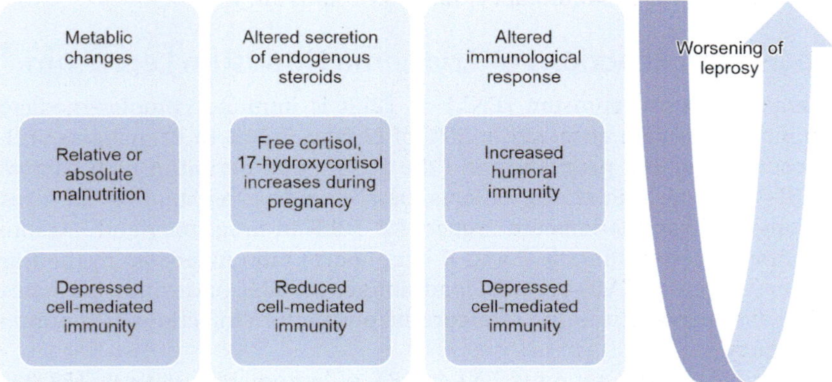

FIG. 1: Pregnancy worsens or downgrades leprosy.

The dapsone resistance was presumed as the primary cause of relapse during pregnancy. Studies on relapse and reactivation in the MDT era are lacking although a case of lepromatous relapse in a pregnant patient who had taken 20 months of daily rifampicin and dapsone is well reported.

PREGNANCY AND LEPRA REACTIONS

- Downgrading reactions are supposed to occur in pregnancy (low CMI) and reversal reactions develop in postpartum period due to rapid regain of CMI.
- T2LR depends on antigenic load, stress, and infections so they can occur throughout pregnancy and the postpartum period.
- In pregnancy, there is worsening of leprous neuritis.

Lepra reactions are immunologically mediated episodes of inflammation seen in 20–50% of leprosy patients. They are divided into type 1 and type 2 LR and both types are altered in pregnancy because of immunological changes and disease progression. Type 1 lepra reactions (T1LRs) are divided into upgrading/reversal and downgrading types as per alteration in CMI. Downgrading reactions are supposed to occur in pregnancy (low CMI) and reversal or upgrading reactions develop in postpartum due to rapid regain of CMI. T2LRs are immune complex-mediated and depend on antigen-antibody excess as observed in MB patients and has been reported throughout the pregnancy and puerperium.

Type 1 Lepra Reaction or Reversal Reaction

Type 1 lepra reaction may be less frequent in pregnancy due to suppressed CMI and reported more after delivery or in lactation due to regain of CMI. The Ethiopian study of 114 pregnant women reported 44% RR during pregnancy and 60% during lactation. The new and recurrent episodes involving nerves are reported late in lactation due to the recognition of bacillary antigens which were unrecognized in pregnancy due to deficient CMI. Cutaneous involvement is a more common presentation than neuritis in T1LR during pregnancy. The deficient CMI in pregnancy results in *M. leprae* antigen expression only in the skin not in nerves so predominant cutaneous lesions are seen.

Type 2 Lepra Reactions or Erythema Nodosum Leprosum

Erythema nodosum leprosum (ENL) or T2LR is immune complex-mediated inflammatory episode observed in 50% of LL and 5–10% of BL patients. T2LR can occur throughout pregnancy and the postpartum period. A high bacterial load (BI 4 or more), untreated patients, persisting drug-resistant bacilli, stress, infections, and vaccinations are triggers for T2LR in pregnancy and lactation. In the first trimester, there is T and B lymphocyte ratio inversion, in the third trimester (decreased CMI) bacterial load/antigens is high, parturition is a state of physical and mental stress and intercurrent/postpartum infections are common in pregnancy.

An Ethiopian study reported ENL in 38% of lepromatous patients (BL 22%; LL 59%) with a peak incidence in the third trimester. From the third trimester to the 15-month postpartum period, ENL was noted in 15% of females. A high BI of 4+ or higher was associated with ENL in pregnancy in 65% of females. Unusual cases like bullous ENL, Lucio phenomenon, and coexistence of type 1 and T2LR have also been seen in pregnancy.

LEPROUS NEURITIS IN PREGNANCY

Leprous neuritis is inflammation of nerves which may present acutely or silently at any stage of leprosy. At least 50% of females are at risk of developing neuritis or nerve function impairment during pregnancy. The disease and reaction-mediated nerve damage progress in pregnancy because immunosuppression increases lepromatous granulomas as well as *M. leprae* antigenic load in the affected nerves. Neuritis is the main complication of T1LR but may be seen with T2LR or as a sole manifestation of LRs. T1LR-related neuritis is mostly seen during the treatment (BL patients) while recurrent episodes of T2LR can involve nerves throughout the pregnancy and lactation. Neuritis of T2LR is more common in the first and third trimesters and severity is higher in untreated, drug-resistant, and BL/LL patients due to high antigenic load in these patients.

TREATMENT OF LEPROSY IN PREGNANCY AND LACTATION (TABLE 2)

- MDT is safe in pregnancy and lactation.
- Minor side effects may occur due to MDT but they are reversible and manageable.
- In cases with rifampicin resistance, clarithromycin, minocycline, and ofloxacin are not safe in pregnancy.
- Lepra reactions are best managed by corticosteroids.
- Immunosuppressants and thalidomide are contraindicated in pregnancy.

TABLE 2: Treatment of leprosy in pregnancy and lactation.

Drug safety profile	Risks during pregnancy and lactation	Management and advice
Rifampicin—Safe	Minor risk of neonatal bleeding when given in 3rd trimester	Intramuscular administration of 1 mg of vitamin K
Dapsone—Safe	• Small decrease in folate absorption • Minor risk of neonatal hemolysis and methemoglobinemia when given in 3rd trimester	• Advise 5 mg of folic acid daily with dapsone throughout pregnancy • Testing for G6PD deficiency to avoid severe hemolysis
Clofazimine—Safe	Darkening of baby's skin color at birth	It disappears within 6 months or a year after stopping the clofazimine or discontinuing breastfeeding

Continued

Continued

Drug safety profile	Risks during pregnancy and lactation	Management and advice
Quinolones/ ofloxacin—Unsafe	Arthropathy and osteochondrosis in animal studies	Avoid during pregnancy and lactation
Minocycline—Unsafe	• Teratogenic in pregnancy • Secreted in breast milk and causes infant teeth discoloration and damage	Avoid during pregnancy and lactation
Prednisolone—Usually safe	• A small increase in the incidence of cleft palate in the first trimester and a theoretical risk of hormonal disturbance in the fetus • It is secreted in breast milk but safe in lactation • The risk–benefit ratio favors use in moderate-to-severe lepra reaction	• Avoid in 1st trimester • Monitor for adverse effects in mothers like hypertension and hyperglycemia • Defer breastfeeding until 4 hours after ingestion of the drug to reduce the infant's exposure to the peak concentration of the drug
Thalidomide—Unsafe	Contraindicated due to teratogenicity	Avoid in childbearing age group
Immunosuppressants, e.g., cyclosporine, methotrexate, and azathioprine	• Methotrexate contraindicated due to teratogenicity • Azathioprine may lead to hematological toxicity in fetus • Cyclosporine-growth retardation in fetus	Avoid during pregnancy and lactation
NSAIDs—Usually safe	Can lead to premature closure of ductus arteriosus, premature births and renal adverse effects	Avoid in 3rd trimester
Bacillus Calmette–Guerin vaccine (BCG)	No harmful effects have been observed on the fetus but it should not be given	Further studies are needed to prove its safety
Antibiotics for ulcer-related infections	Decide safe antibiotic as per known microbiology and resistance pattern	Antibiotics are given as per the benefit ratio
(G6PD: glucose-6-phosphate dehydrogenase; NSAID: nonsteroidal anti-inflammatory drug)		

The standard MDT consisting of dapsone, rifampicin, and clofazimine is highly effective and considered safe during pregnancy/lactation. Although antileprosy drugs can cross the placental barrier and secreted into breast milk, they are neither teratogenic nor toxic. Rifampicin may increase the risk of neonatal bleeding when given in the third trimester. Dapsone-induced methemoglobinemia and hemolysis have been reported in mother and their babies. Testing for glucose-6-phosphate dehydrogenase (G6PD) levels can avoid the risk of severe hemolysis and continued intake of iron folic acid (5 mg) prophylaxis is beneficial to combat anemia. Clofazimine-induced skin discoloration in fetus/infants is another issue but it is reversible.

Rifampicin Resistance

In rare cases with rifampicin resistance, second-line drugs may be needed to treat leprosy. The childbearing woman may be advised to use strict contraception because second-line drugs should be avoided in pregnancy. Minocycline is teratogenic, ofloxacin leads to arthropathy, and clarithromycin is associated with a fetal loss if used in the first trimester (not teratogenic).

Treatment of Lepra Reactions during Pregnancy and Lactation

Corticosteroids are safe to manage LRs/neuritis in pregnancy and lactation. In the antenatal period, females should be monitored for steroid-induced diabetes and hypertension. Although steroids are nonteratogenic, an increased incidence of fetal cleft palate in the first trimester and a theoretical risk of hormonal imbalances in a fetus are reported. Breastfeeding is safe but mothers should be advised to defer feeding by 4 hours to prevent infants' exposure to peak concentrations of prednisolone.

Thalidomide and immunosuppressants (azathioprine, methotrexate, or cyclosporine) are contraindicated in pregnancy. Antimalarials may be given as per the risk-benefit ratio but their safety is unestablished. A high dose of clofazimine is not teratogenic and is usually well tolerated during pregnancy.

COUNSELING

All pregnant mothers should be advised to have regular antenatal check-ups, take 5 mg of folic acid daily and complete antileprosy treatment without any fear of harmful effects on the fetus. Explain that clofazimine will darken the skin color of the baby, but it will fade away when breastfeeding ceases or earlier if the mother discontinues clofazimine. Exclusive breastfeeding is safe without any fear of leprosy transmission to infants but MDT must be continued by the mother.

SUGGESTED READINGS

1. Kumar KH, Kumar B. IAL Textbook of Leprosy, 2nd edition. New Delhi: Jaypee Brothers Medical Publisher; 2016.
2. Sardana K, Khurana A. Jopling's Handbook of Leprosy, 6th edition. New Delhi: CBS Publishers and Distributors; 2020.
3. Scollard D, Gillis T. International Textbook of Leprosy. Greenville: American Leprosy Missions; 2019.
4. King JA, Marks RA. Pregnancy and Leprosy-A Review of 52 Pregnancies in 26 Patients with Leprosy. Am J Obstet Gynecol. 1958;76(2):438-42.
5. Duncan ME. An Historical and Clinical Review of the Interaction of Leprosy and Pregnancy: A Cycle to be Broken. Sot Sci Med. 1993;37(4):457-72.
6. Lockwood DNJ, Sinha HH. Pregnancy and Leprosy: A Comprehensive Literature Review. Int J Leprosy. 1999;67(1):6-12.
7. Sarkar R, Pradhan S. Leprosy and women. Int J Women's Dermatol. 2016;2:117-21.
8. Ozturk Z, Tatliparmak A. Leprosy treatment during pregnancy and breastfeeding: A case report and brief review of literature. Dermatologic Therapy. 2017;30:e12414.

9. Prakoeswa FRS, Maharani F, Puspitasari E, Listiawan MY, Endaryanto A, Prakoeswa CRS. The differences in maternal and child health factors amongst leprosy patients in endemic and non-endemic areas. Bali Med J. 2021;10(3):1403-7.
10. Amorim GM, Maestri T, Oppitz A, Leye M, Merini FL, Vignatti LJ. Virchowian leprosy and erythema nodosum leprosum in a 34-week pregnant woman without any previous diagnosis. Rev Med (São Paulo). 2022;101(1):1-6.
11. Bharucha J, Saito-Tom L. Postpartum sepsis-like illness and rash associated with Hansen's disease. Case Rep Perinat Med. 2022;11(1):20210046.
12. Vijay N, Swati Sarma S. Leprosy with Erythema Nodosum Leprosum in Pregnancy: A Rare Phenomenon! J South Asian Feder Obstet Gynaecol. 2019;11(5):329-30.

11.2 Fungal Infections and Pregnancy

Ritu Rani, Mudita Gupta

INTRODUCTION

Pregnancy induces a myriad of physiological changes that significantly alter the behavior of many diseases. Superficial fungal infections likewise become more prevalent and require special attention. Superficial fungal infections include candidal and dermatophytic infections. These infections can cause significant discomfort and may lead to further complications if not properly managed.

The heightened susceptibility to these infections during pregnancy is primarily due to hormonal fluctuations, such as increased estrogen and progesterone levels, which create an environment conducive to fungal growth. Additionally, the immune system undergoes modulation to support the developing fetus, often reducing the body's ability to combat these pathogens. Weight gain and increased sweating add to these risk factors. Understanding the prevalence, pathogenesis, and safe treatment options for these infections is helpful for improving the health and well-being of both the mother and the fetus.

- Pregnant patients are more susceptible to superficial fungal infections.
- Immune hormonal changes, weight gain, increased sweating, and barrier disruption are predisposing factors for dermatophytosis and candidiasis.
- Immunohormonal changes, alteration of local microflora, and pH predispose for candidal infection.

DERMATOPHYTIC INFECTIONS

Dermatophytes are the most common cause of superficial fungal infections of the skin. They may affect up to 20–25% of world's population. Broadly dermatophytes are divided into *Epidermophyton, Microsporum*, and *Trichophyton*. They may infect skin, hair, and nail. In India, dermatophytic infections have become very common to attain epidemic proportion.

Immunopathogenesis of Dermatophytoses

Predisposing factors of dermatophytic infections are immunosuppression, maceration in intertriginous areas due to sweat, rubbing and alkaline pH, tight-fitting clothes, occluded footwear, increased environmental temperature, and humidity. Body's defenses against dermatophytic infections include heightened cell turnover, production of antimicrobial peptides (AMPs), phagocytosis by neutrophils and macrophages, and a robust immune response, especially cell-mediated immunity. Increased occlusion due to gain in weight leads to maceration in intertriginous areas. Also, pruritus which is common in pregnancy further damages skin barrier. These changes are favorable for fungal growth.

During pregnancy, significant alterations occur in toll-like receptors (TLRs), which are crucial components of the innate immune system responsible for recognizing pathogen-associated molecular patterns (PAMPs) and initiating immune responses. These changes are necessary to balance immune tolerance toward the fetus and the need to protect the mother from infections. Studies suggest that the expression of certain TLRs, such as TLR2 and TLR4, may increase in specific tissues, enhancing the immune response against fungal pathogens.

- Dermatophytic infections are most common superficial fungal infections.
- During pregnancy, there are various risk factors on one hand and certain immunomodulations have a protective effect.
- Lack of taking timely treatment for fear of adverse effects to fetus, decreased Th1 activity, and functional modulation of innate immunity lead to severe and persistent infection.

During pregnancy, the production of AMPs such as β-defensins, psoriasin, and RNase7 can be upregulated to compensate for the altered immune response. β-defensin 2 and 3 levels may increase, enhancing the skin's ability to combat fungal pathogens. Similarly, the upregulation of psoriasin and RNase7 contributes to the overall antimicrobial defense, protecting the skin and mucous membranes from infections. These changes help bolster the body's defenses during a time of immunological compromise and other predisposing factors of fungal infections of skin.

The alterations in neutrophil and macrophage function during pregnancy can increase susceptibility to fungal infections. Although the numbers of these immune cells are elevated, their functional modulation, aimed at reducing inflammation and protecting the fetus, can diminish their effectiveness in clearing infections. Th1 type of cell-mediated immunity is normally responsible for increasing epidermal turnover and hence eliminating the dermatophyte. Consequently, fungal infections may become more prolonged or severe due to this dampened immune response. The shift toward an anti-inflammatory state, while essential for fetal protection, can impede the body's ability to mount an effective defense against dermatophytes **(Table 1)**.

TABLE 1: Protective and causative factors predisposing for dermatophyte infection in pregnancy.	
Protective factors	**Causative factors**
	• Increased sweating
• Increased TLR-2, 4	• Barrier disruption
• Increased antimicrobial peptides • β-defensins • Psoriasin • RNase7	• Decreased Th1 • Altered macrophage and neutrophil function
(TLR: toll-like receptor)	

CANDIDAL INFECTIONS

Vulvovaginal Candidiasis

Vulvovaginal candidiasis (VVC) is candidal infection involving vagina, vestibule, labia majora/minora, and perianal region. Lifetime prevalence of VVC in women is 75% with 8% of these have recurrent VVC. Recurrent VVC is defined as having ≥3 episodes of VVC per year. VVC is the second common cause of vaginal infection. Pregnancy is a risk factor for VVC; up to 20% of women experience candidiasis during pregnancy while this figure increases to 30% in third trimester. Broadly, VVC is classified into uncomplicated and complicated type. Latter includes recurrent VVC, immunocompromised state, those who have severe symptoms, infection with nonalbicans, and pregnancy. *Candida albicans* is the predominant species in 90% of the cases followed by nonalbicans species like *Candida glabrata, C. tropicalis, C. krusei,* and *C. parapsilosis.*

Pregnancy is considered a complicated VVC because longer course of treatment is required, choice of antifungal which can be prescribed is limited, and fetal outcome may get compromised. Pregnancy is a dynamic state where female genital tract is a point of entry for number of pathogens for various sexually and nonsexually transmitted diseases. Vaginal discharge is the most common complaint and presents as curdy white discharge, itching, burning, erythema, swelling, irritation of vulva and vagina with dysuria and dyspareunia. At times, this infection may be asymptomatic. The infection can be acute, chronic, superficial, or deep and has broad clinical spectrum. Any physiological changes that affect the beneficial *Lactobacillus* species microflora in the vagina would alter the acidity of the vagina enhancing the establishment of pathogenic organisms such as *Candida* **(Box 1)**.

Immunosuppression: Epithelial cells and resident immune cells, such as neutrophils and macrophages, play crucial roles in the initial defense against *Candida*. However, hormonal changes during pregnancy can alter their function.

Effects on hormones: Increased progesterone inhibits neutrophil activity against *Candida*. Estrogen disrupts the normal vaginal microflora, resulting in increased yeast colonization. It also enhances *Candida*'s ability to adhere to the vaginal

BOX 1 Various factors leading to vulvovaginal candidiasis.

- Immunosuppression
- Effect of hormones
- Increased vaginal glycogen content
- Alteration in vaginal pH
- Effect on cell-mediated immunity

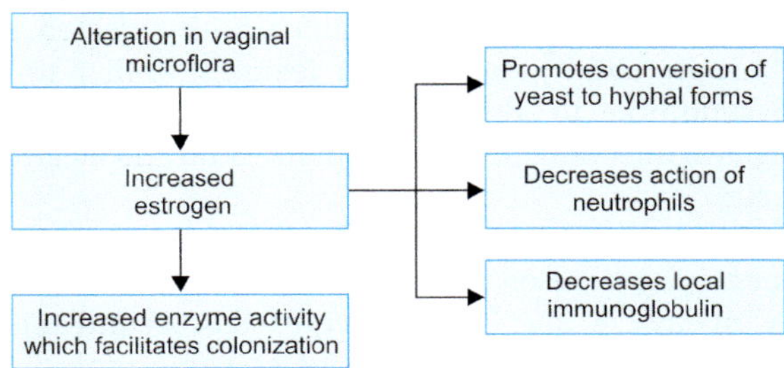

FIG. 1: Estrogen-induced changes in vagina.

epithelium and promotes its transition from the yeast form to the pathogenic hyphal form. Additionally, estrogen weakens the vaginal epithelial defenses and suppresses the production of locally secreted immunoglobulins. The enzymes aspartyl proteinases and phospholipases produced by *Candida* further facilitate colonization **(Fig. 1)**.

Increased vaginal glycogen content: Elevation of vaginal glycogen content provides an additional source of carbon which facilitates candidal colonization.

Alteration of vaginal pH: Normal vaginal has pH of 4.0–4.5. In pregnancy, this pH increases to 5.0–6.5. This loss of acidic environment favors candidal colonization.

Conversion of Th1 to Th2 response: This leads to suppression of cytotoxic T cell response.

- Vulvovaginal candidiasis is common in pregnancy.
- Immunosuppression, hormonal influences, and altered microflora in vagina are causative factors.
- VVC during pregnancy is a complicated type of VVC.
- VVC may be recurrent.
- VVC affects both mother and fetus.

Complications of Vulvovaginal Candidiasis

Maternal

Vulvovaginal candidiasis can cause increased discomfort, pain, and secondary bacterial infections, potentially leading to recurrent infections that impact her quality of life and emotional well-being.

Impact on Newborn

- *Preterm birth*:
  Ascending intrauterine infection results in preterm birth. Increase in the levels of interleukins in vaginal fluid causes a higher inflammatory response in symptomatic VVC.
- Fetal growth restriction
- Vertical and horizontal transmission
- *Congenital cutaneous candidiasis (CCC)*: This occurs when fetus/newborn during delivery/in utero comes in contact with infected mother's fluid/mucosa. Clinically child presents with features similar to *Staphylococcus* scalded skin syndrome. In addition to skin, umbilical cord and placenta may also show signs of infection. In preterm infant, fluid and electrolyte imbalance may also occur.

In VVC, topical agents should be used for 7 days episodically. Longer episodic treatment may be used in resistant cases or recurrent VVC. At times, oral fluconazole on day 1, 4, and 7 may be required in second and third trimester recurrent VVC. At times, longer duration of episodic topical treatment with systemic fluconazole 150 mg/week for 6 months may be required in recurrent VVC.

Oral thrush: Dryness of mouth, altered oral microflora, and immunosuppression may increase risk of oral thrush in pregnancy.

INVESTIGATIONS

Potassium hydroxide (KOH): Scrapings from skin, nail, vaginal swab, oral mucosal swab, or hair can be taken and dissolved in 10–40% KOH. Candidal infection is suggested when budding hyphae can be seen. Dermatophytes appear as long, smooth, refractile, branching, undulating, and septate hyphal filaments.

Fungal culture: It is the gold standard but has a low sensitivity. Sabouraud dextrose agar (SDA) is used as culture medium.

Polymerase chain reaction: It is a highly sensitive technique to detect fungal DNA in clinical samples.

Histopathology: A tissue sample from the infected area can be examined under a microscope to identify fungal hyphae or yeast cells. Histopathological examination can provide definitive evidence of fungal infection and its impact on tissues.

ANTIFUNGAL AGENTS IN PREGNANCY

Fungi are eukaryotic organisms, with a true nucleus and organelles. They have a cell wall which comprises chitin, glucans, and mannoproteins and a cell membrane made up of ergosterol. Antifungal agents exploit the difference in structure between a fungal cell and human cell. Instead of the cholesterol in human cells, fungal cells have ergosterol. Antifungal drugs target cell wall, cell membrane, microtubules, and nucleus **(Fig. 2)**. There are multiple antifungal agents but there are only a few which are safe in pregnancy.

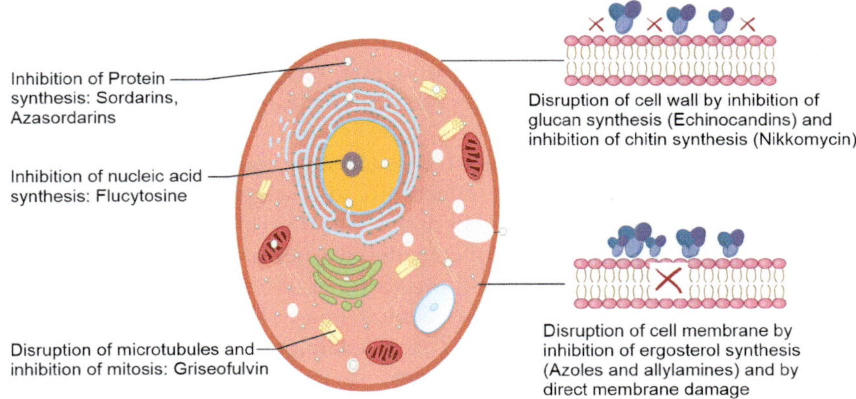

FIG. 2: Mechanism of action of antifungal drugs.

TABLE 2: Categorization of topical and systemic antifungal drugs according to US FDA.

US FDA category	Oral agents	Topical agents
A		Nystatin (10%)
B	Terbinafine (250 mg/day)	• Ciclopirox olamine (1%) • Naftifine (1%) • Terbinafine (1%) • Clotrimazole (1% or 2%) • Miconazole (2%) • Oxiconazole
C	• Fluconazole (150 mg/day) • Itraconazole (200 mg/day) • Griseofulvin (500 mg/day) • Flucytosine • Posaconazole	• Econazole (1%) • Terconazole (0.4% and 0.8%) • Tioconazole (6.5%) • Butoconazole (2%) • Selenium sulfide (1% and 2.5%)
D	• Fluconazole (400–600 mg/day) • Voriconazole	
X		

(US FDA: United States Food and Drug Administration)

The classification of common antifungal drugs and their conventional FDA categorizations are listed in **Table 2**.

Systemic Drugs

Azoles

Azoles bind to the heme group of enzyme 14-α-demethylase, blocking the conversion of lanosterol to ergosterol. Without ergosterol, the fungal cell membrane becomes less fluid and more permeable, leading to cell dysfunction and death. This disruption in membrane integrity affects numerous membrane-bound enzymes, leading to impaired cell growth and replication, eventually causing cell death. They are fungistatic in nature. Azoles are further of two types imidazoles (topical only) and triazoles (ketoconazole, itraconazole, fluconazole, voriconazole, and posaconazole).

Fluconazole is a systemic triazole which is effective against yeasts like *Candida* and *Cryptococcus*. Its teratogenic effects are dose-dependent, with 150 mg considered FDA Category C and higher doses (>300 mg) classified as Category D. Doses below 300 mg are generally considered safer after the first trimester. Fluconazole crosses the placenta and can cause craniofacial and rib abnormalities. Its use has been linked to congenital heart defects (such as cardiac septal defects), spontaneous abortions, cleft palate or lip, and musculoskeletal malformations. Reports also include cases of trapezoidocephaly, mid-facial hypoplasia, cartilage abnormalities with multiple synostoses, and skeletal fractures associated with fluconazole use.

Itraconazole, another commonly prescribed antifungal is not considered safe in pregnancy (FDA category C). It has been reported to increase risk of abortions but is nonteratogenic.

Ketoconazole has been shown to be teratogenic in animal studies, causing musculoskeletal malformations, liver toxicity, and endocrine-related side effects. Therefore, it is generally advised to avoid using it for superficial fungal infections during pregnancy.

Voriconazole has also been found to be teratogenic in rodent studies, even at low doses (equivalent to 0.3 times the recommended human dose), leading to skeletal and internal organ abnormalities. Due to insufficient data in humans, voriconazole is classified as a Category D drug and should be strictly avoided during pregnancy.

Griseofulvin

Griseofulvin inhibits fungal cell division by disrupting the microtubules necessary for mitosis, and it accumulates in keratinized tissues to provide targeted antifungal activity. It is an orally administered fungistatic drug. It is used in dermatophytosis but not effective against yeasts, molds, or systemic fungi. It crosses the placenta and is teratogenic in rodents. It has been classified as pregnancy category C and its use is restricted in pregnancy.

Allylamines

Terbinafine is a squalene epoxidase inhibitor which is extensively used in practice, both in oral and topical preparations. These are fungicidal and have a broad spectrum of activity. They are effective against dermatophytic skin infections, onychomycosis and other cutaneous dermatophytoses, including chromomycosis and mycetoma. It is recommended as FDA pregnancy category B and is considered the safest oral antifungal.

Flucytosine

Flucytosine is an antifungal medication primarily used in combination with other antifungals, such as amphotericin B, to treat severe fungal infections, including cryptococcal meningitis and systemic candidiasis. It functions by disrupting fungal DNA and RNA synthesis, ultimately inhibiting cell growth and replication. However, flucytosine is classified as an FDA Category C drug. It is used in mothers only in case of life-threatening infections.

Topical Agents

Topical antifungals are applied directly to the site of infection, ensuring a high concentration of the medication where it is needed. They are absorbed minimally into the bloodstream; the risk of systemic side effects is significantly reduced. This makes them safer for use in pregnancy. They have additional anti-inflammatory activity. But topical agents may be inadequate for large surface areas and they may cause contact dermatitis due to the vehicle used. Nanocarriers have helped to improve efficacy of topical antifungal medication. Various nanocarriers available are solid lipid nanoparticles, microemulsions, liposomes, niosomes, microsponge, nanogel, nanoemulsion, micelles, etc.

Topical Azoles

Topical azoles like miconazole, clotrimazole, oxiconazole, and sulconazole are category B drugs. While other commonly prescribed topical antifungals like luliconazole, sertaconazole, and econazole are category C drugs. Other topical agents like bifonazole, fenticonazole, isoconazole, and tioconazole indicated for superficial fungal infections are also included in pregnancy category C. So if at all these topical drugs are used, a lowest effective dose for the shortest duration should be used.

Topical Allylamines

Naftifine, terbinafine, and butenafine are various topical allylamines. All of them are category B drugs.

Polyenes

They bind to ergosterol of fungal cell membrane → depolarization of the membrane → formation of pores → leakage of intracellular contents. Nystatin and amphotericin B both are considered safe in pregnancy (Category B). They are effective against candidal infection but not against dermatophytes.

Echinocandins

They act by inhibiting synthesis of 1,3-β-d-glucan, a key component fungal cell wall. Various echinocandins are anidulafungin, caspofungin and micafungin. They are usually not required for superficial infections of skin. They belong to pregnancy category C agents.

Ciclopiroxolamine

Ciclopiroxolamine acts by disrupting multiple biochemical processes within the fungal cells. It inhibits the uptake of essential substrates and ions, particularly iron, which is crucial for the metabolic functions of the fungus. This disruption leads to the inhibition of fungal growth and eventually causes cell death.

Additionally, ciclopiroxolamine has anti-inflammatory properties, which help in reducing the symptoms of fungal infections. It is available in several formulations, including creams, gels, shampoos, and nail lacquers. Ciclopiroxolamine is generally considered safe for use during pregnancy. Some patients may experience mild side effects such as redness, itching, or burning at the application site.

Amorolfine

It belongs to the class of antifungal agents known as morpholines and works by inhibiting the synthesis of ergosterol by inhibiting D14α reductase and D7–D8 isomerase. It has both fungistatic and fungicidal action. Amorolfine is available as a nail lacquer (5%) and is applied once or twice a week to the affected nails. It is also available as 0.5% cream which can be used in superficial fungal infections. Common side effects include mild skin irritation, redness, itching, or a burning sensation at the application site.

Tavaborole

Tavaborole (family oxaborole) is a new drug used specifically for onychomycosis. It acts by inhibiting cytosolic leucyl-transfer RNA synthetase involved in protein synthesis.

It is available as 5% solution and has to be applied daily for 48 weeks. There is no data on safety of this drug in pregnancy. Oral formulation of tavaborole has been found to be embryotoxic and causing birth defects in rabbits, though topical formulation did not cause such adverse effects.

SPECIAL CONSIDERATION

Onychomycosis in Pregnancy

Onychomycosis may act as a nidus of other superficial fungal infections both to the mother and the fetus. Also esthetically, the discoloration, thickening, and disfigurement of nail may not be acceptable to a woman during this beautiful phase of life. It may cause increased stress to her. Systemic antifungal agents are usually avoided in pregnancy because they have to be given for a long period. Throughout pregnancy, use of topical therapy is preferred. Topical ciclopirox (FDA category B) and amorolfine (not FDA approved) are considered safe throughout pregnancy. Tavaborole topically is effective in onychomycosis but safety in pregnancy is not well documented (category C). Topical formulations in onychomycosis may not be effective as monotherapy. At times, decreasing the load of fungal elements by trimming nail, abrading, filing and nail avulsion may be helpful. Though usually onychomycosis may be asymptomatic and may not require any urgent intervention but partial nail avulsion is required in painful onychomycosis.

Tinea Capitis in Pregnancy

Tinea capitis is an infection of hair shaft or scalp caused by *Trichophyton and Microsporum* species. It is usually seen in adolescents but close contact may lead to infection in a pregnant female. Associated hair loss and scaling may be distressing to the patient. Topical antifungals are prescribed but are less effective. *T. capitis* being less common during pregnancy, no studies or guidelines are available for the management.

Prevention of Superficial Fungal Infections during Pregnancy

Preventing fungal infections during pregnancy involves a combination of good hygiene practices, proper clothing choices, dietary adjustments, and regular health monitoring. Maintaining clean and dry skin is essential, particularly in areas prone to moisture accumulation such as under the breasts, in the groin, and between the toes. Using mild, fragrance-free soaps, and avoiding harsh scrubbing can help prevent skin irritation. Wearing loose-fitting, breathable fabrics like cotton and changing underwear and socks frequently can reduce moisture buildup and discourage fungal growth. After bathing, it is important to dry the skin thoroughly, especially in skin folds. For those with gestational diabetes, closely monitoring and managing blood sugar levels is vital to reducing the risk of infections.

- Keep the skin clean and dry with gentle cleaning.
- Wearing loose clothes made of breathable fabrics.
- Avoid irritants.
- Good oral hygiene, rinsing mouth after inhaled steroids.
- Judicious use of antibiotics

Using antibiotics only when necessary and rinsing the mouth after using inhaled corticosteroids can help maintain normal flora and prevent fungal overgrowth. Early intervention and adherence to prescribed treatments for fungal infections are important to ensure complete resolution and prevent recurrence.

SUGGESTED READINGS

1. Messina A, Mariani A, Brandolisio R, Tavella E, Germano C, Lipari G, et al. Candidiasis in Pregnancy: Relevant Aspects of the Pathology for the Mother and the Fetus and Therapeutic Strategies. Trop Med Infect Dis. 2024;9:114.
2. Disha T, Haque F. Prevalence and Risk Factors of Vulvovaginal Candidosis during Pregnancy: A Review. Infect Dis Obstet Gynecol. 2022;20:6195712.
3. Pilmis B, Jullien V, Sobel J, Lecuit M, Lortholary O, Charlier C. Antifungal drugs during pregnancy: an updated review. J Antimicrob Chemother. 2015;70:14-22.
4. Jartarkar SR, Patil A, Goldust Y, Cockerell CJ, Schwartz RA, Grabbe S, et al. Pathogenesis, Immunology and Management of Dermatophytosis. J Fungi (Basel). 2021;8(1):39.
5. Prabhu SS, Sankineni P. Managing Dermatophytoses in Pregnancy, Lactation, and Children. Clin Dermatol Rev. 2017;1(Suppl 1):34-7.
6. Patel MA, Aliporewala VM, Patel DA. Common Antifungal Drugs in Pregnancy: Risks and Precautions. J Obstet Gynaecol. 2021;71(6):577-82.

11.3 Varicella and Pregnancy

Devyani Sapra, Biju Vasudevan, Vishal Sharma

INTRODUCTION

Varicella, commonly known as chickenpox, is a highly contagious disease caused by the varicella zoster virus (VZV), a member of the herpesvirus family. VZV is a double-stranded DNA virus. The primary infection typically manifests as an itchy, vesicular rash accompanied by fever, malaise, and fatigue **(Fig. 1)**. Rash generally heals with crusting in 5 days. The incubation period varies between 1 and 3 weeks and the disease is infectious 2 days before the onset of rash until the vesicles get crusted. Primary infection usually confers lifelong immunity and second attacks are uncommon, especially in immunocompetent individuals. After the initial infection, VZV establishes latency in the sensory nerve root ganglia and can get reactivated decades later in response to stress or immunosuppression, resulting in a painful vesicular rash in a dermatomal pattern called shingles or herpes zoster.

Varicella is generally a mild illness in children, but it can have more severe consequences in adults, particularly in pregnant women, due to the altered immune response during pregnancy. This increased susceptibility leads to a heightened risk of complications, making varicella in pregnancy a serious concern. The most dangerous period for the fetus is during the first 20 weeks of gestation, where infection can result in congenital varicella syndrome (CVS), characterized by a range of developmental abnormalities.

EPIDEMIOLOGY

Women who do not harbor immunity to varicella till the childbearing age are at a risk of developing the disease during pregnancy (0.05–0.07%). Incidence of

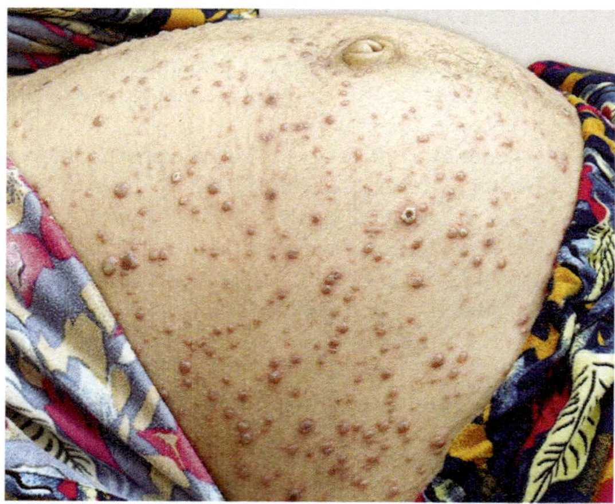

FIG. 1: A pregnant patient with extensive varicella lesions.

varicella in pregnancy is calculated to be 2–3/1,000 pregnancies. Infection with VZV in pregnancy may result in adverse outcomes in both the mother and fetus. Lower socioeconomic status can be associated with higher risk of infection due to the factors like overcrowding and limited access to healthcare. Healthcare workers and teachers may have increased exposure risk. In countries with high vaccination coverage, the incidence of varicella in pregnancy has significantly decreased. However, even in these countries, outbreaks can occur among unvaccinated individuals or those with weakened immune systems.

Maternal Complications

Although varicella infection is much less common in adults than in children, it is associated with a greater morbidity, such as pneumonia, hepatitis, and encephalitis. Varicella infection can lead to premature birth. The pregnant women may present with respiratory symptoms, neurological symptoms such as photophobia, seizures, or drowsiness, a hemorrhagic rash or bleeding, or a dense rash with or without mucosal lesions, etc., which may be indicative of potentially life-threatening chickenpox warranting intensive care at a hospital. The mortality rate of chickenpox increases with age. Mortality in early adulthood is 15 times higher than childhood mortality rate. VZV pneumonia can occur in up to 10–20% of pregnant women with chickenpox, and the severity of complication seems to increase as the pregnancy advances leading to a mortality rate of 14%, whereas in the general population, varicella pneumonia has a mortality rate of 10–11%. The effects of the gravid uterus on respiratory function in later gestation add to the severity. Other risk factors for varicella pneumonitis in pregnancy include smoking, chronic obstructive lung disease, immunosuppression, and presence of more than 100 skin lesions or hemorrhagic lesions.

Maternal complications:
- Severe rash (>100 lesions)
- Pneumonitis
- Hepatitis
- Encephalitis

Varicella pneumonitis in pregnancy carries a higher mortality.

Fetal Complications

The effects of maternal varicella on the fetus vary with the gestational age at time of infection.

First and Second Trimester

The risk of miscarriage does not increase with primary VZV infection in the first trimester. However, viremia or serological conversion in the first 28 weeks of pregnancy may cause fetal varicella syndrome (FVS). The risk of incidence of FVS prior to the 13 weeks' period of gestation is 0.4% and increases to 2% between 13 and 20 weeks. It also has a mortality rate of 30% in the 1st month of life.

Clinical presentation of FVS is characterized by one or more of the following:
- Skin scarring in a dermatomal distribution
- Eye defects (microphthalmia, chorioretinitis, or cataracts)

- Hypoplasia of the limbs
- Neurological abnormalities (microcephaly, cortical atrophy, mental retardation or dysfunction of bowel and bladder sphincters)

The pathogenesis behind development of FVS seems to be subsequent to herpes zoster reactivation in utero rather than the primary infection itself. So, a time lag of at least 5 weeks after the primary infection is advised for a detailed ultrasound examination of the fetus.

- Fetal varicella syndrome (due to reactivation of VZV in utero)
- Scarring in dermatomal pattern
- Eye defects
- Neurological abnormalities
- Hypoplasia of limbs

Third Trimester

Maternal varicella in the last trimester till 36 weeks' gestation carries a very low risk of developing fetopathy and outcome is usually good.

Peripartum VZV

Last 3 weeks to >5 days before delivery: Despite high titers of passively acquired maternal antibody, almost 23% babies develop clinical varicella. The route of infection can be transplacental, ascending vaginal or due to direct contact with lesions during or after delivery.

5 days before delivery to 2 days after delivery: As the fetus is exposed to a high viral load without getting enough time to acquire passively transferred maternal antibody, around 20–50% of the newborns contract "neonatal varicella," and 30% of them develop fulminant infection with disseminated cutaneous lesions and visceral involvement. However, with the use of antivirals and varicella zoster immunoglobulin (VZIG), the mortality rate has declined from 30 to 7% among neonates with severe varicella infection.

- *First trimester*: Minimal risk
- *13–28 weeks*: Fetal varicella syndrome
- *28–36 weeks*: Low risk
- *37–39 weeks + 2 days*: 23% incidence of neonatal varicella
- *5 days before delivery*: 2 days after delivery 20–50% chances of neonatal varicella (also systemic involvement and severity is more)

Fetal loss: In some cases, varicella infection can result in miscarriage or stillbirth.

Neonatal varicella: If the mother develops varicella shortly before or after delivery, the newborn is at risk of developing severe neonatal varicella.

TRANSMISSION

Varicella is highly contagious, spreading primarily through direct contact with the characteristic vesicular rash. However, transmission can also occur via airborne droplets containing viruses and can be inhaled by others. The virus can also be shed from the respiratory tract before the onset of the rash, increasing the risk of undetected transmission.

Contaminated objects, such as toys or shared utensils, can serve as indirect sources of infection. The virus can survive on surfaces for short periods, allowing for potential transmission through contact with these objects.

The incubation period for varicella is typically 10–21 days, during which the infected individual is asymptomatic but contagious. This prolonged incubation period contributes to the ease with which the virus spreads within communities.

Modes of transmission of VZV:
- Contact with vesicular fluid
- Droplet
- Fomites

Incubation period 10–21 days

PREVENTION

Primary Prevention

This includes vaccination prepregnancy and postexposure prophylaxis (PEP) in pregnant women. The RCOG recommends that all pregnant women should be asked about previous chickenpox/shingles during booking and this to be documented. Women who have not had chickenpox, or are known to be seronegative for chickenpox, should be advised to avoid contact with chickenpox and shingles case during pregnancy and to inform healthcare workers of a potential exposure without delay.

Vaccination

Vaccination is the cornerstone of varicella prevention in pregnancy. It helps in preventing the disease and its complications. In India, varicella vaccine is not included in the universal immunization program due to the cost and lifelong immunity which occurs after primary infection. A previous history of chickenpox infection has a 97.9–99.7% positive predictive value for the presence of serum varicella antibodies. If a woman is unsure of her immunity status, a blood test can be performed to check for antibodies against VZV. The nonimmune, nonpregnant women can be offered varicella vaccine 2 doses given 4–8 weeks apart with advice to avoid pregnancy for 4 weeks after completing the vaccine schedule. Vaccination can also be done postpartum and mothers should be advised that breastfeeding can be safely continued.

Postexposure Prophylaxis (Flowchart 1)

If a nonimmune pregnant woman has a significant exposure to chickenpox, she should be offered VZIG within 96 hours of exposure or as soon as possible. The RCOG recommends offering VZIG to susceptible women up to 10 days after exposure. These women should be managed as potentially infectious from 8 to 28 days after exposure if they receive VZIG and from 8 to 21 days after exposure if they do not receive VZIG. Significant contact is defined as contact with the

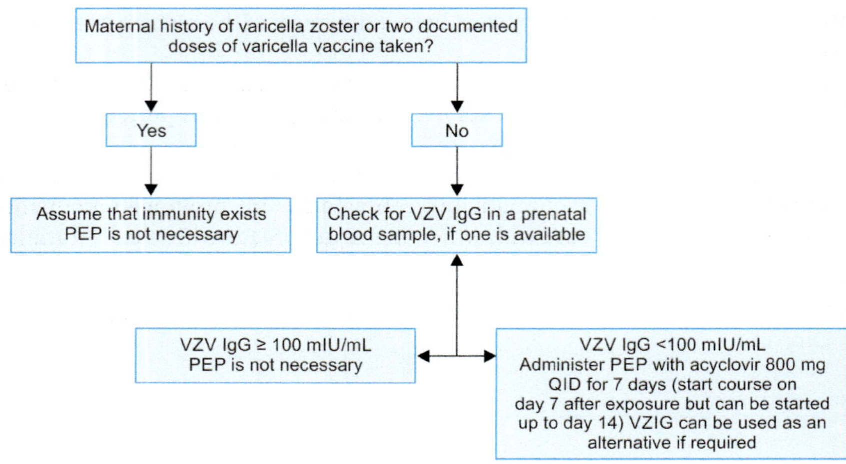

FLOWCHART 1: Management protocol of postexposure prophylaxis (PEP).
(VZV: varicella zoster virus; VZIG: varicella zoster immunoglobulin)

infected case in the same room for 15 minutes or more, face-to-face contact or contact in the setting of a large open ward.

Varicella zoster immunoglobulin is a human immunoglobulin derived from the plasma of donors with high VZV antibody titers. Hence, the patient consent is required as it is associated with theoretical risk of blood products derived infection. The recommended dose of VZIG is 125 U/10 kg of body weight up to a maximum of 625 U. As the maternal viremia may still occur despite immunoprophylaxis with VZIG, it plays a significant role in reducing severity of varicella in mother and the neonate, as well as in decreasing the risk of FVS. The side effects include injection site reaction (pain, erythema, and swelling) reported in 1% of patients, and rarely rash, malaise, headache, and gastrointestinal symptoms may occur. Anaphylaxis is extremely rare.

Immediate evaluation of immunity status is essential following potential varicella exposure. If immunity is uncertain or absent, a varicella IgG test should be performed. Nonimmune pregnant women should be isolated to prevent disease spread. PEP with oral acyclovir is the preferred treatment, with VZIG as an alternative. Close monitoring for varicella symptoms is necessary for at least 4 weeks postexposure. Women with underlying medical conditions may require tailored management based on individual risk factors **(Flowchart 1)**.

Early detection and management are crucial for minimizing the risks associated with varicella in pregnancy. If a pregnant woman is exposed to varicella, she should consult with her healthcare provider immediately.

- *Prepregnancy (at least 4 weeks prior to conception or postpartum)*: Varicella vaccine
- *During pregnancy*: VZIG (within 10 days of exposure to infected person)

Education and awareness are essential for preventing varicella in pregnancy. Healthcare providers should educate women of childbearing age about the importance of vaccination and the risks of varicella during pregnancy. Public health campaigns can also help raise awareness about the disease and its prevention.

MANAGEMENT

Diagnosis

The diagnosis of a classical uncomplicated case of varicella is based on its clinical features at presentation, and laboratory testing is unwarranted. However, in cases in which clinical manifestations are not classic but infection is suspected, polymerase chain reaction (PCR) testing for VZV DNA (if available) can be performed on samples obtained from the bases of unroofed vesicles. In severe or complicated cases of chickenpox, organ-specific investigations should be done. Clinically, the characteristic itchy rash with fluid-filled blisters is often indicative, but laboratory confirmation is crucial. Blood tests are the mainstay of diagnosis but are not done in routine practice. The VZV IgM antibody test specifically detects a recent infection, while the VZV IgG antibody test confirms past immunity. All pregnant women with varicella and any respiratory symptom, however mild, should undergo chest radiography with abdominal shielding to confirm varicella pneumonia. The diagnosis is based on the characteristic radiographic findings of bilateral peribronchial nodular infiltrates in a woman with chickenpox. A complete baseline workup including hematological and biochemical investigations should be ordered. Liver function tests including transaminases should be done. Serologic tests for antibodies against VZV are significant in a pregnant woman who is exposed to varicella and has no history of chickenpox in the past. The test holds minimal value during acute varicella infection.

Investigations:
- Clinical features are usually sufficient to make a diagnosis
- Deroofing vesicle followed by:
  - Tzanck (multinucleated giant cells)
  - PCR
- *Serology*:
  - IgM—recent infection/vaccination
  - IgG—past infection (usually done to test if mother has ever been exposed to VZV in the past)
- Liver function test especially transaminases
- Hematological especially if bleeding manifestations
- Chest radiography—if features suggestive of pneumonia

Treatment of Varicella in Pregnancy

Pregnant women developing chickenpox rash should immediately report to the medical caregiver. Most of these women do not require hospitalization. Until all the lesions are crusted, they should avoid contact with other susceptible people, such as other pregnant women and neonates. If the pregnant women present within 24 hours of onset of rash and are 20 weeks of gestation or beyond, oral acyclovir should be prescribed in the dose of 800 mg five times a day for 7 days. Though acyclovir in first trimester is associated with theoretical risks of teratogenesis, however, usage of drug before 20 weeks of gestation should also be considered as the literature does not suggest any significant risk in neonates exposed to the drug in utero. The drug is given mainly for maternal benefit as it reduces the duration of fever and other symptoms of varicella infection if commenced within 24 hours of developing the rash. Although acyclovir does not protect the fetus from FVS or the newborn from neonatal varicella, it exerts some positive effects as drug migration across placenta may result in reduced transplacental transmission and lower fetal viremia.

Indication for acyclovir in pregnancy:
- Before 20 weeks—for reducing maternal symptoms
- After 20 weeks: It does not protect fetus from fetal varicella syndrome or neonatal varicella, but as it can cross placenta, it decreases severity.

Acyclovir is a synthetic nucleoside analog that inhibits replication of the VZV. The drug is specific for herpes simplex viruses (HSV) and VZV infected cells as it is converted to acyclovir monophosphate by viral thymidine kinase (TK), and further steps of phosphorylation are catalyzed by human cellular guanylate cyclase. It results in formation of acyclovir triphosphate which inhibits the viral DNA polymerase. In addition, it is mistaken for deoxyguanosine triphosphate and gets incorporated into newly synthesized viral DNA, leading to obligate chain termination since the molecule lacks the 3'-hydroxyl group required for further DNA chain elongation. After oral administration, it is incompletely absorbed with bioavailability of about 15–30%. The drug penetrates well into most tissues, including the CNS. More than 80% of the administered dose is excreted unchanged in the urine by glomerular filtration and tubular secretion. An orally administered prodrug of acyclovir, valacyclovir, has better oral bioavailability and improved pharmacokinetics. The recommended dose for immunocompetent adults with varicella is 1,000 mg three times daily for 7 days **(Table 1)**.

Penciclovir is also an acyclic guanine derivative resembling acyclovir in chemical structure, mechanism of action, poor absorption, and antiviral

TABLE 1: Dosage of antiviral drugs used in varicella in pregnancy.

Antiviral treatment for varicella in pregnancy		
	Drug	**Pregnancy prescribing status (US FDA)**
Uncomplicated Chickenpox	• Acyclovir 800 mg 5 times a day or, • Valacyclovir 1,000 mg 3 times a day or, • Famciclovir 500 mg 3 times a day	• Category B • Category B • Category B
Varicella pneumonia	Intravenous acyclovir 10–15 mg/kg 8 hourly	Category B

(US FDA: United States Food and Drug Administration)

spectrum. With famciclovir as a prodrug, the bioavailability of penciclovir increases up to 77%. Famciclovir is administered in the dosage of 500 mg three times daily in chickenpox as well as herpes zoster. Adequate hydration of the patient must be maintained during the antiviral therapy. Major organ toxicities associated with acyclovir/valacyclovir/famciclovir include renal failure due to rapid IV administration, thrombotic angiopathy in immunocompromised, and neurotoxicity with higher doses and deranged renal function.

Foscarnet is another antiviral drug which may be used in acyclovir-resistant VZV infections. The drug does not require intracellular activation by TK, as it is a pyrophosphate analog that inhibits the viral DNA polymerase by blocking the pyrophosphate-binding site. Foscarnet is administered by the intravenous route and 80–90% of an administered dose is excreted unchanged in the urine. The appropriate dose of drug in VZV infections has not been assessed systematically, but doses ranging from 40 mg/kg every 8 hours to 100 mg/kg every 12 hours have been used. The most important adverse effect associated with foscarnet therapy is nephrotoxicity.

Immunocompromised women, or with respiratory symptoms, CNS symptoms like photophobia, seizures or drowsiness, hemorrhagic or a dense rash, continued lesions beyond the 6th day or renewed fever should be managed in intensive care unit. Intravenous acyclovir (10–15 mg/kg IV 8 hourly) should be given to all pregnant females with severe or complicated chickenpox. VZIG has no therapeutic benefit after the development of rash, hence is not recommended. Symptomatic treatment for fever and pruritus should be given to all the affected women, along with advice to maintain hygiene so as to prevent secondary bacterial infection **(Table 1)**.

Women should have their immunity to varicella discussed and documented at their booking visit. Their immunity can be confirmed by either reliable history of varicella, two varicella vaccines, or by a laboratory test (varicella IgG) following exposure in line with National Immunization Advisory Committee (NIAC) guidance. Laboratories may choose to only send varicella IgG if a woman is exposed, rather than on all women with an uncertain varicella history.

Perinatal Varicella

As the VZV infection in the last 4 weeks of pregnancy poses a high risk of varicella infection of newborn along with significant morbidity and mortality, supportive treatment along with oral/intravenous acyclovir should be initiated without any delay. The patient should be isolated and a planned delivery must be delayed for at least 7 days since the onset of rash to facilitate crusting of active vesicles as well as passive immunity of the neonate. Delivery during viremia period with active vesicles may precipitate maternal hemorrhage and coagulopathy due to thrombocytopenia or hepatitis. However, if the delivery is indicated for obstetric reasons or life-threatening complications, a multidisciplinary approach should be warranted, including the respiratory physician, intensivist, and infectious disease specialist.

Amniocentesis can be performed to detect varicella DNA in the amniotic fluid, providing valuable information about the potential impact on the fetus. However, it is important to weigh the risks and benefits of this procedure carefully, as it carries inherent risks to both the mother and fetus.

A vaginal delivery is not indicated in the presence of active disease. During a cesarean section, an epidural anesthesia may be safer as the dura is not penetrated which may be theoretically associated with risk of transmission of VZV from skin lesions to the central nervous system via spinal anesthesia. A site free of lesions should be chosen for needle placement.

If the mother develops primary varicella infection, close collaboration with a neonatologist is vital to ensure optimal care for the newborn. The risk of severe disseminated varicella in the infant is significantly increased in these cases.

Perinatal varicella precautions to be taken:
- If possible delivery should be delayed for at least 7 days.
- Thrombocytopenia and hepatitis should be ruled out.
- Amniocentesis may be performed to detect viral DNA (but risk associated with procedure should be considered).
- Mode of delivery should be individualized on case-to-case basis.
- Cesarean should be done under epidural anesthesia.

Neonatal Varicella

If the onset of maternal rash is 5 days before delivery till 2 days after delivery, VZIG should be administered to the neonate within 72 hours of birth. It is given as 62.5 IU intramuscular for infants <2 kg and 125 IU for infants >2 kg. The RCOG does not recommend testing the neonate prior to VZIG. In a resource-poor setting or if VZIG is unavailable, IVIG can also be administered at a dose of 400 mg/kg. Acyclovir is indicated in case the neonate develops a rash of varicella, irrespective of VZIG administration. Management of neonate is as described in **Table 2**. VZIG may not prevent the infection, it can reduce the severity of the

TABLE 2: Summary of management of VZV in pregnancy.

Management of varicella in pregnancy			
Situation	**Maternal management**	**Fetus management**	**Neonatal management**
Pregnant women with significant exposure	Depends on history of chickenpox in past or vaccination or serological testing	None if no clinical features	None if no clinical features
Varicella before 20 weeks of gestation	• Symptomatic treatment • Consider oral acyclovir • Intravenous acyclovir 10–15 mg/kg every 8 hours if severe varicella	• Risk of FVS • Detailed sonography at 16–20 weeks and/or 5 weeks after onset of rash	30% mortality risk

Continued

Continued

Situation	Maternal management	Fetus management	Neonatal management
Varicella from 20 to 36 weeks' gestation	• Symptomatic treatment • Oral acyclovir if onset of rash within 24 hours • Intravenous acyclovir 10–15 mg/kg every 8 hours if severe varicella	Detailed sonography 5 weeks after onset of rash	Increased risk of herpes zoster in infancy and childhood
Varicella between last 3 weeks to >5 days before delivery	• Symptomatic treatment • Oral acyclovir if onset of rash within 24 hours • If possible, delay elective delivery for 7 days from onset of rash	No additional monitoring	• Neonatal varicella (risk 23%) • No VZIG • Acyclovir if clinical symptoms appear
Varicella between 5 days antepartum and 2 days postpartum	• Symptomatic treatment • Oral acyclovir if onset of rash within 24 hours • If possible, delay elective delivery for 7 days from onset of rash	No additional monitoring	• Neonatal varicella (risk 20–50%, mortality 20–23%) • Severe neonatal varicella (risk 17–30%, mortality 31%) • VZIG/IVIG should be administered within 72 hours of birth • IV acyclovir if clinical symptoms appear

(FVS: fetal varicella syndrome; IVIG: intravenous immunoglobulin; VZIG: varicella zoster immunoglobulin; VZV: varicella zoster virus)

disease in the neonate. Management of neonatal varicella has been described in **Flowchart 2**.

Women with varicella may continue breastfeeding. Expressed breast milk can also be fed to the neonate if there are active lesions around the nipple. Breastfeeding is strongly encouraged for women with varicella. The benefits of breastfeeding typically outweigh the potential risks of viral transmission. To minimize the risk of transmission, it is essential to cover any blisters on the breast with a sterile dressing. If blisters are near the nipple, expressing milk from that side until they scab over is recommended.

The expressed milk can be safely fed to the baby if they are receiving VZIG and/or antiviral treatment like acyclovir. However, if the infant is not on these treatments, the expressed milk should be discarded.

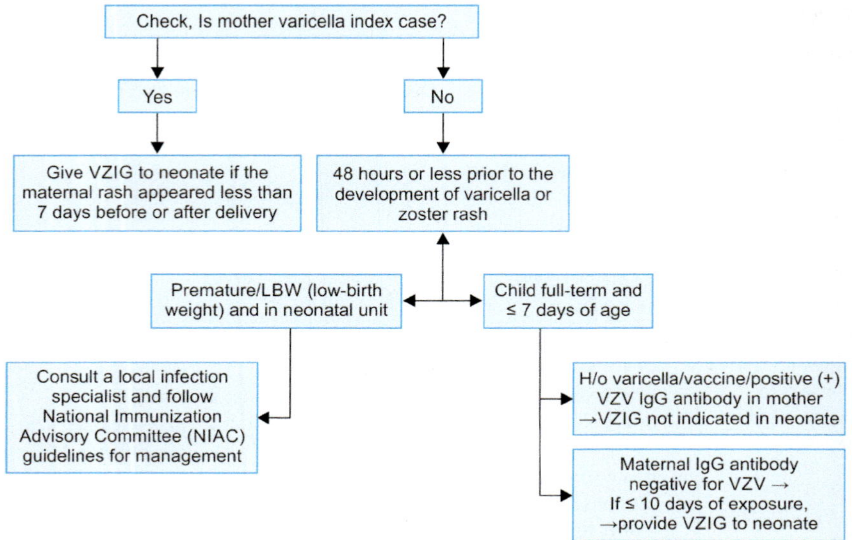

FLOWCHART 2: Management of mother and baby when exposure occurs near to delivery.
(VZIG: varicella zoster immunoglobulin; VZV: varicella zoster virus)

CONCLUSION

Varicella is a highly contagious viral infection caused by the VZV, and confers lifelong immunity. Pregnant women infected with the VZV are at increased risk for severe complications, including varicella pneumonia, hepatitis, and encephalitis. Fetal exposure, particularly during the first and second trimesters, can result in CVS, characterized by limb hypoplasia, cutaneous scarring, ocular anomalies, and central nervous system abnormalities. Perinatal infection poses a high risk for neonatal varicella, especially if maternal rash onset occurs within the critical window of 5 days before to 2 days after delivery. Preventive strategies are paramount, with preconception varicella vaccination being the most effective measure for nonimmune women. For those exposed during pregnancy, VZIG administration within 10 days can attenuate disease severity. Prompt antiviral therapy with acyclovir is recommended for pregnant women manifesting varicella symptoms to reduce the risk of complications. These women should be closely monitored, and appropriate neonatal care should be planned if delivery occurs near the time of maternal infection. The financial burden associated with medical care, long-term disability, and lost productivity can be substantial for families and healthcare systems. Additionally, the psychological impact of having a child with CVS or experiencing severe complications of pregnancy can be profound. It is essential to continue efforts to increase vaccination rates among women of childbearing age and to promote awareness of the risks of varicella during pregnancy. Further research is needed to develop new and effective prevention and treatment strategies for varicella infection in pregnancy.

SUGGESTED READINGS

1. Enders G, Miller E, Cradock-Watson J, Bolley I, Ridehalgh M. Consequences of varicella and herpes zoster in pregnancy: prospective study of 1739 cases. Lancet. 1994;343:1548-51.
2. Harger JH, Ernest JM, Thurnau GR, Moawad A, Momirova V, Landon MB, et al. Risk factors and outcome of varicella zoster virus pneumonia in pregnant women. J Infect Dis. 2002;185: 422-7.
3. Tan MP, Koren G. Chickenpox and pregnancy: Revisited. Reprod Toxicol. 2005;21:410-20.
4. Shrim A, Koren G, Yudin MH, Farine D; Maternal Fetal Medicine Committee. Management of varicella infection (chickenpox) in pregnancy. J Obstet Gynaecol Can. 2012;34:287-92.
5. Nathwani D, Maclean A, Conway S, Carrington D. Varicella Infections in pregnancy and the newborn. J Infect. 1998;36:59-71.
6. Pastuszak AL, Levy M, Schick B, Zuber C, Feldkamp M, Gladstone J, et al. Outcome after maternal varicella infection in the first 20 weeks of pregnancy. N Engl J Med. 1994;330:901-5.
7. Grose C. Congenital varicella-zoster virus infection and the failure to establish virus-specific cell-mediated immunity. Mol Biol Med. 1989;6:453-62.
8. Schulze A, Diätisch HJ. The natural history of varicella embryopathy: a 25-year old follow-up. J Pediatr. 2000;137:871-4.
9. Ghosh S, Chaudhuri S. Pregnancy and varicella infection: A resident's quest. Indian J Dermatol Venereol Leprol. 2013;79:264-7.
10. Nanthakumar MP, Sood A, Ahmed M, Gupta J. Varicella Zoster in pregnancy. Eur J Obstet Gynecol Reprod Biol. 2021;258:283-7.
11. Gardella C, Brown ZA. Managing varicella zoster infection in pregnancy. Cleveland Clin J Med. 2007;74(4):290.
12. Royal College of Obstetricians and Gynaecologists. (2015). Chickenpox in pregnancy. RCOG green-top guideline No.13. January 2015. [online] Available from https://www.rcog.org.uk/guidance/browse-all-guidance/green-top-guidelines/chickenpox-in-pregnancy-green-top-guideline-no-13/. [Last accessed January, 2025].
13. Watson B, Civen R, Reynolds M, Heath K, Perella D, Carbajal T, et al. Validity of self-reported varicella disease history in pregnant women attending prenatal clinics. Public Health Rep. 2007;122:499-506.
14. Public Health England. Varicella: the green book, Chapter 34. London: Public Health England; 2012.
15. Shrim A, Koren G, Yudin MH, Farine D. No. 274- Management of varicella Infection (Chickenpox) in Pregnancy. J Obstet Gynaecol Can. 2018;40(8):e652-7.
16. Cohen A, Moschopoulos P, Stiehm RE, Koren G. Congenital varicella syndrome: the evidence for secondary prevention with varicella-zoster immune globulin. Can Med Assoc J. 2011;183:204-8.
17. Levin MJ, Duchon JM, Swamy GK, Gershon AA. Varicella zoster immune globulin (VARIZIG) administration up to 10 days after varicella exposure in pregnant women, immunocompromised participants, and infants: varicella outcomes and safety results from a large, open-label, expanded access program. PLoS One. 2019;14:e0217749.
18. Koren G, Money D, Boucher M, Aoki F, Petric M, Innocencion G, et al. Serum concentrations, efficacy, and safety of a new, intravenously administered varicella zoster immune globulin in pregnant women. J Clin Pharmacol. 2002;42:267-74.
19. Stone KM, Reiff-Eldridge R, White AD, Cordero JF, Brown Z, Alexander ER, et al. Pregnancy outcomes following systemic prenatal acyclovir exposure: conclusions from the international acyclovir pregnancy registry, 1984–1999. Birth Defects Res A Clin Mol Teratol. 2004;70: 201-7.
20. Gnann Jr JW. (2011). Antiviral therapy of varicella-zoster virus infections. [online] Available from https://www.ncbi.nlm.nih.gov/books/NBK47401/. [Last accessed January, 2025].
21. Brown NW, Parsons AP, Kam PC. Anesthetic considerations in a parturient with varicella presenting for Caesarean section. Anesthesia. 2003;58:1092-5.

22. Health Protection Agency. Guidance on viral rash in pregnancy: investigation, diagnosis and management of viral rash illness, or exposure to viral rash illness, in pregnancy. London: Health Protection Agency; 2011.
23. Bertelli A, Carta V, Mangeri L, Caruso A, De Francesco MA. Varicella-Zoster virus prevalence among pregnant women: A European epidemiological review. Life. 2023;13(2):593.

11.4 Vulvovaginal Candidiasis

Diksha Goyal, Sanjeev Gupta, Gagandeep Kaur

INTRODUCTION

Vulvovaginal candidiasis (VVC) is a common and often difficult condition that many women experience during pregnancy. This yeast infection primarily affects the vagina but can also spread to the labia minora, labia majora, and occasionally the perianal region. The physiological changes that occur during pregnancy, particularly in the second and third trimesters, increase the risk of developing VVC. Often overlooked by women, this can lead to delays in diagnosis and treatment, complicating the condition further.

EPIDEMIOLOGY

Approximately 75% of pregnant women experience at least one episode of vaginal candidiasis, with recurrence occurring in about 50% of these cases. *Candida* species are present as commensals in 25–50% of healthy women. Vaginal candidiasis is more common among young adults, particularly those between 20–25 years of age, an early reproductive stage. Recurrent vulvovaginal candidiasis (RVVC) is defined as three or more symptomatic episodes within a 12-month period, affecting approximately 138 million women worldwide annually.

A study by Fardiazar et al. found a statistically significant increase in RVVC during the second and third trimesters of pregnancy. Among all *Candida* species, *Candida albicans* is the most common cause, responsible for 85–95% of cases. *C. glabrata* is the second leading cause of VVC (~8% of cases). Other candidal species such *Candida tropicalis, Candida krusei,* and *Candida parapsilosis* are implicated. Rarely, *Saccharomyces cerevisiae* can cause vulvo-vaginitis, though it typically presents with milder clinical signs and symptoms.

- Vulvovaginal candidiasis is a common infection of vagina and adjoining structures.
- Risk increases in pregnancy.
- *Candida albicans* is the most common cause followed by *C. glabrata*.

PREDISPOSING FACTORS

Several factors contribute to the development of VVC during pregnancy:

- *Hormonal changes*: Elevated estrogen levels during pregnancy enhance yeast adherence to the vaginal mucosal epithelium and promote hyphal formation through the activation of cytoplasmic estrogen receptors. This explains the increased risk of VVC in women of childbearing age.

- *Weakened immune system*: During pregnancy, the immune response shifts from Th1 to Th2 dominance, resulting in decreased cell-mediated immunity. Higher levels of interleukin-4 (IL-4), IL-5, and IL-13 further contribute to the recurrence of VVC by weakening the body's ability to combat the infection.
- *Acidic pH*: While a low pH generally inhibits the growth of many pathogens, some *Candida* species thrive in acidic environments.
- *Increased vaginal discharge*: Increased vaginal mucosal glycogen production of pregnancy can create moist and favorable environment.
- *Use of antibiotics*: Prolong use of antibiotics can disrupt the natural balance of beneficial *Lactobacillus* species, microflora in the vagina, allowing *Candida* infection.
- *Diabetes*: Elevated levels of glucose provide ideal environment for fungal growth.
- *Tight clothing*: Tight clothing can trap moisture and heat, creates conditions favorable for yeast growth.
- *Poor hygiene*: Inadequate hygiene and use of scented products can increase the risk of yeast infection during pregnancy.

Increased risk of vulvovaginal candidiasis in pregnancy:
- *Hormonal changes*: Gestational diabetes
- *Immunomodulation*: Tight clothing
- *Altered vaginal pH*: Decreased ability to maintain genital hygiene
- Increased glycogen

Key stages and factors involved in VVC development:

Colonization:
- *Candida albicans* is a commensal in vagina. However, when the balance of the vaginal environment is disrupted, *Candida* shows transition from a harmless commensal (yeast form) to a pathogenic (hyphal) form.
- Factors such as antibiotics use, hormonal changes (e.g., during pregnancy or oral contraceptive use), diabetes, or immunosuppression can lead to an overgrowth of *Candida*.

Adhesion and invasion:
- Hyphae can invade epithelial cells and trigger an immune response.
- Hyphal cells produce virulence factors, such as secreted aspartyl proteinases (SAPs), phospholipases, and mannoproteins which degrade host tissues and enhance fungal adhesion and invasion.
- The adhesion of *Candida* to vaginal epithelial cells is a critical step in pathogenesis. Specific adhesions on the fungal cell surface, such as ALS (agglutinin-like sequence) proteins, facilitate binding to host tissues.
- After adhering, *Candida* invades epithelial cells either through direct penetration or by inducing the host cells to take up the fungus. The hyphal form is particularly important in this invasive process.

Evasion of host defenses:
- *Candida* employs several strategies to evade the host immune response. These include altering its cell wall components to avoid detection by immune cells and secreting enzymes that degrade host immune molecules.
- Additionally, *Candida* biofilm formation provides a protective niche that enhances resistance to immune attack and antifungal treatments.

Inflammatory response:
- Vaginal epithelial cells recognize *Candida* through pattern recognition receptors (PRRs), such as toll-like receptors (TLRs) and dectin-1, leading to the activation of immune signaling pathways.
- Inflammasome receptors have important role in the acute infection. These are activated by the inflammatory factors and fungal components such as glucan, chitin, and mannan. Fungal components bind to macrophage receptors which lead to activation of innate immunity and inflammasomes, particularly NLRP3. NLRP3 plays a crucial role in the pathogenesis of VVC.
- The immune response includes the release of proinflammatory cytokines [e.g., IL-1β, IL-6, and tumor necrosis factor-α (TNF-α)], recruitment of neutrophils, and production of antimicrobial peptides.
- In symptomatic VVC, this immune response leads to inflammation, which manifests as the characteristic signs of infection—itching, redness, swelling, and discharge.
- Candidalysin is a secreted cytolytic peptide toxin and plays role in the initiating infection from the hyphal form. Candidalysin plays a pivotal role in the pathogenesis of *Candida albicans* infections by damaging host epithelial cells, triggering an immune response, and contributing to tissue inflammation. It also helps in formation of biofilm. Its dual role in promoting fungal invasion and modulating host defenses makes it a critical factor in both acute and chronic forms of candidiasis. It induces a dysfunctional immune response which is not protective despite of recruitment of large number of neutrophils. To modulate inflammatory response, neutralization of candidalysin plays a crucial role in the therapeutic strategy and prevention from vaginal candidiasis.
- Hyperglycemia favors adhesions and proliferation of *Candida* species. It increases the expression of C3 fungal receptors and growth of biofilm in glucose concentration of >200–240 mg/dL.

Recurrent and chronic VVC:
- Recurrent vulvovaginal candidiasis occurs in some women and is associated with various factors, including genetic predispositions, impaired immune responses, or persistent disruption of the vaginal microbiome.
- Chronic infections may also be associated with biofilm formation, which makes the infection more resistant to antifungal therapies.

A biofilm is characterized as a complex, multicellular, and multilayered three-dimensional structure where cells are encased in an extracellular matrix (ECM), perform specialized functions, and interact with one another. *Candida albicans* and other species have the ability to make biofilms, hence fungus produces a protective environment to which antimicrobials are not able to penetrate and they remain adhered to the vaginal epithelium. There are two types of biofilm involved to cause VVC—abiotic biofilms and biotic films. Abiotic films require a substrate (plastic or metal), such as intrauterine devices which are placed for contraception. Biotic film utilizes the vaginal epithelium and provides the favorable conditions for formation of persister cells, which can cause antifungal resistance.

Polymicrobial biofilms: In some cases, *Candida* can form biofilms alongside bacteria, which can further complicate treatment due to the mixed microbial environment.

CLINICAL FEATURES

- Itching and irritation
- *Burning sensation*: Burning sensation can occur particularly during urination or intercourse.
- *Discharge*: Thick, white, and odorless vaginal discharge (consisting of sloughed epithelium, immune cells, yeast, and vaginal fluid)
- *Redness and swelling*: Redness, swelling, and inflammation of the vulva and vaginal tissues
- Soreness and pain

CLASSIFICATION OF VULVOVAGINAL CANDIDIASIS

Classification of vulvovaginal candidiasis is described in **Table 1**.

COMPLICATIONS

- Premature rupture of membrane
- Preterm labor
- Chorioamnionitis

TABLE 1: Classification of vulvovaginal candidiasis (VVC).

Uncomplicated	Complicated
Sporadic or infrequent	Recurrent (three or more episodes of symptomatic VVC in <1 year)
Mild to moderate	Severe
Likely to be *Candida albicans*	Non-*albicans* candidiasis
Immunocompetent	Women with diabetes, or immunocompromising conditions (e.g., HIV, pregnancy), or immunosuppressive therapy

Source: Sobel JD, Faro S, Force RW, Foxman B, Ledger WJ, Nyirjesy PR, et al. Vulvovaginal candidiasis: epidemiologic, diagnostic, and therapeutic considerations. Am J Obstet Gynecol. 1998;178:203-11.

IMPACT ON NEWBORN

- *Preterm birth*: Roberts et al. studied pregnant women of <20 weeks of gestation who were asymptomatic and *Candida* culture positive. They found increased rate of preterm birth in untreated asymptomatic women as compared to those without candidiasis (6.25 vs. 2.99%). There was decrease of preterm birth in the women treated with topical therapy. It can occur spontaneously following premature rupture of amniotic membranes or induced labor due to detection of infection. There is a high risk of mortality as compared to those born full-term. There is potential risk to various organs such as central nervous system, cardiovascular system, and lungs.

  Inflammatory cascade stimulation in the amniotic cavity involves proinflammatory cytokines, chemokine and prostaglandins contribute for cervical maturation and induction of contractions.
- *Fetal growth restriction*: Growth restriction can be the adverse outcome of intrauterine inflammation.
- *Vertical and horizontal transmission*: Neonate can get *Candida* species infection through either vertical transmission or horizontal transmission during perinatal period. Vertical transmission can take place through mother colonized with *Candida* infection via hematogenous dissemination from mother to fetus, direct invasion of membranes or ascending infection after spontaneous rupture of membranes. Studies have shown detection of *Candida albicans* in 33% of preterm infants born to mother with VVC.

  In case of horizontal transmission, neonate can acquire infection through parents colonized with *Candida* species, nursery and healthcare workers such as neonatal intensive care unit. Most common mode of infection is neonatal intensive care unit.
- *Congenital cutaneous candidiasis (CCC)*: CCC is a very rare condition which can occur in both term and preterm infants. It can occur in utero or during the passage through birth canal due to contact of the fetus with infected maternal fluids or mucosa which can result in systemic infection.

  Vulvovaginal candidiasis, premature rupture of membrane, chorioamnionitis, cervical cerclage suture, and intrauterine foreign bodies are the risk factors for CCC. It is difficult to diagnose and may go unnoticed.

  Clinical features include widespread maculopapular rash with desquamation which can resemble staphylococcal scalded skin syndrome. Other features include pustules, cracking skin, funisitis, diffuse erythema, desquamation, abscess, and yellow plaques secretion in placental infection. Preterm infants are more prone for fluid and electrolyte imbalance and end-organ dissemination such as meningitis, bronchopneumonia, arthritis, and endocarditis. It leads to very high mortality in infants.

  Candida albicans is the most common isolate from blood, skin, and cerebrospinal fluid culture. Treatment includes administration of intravenous amphotericin B deoxycholate at a dosage of 1 mg/kg daily as initial therapy. Fluconazole can be used if no prior exposure. Duration of treatment should not be <20 days and it should be extended by 2 weeks after culture negativity.

DIAGNOSIS

A diagnosis of VVC involves clinical features such as presence of external dysuria, vulval pruritus, pain, swelling, and redness. Pruritus without discharge is the most specific symptom of VVC. Examination findings include vulvar edema, fissures, excoriations, and thick curdy vaginal discharge.

Wet saline mount [10% potassium hydroxide (KOH)] of vaginal discharge demonstrates budding yeasts, hyphae, or pseudohyphae **(Fig. 1)**. KOH enhances visualization of yeast and mycelia by lysis of cellular material that obscure the yeast or pseudohyphae.

Potassium hydroxide should be done in all the symptomatic women in VVC, not only to diagnose VVC but also to look for mixed infection. A 10% KOH wet mount has high sensitivity for germinating yeast, around 90%. Positive results in KOH indicate high yeast concentration in vaginal secretions and severity of signs and symptoms. Large number of white cells indicate mixed infection as these are absent in VVC. Women with positive results should be treated.

Vaginal pH remains normal in VVC (4.0–4.5). If vaginal pH test shows the value of >5.0, we should suspect bacterial vaginosis, trichomoniasis, or a mixed infection.

Fungal culture is the most sensitive and specific method for the diagnosis of VVC **(Fig. 2)**. It should be performed in symptomatic women with negative KOH wet mount microscopy and normal vaginal pH. Routine cultures are not required for the diagnosis of VVC. If fungal culture is not feasible then empiric treatment can be given. Identification of candidiasis by culture in asymptomatic women is not recommended because 10–15% of the women harbor *Candida* species in vaginal mucosa.

Polymerase chain reaction (PCR) test can be done to detect *Candida* species but not readily available.

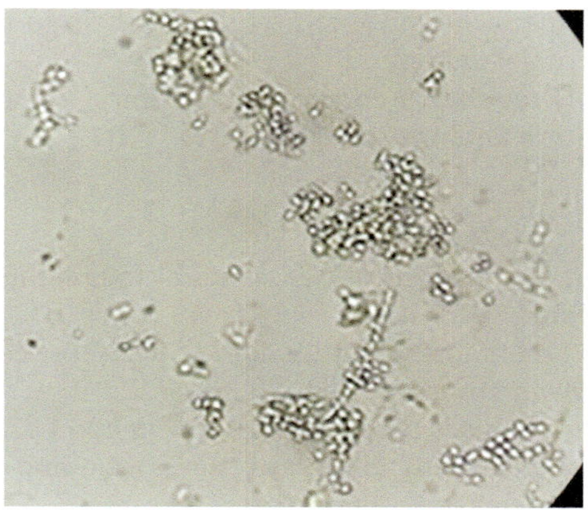

FIG. 1: KOH mount displaying pseudohyphae and budding yeast.
(KOH: potassium hydroxide)

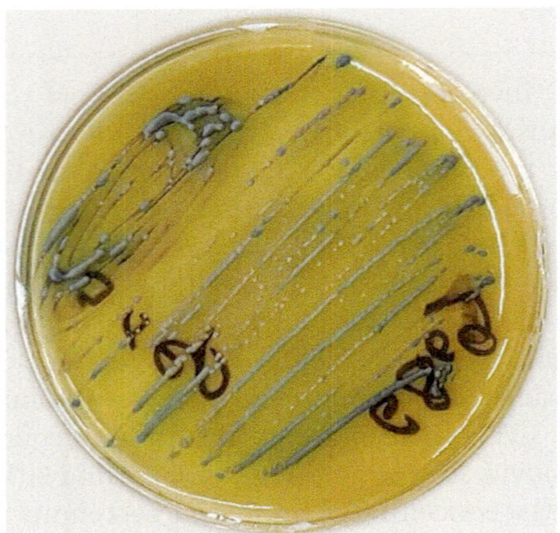

FIG. 2: HiCrome culture agar with colored colonies of *Candida albicans*.

TABLE 2: Quantitative method for diagnosing vulvovaginal candidiasis.

Variable parameter	Minimal score	Maximum score	Extent	Points
Growth on CHROMagar *Candida*	0	5		
Average number of yeasts in direct microscopy (at least 10 fields, 1,000×)	0	2	0–1 (0 point) 2–3 (1 point) ≥4+ (2 point)	0 1 2
Pruritus	0	2		
Vaginal discharge	0	1		
Total	0	10		

Immunochromatography is a sensitive and specific test for rapid diagnosis of VVC. It is easy to perform and interpret. It may help in timely initiation of appropriate antimicrobial therapy.

Diagnosis of VVC requires a correlation of clinical symptoms, wet mount microscopy, and culture findings.

Quantitative Method

Quantitative method for diagnosis of VVC contains four components, combined into three criteria **(Table 2)**.

- *Clinical criteria*: It contains the evaluation of two most common symptoms (vaginal discharge and pruritus).
- *Microscopic criteria*: This is based on Gram-stain and Lőffler stained vaginal smears estimate average number of blastospores (budding yeasts and mycelial elements) per visual field.
- *Cultural criteria*: It is based on fungal culture using CHROMagar. Less than 10 CFU is given 0 point.

If there are 10-100 CFU it is considered as a moderate growth and is given 5 points.

Interpretation

- *Total score*: 0–5 points—lack of VVC
- *Total score*: 6–10—presence of VVC
- *Sensitivity*: 71%, *specificity*: 98%

Differential Diagnosis

- Trichomoniasis
- Bacterial vaginosis
- Unrecognized genital herpes
- Hypersensitivity
- Irritant vulvovaginitis
- Allergic vulvovaginitis
- Physiological leukorrhea
- Idiopathic focal vulvar vestibulitis

TREATMENT

Majority suggest that it is unnecessary to treat asymptomatic healthy female with vaginal colonization. In Germany, it is recommended to screen for vaginal candidal colonization in third trimester of pregnancy. It results in significant reduction in congenital *Candida* colonization after maternal treatment.

Treatment for vaginal candidiasis during pregnancy typically involves topical antifungal agents. Oral antifungal medications should be avoided during pregnancy due to potential risk to the developing fetus.

According to Cochrane review (2001) for topical therapy in vaginal candidiasis, imidazoles were more effective than nystatin.

Oral fluconazole might cause spontaneous abortion or congenital anomalies, so it should be avoided in case of pregnant women.

Short-course topical antifungal drugs can treat uncomplicated VVC effectively **(Table 3)**.

TABLE 3: Topical treatment for vulvovaginal candidiasis.

Over the counter (OTC) topical agents	Prescription-based topical agents
Cream clotrimazole (1%) 5 g daily for 7–14 days	Cream butoconazole (2%) 5 g single application
Cream clotrimazole (2%) 5 g daily for 3 days	Cream terconazole (0.4%) 5 g daily for 7 days
Cream miconazole (2%) 5 g daily for 7 days	Cream terconazole (0.8%) daily for 3 days
Cream miconazole (4%) 5 g daily for 3 days	Vaginal suppository terconazole 80 mg daily for 3 days
• Vaginal suppository miconazole 100 mg daily for 7 days • Vaginal suppository miconazole 200 mg daily for 3 days • Vaginal suppository miconazole 1,200 mg for 1 day	
Ointment tioconazole (6.5%) 5 g, single application	

Non-albicans Vulvovaginal Candidiasis

Specific therapy for non-albicans VVC is no specific, longer duration of therapy for around 7–14 days with nonfluconazole agents might benefit these patents.

Follow-up

According to CDC guidelines 2021, follow-up is not recommended. In case of recurrent and persistent symptoms, follow-up visits are required.

SUGGESTED READINGS

1. Cole AM. Innate host defense of human vaginal and cervical mucosae. Curr Top Microbiol Immunol. 2006;306:199-230.
2. Yano J, Sobel JD, Myirjesy P, Sobel R, Williams VL, Yu Q, et al. Current patient perspectives of vulvovaginal candidiasis: Incidence, symptoms, management and post-treatment outcomes. BMC Womens Health. 2019;19:48.
3. He Y, Tang R, Deng J, Cai T, He P, Wu J, et al. Effects of oestrogen on vulvovaginal candidiasis. Mycoses. 2022;65:4-12.
4. Muzny CA, Schwebke JR. Biofilms: A Underappreciated Mechanism of Treatment Failure and Recurrence in Vaginal infections. Clin Infect Dis. 2015;61:601-6.
5. Wu X, Zhang S, Xu X, Shen L, Xu B, Qu W, et al. RAFT-Derived Polymethacrylates as a Superior Treatment for Recurrent Vulvovaginal Candidiasis by Targeting Biotic Biofilms and Persister Cells. Front Microbiol. 2019;10:2592.
6. Cunha C, Carvalho A, Esposito A, Bistoni F, Romani L. DAMP signalling in fungal infections and diseases. Front Immunol. 2012;3:286.
7. Camilli G, Tabouret G, Quintin J. The complexity of Fungal beta-Glucan in Health and Disease: Effects on mononuclear phagocyte system. Front Immunol. 2018;9:343771.
8. Kalkanci A, Güzel AB, Jabban II, Aydin M, Ilkit M, Kuştimur S. *Candida* vaginitis in non-pregnant patients: A study of antifungal susceptibility testing and virulence factors. J Obstet Gynaecol. 2013;33:378-83.
9. Willems HME, Ahmed SS, Liu J, Xu Z, Peters BM. Vulvovaginal Candidiasis: A Current Understanding and Burning Questions. J Fungi. 2020;6:27.
10. Richardson JP, Willems HME, Moyes DL, Shoaie S, Barker KS, Tan SL, et al. Candidalysin Drives Epithelial Signaling, Neutrophil Recruitment, and Immunopathology at the Vaginal Mucosa. Infect Immun. 2018;86:e00645-17.
11. Romero R, Espinoza J, Kusanovic J, Gotsch F, Hassan S, Erez O, et al. The preterm parturition syndrome. BJOG An Int J Obstet Gynaecol. 2006;11(Suppl. S3):17-42.
12. MacIntyre DA, Sykes L, Teoh TG, Bennett PR. Prevention of preterm labour via the modulation of inflammatory pathways. J Matern Neonatal Med. 2012;25 (Suppl. S1):17-20.
13. Al-Azemi M, Raghupathy R, Azizieh F. Pro-inflammatory and anti-inflammatory cytokine profiles in fetal growth restriction. Clin Exp Obstet Gynecol. 2017;44:98-103.
14. Sánchez-Padilla AP, Valencia-Herrera AM, Toledo-Bahena ME, Mena-Cedillos CA, Duarte-Abdala M, Salazar-García M, et al. Congenital Cutaneous Candidiasis: Uncommon Entity or Underdiagnosed? Curr Fungal Infect Rep. 2019;13:175-80.
15. Kaufman DA, Coggins SA, Zanelli SA, Weitkamp JH. Congenital Cutaneous Candidiasis: Prompt Systemic Treatment Is Associated with Improved Outcomes in Neonates. Clin Infect Dis. 2017;64:1387-95.
16. Zhao Y, Yu Z, Yue X. Evaluating the accuracy and diagnostic value of CFW and a new fluorescent reagent, fluorescent brightener 85, for the diagnosis of vulvovaginal candidiasis. J Clin Lab Anal. 2021;35(8):e23891.

11.5 Pyogenic Infections

Parul Verma, Divya Seshadri

INTRODUCTION

Pyogenic infections of the skin and its appendages are caused mainly by two gram-positive cocci, viz., staphylococci and streptococci. The pregnant females are no exception and may be sometimes more prone in view of changing hormonal and immunological profile The various types of cutaneous infections caused by these two bacteria are listed in **Table 1**.

They can also be classified as purulent and nonpurulent infections. Staphylococci being common cause of purulent infections and nonpurulent infections are more often caused by streptococci. However, there is a degree of overlap and staphylococci are also fairly frequently implicated in nonpurulent infections too. **Table 2** shows some salient points about the two bacteria.

IMPETIGO

This superficial skin infection can be of two types, i.e., nonbullous impetigo (or impetigo contagiosa of Tilbury Fox) and bullous impetigo. **Table 3** compares and contrasts these two entities.

TABLE 1: Cutaneous infections caused by staphylococci and streptococci.

	Direct infection of skin	Bacterial toxin related skin disease
Staphylococcus	• Impetigo • Ecthyma • Folliculitis • Sycosis • Abscess • Furunculosis • Carbuncle • Cellulitis (occasional) • Acute paronychia • Botryomycosis	• Staphylococcal scalded skin syndrome (SSSS) • Toxic shock syndrome (TSS) • Recurrent toxin-mediated perineal erythema • Staphylococcal scarletina
Streptococcus	• Impetigo • Ecthyma • Erysipelas • Cellulitis • Perineal streptococcal dermatitis • Streptococcal intertrigo • Blistering distal dactylitis	• Scarlet fever • Toxic shock-like syndrome • Recurrent toxin-mediated perineal erythema

TABLE 2: Salient points about staphylococci and streptococci.

	Staphylococcus	***Streptococcus***
Arrangement	Clusters resembling grapes	In chains
Species causing majority of human skin infections	*Staphylococcus aureus*	*Streptococcus pyogenes* (group A *Streptococcus* or GAS)
Other species of note		Group B *Streptococcus* (*Streptococcus agalactiae*) colonizes the vagina, gastrointestinal tract, and the upper respiratory tract. It rarely causes skin and soft tissue infections (mainly in the elderly/ immunocompromised), but it is a leading cause of postpartum infection and neonatal sepsis. Screening by vaginal and anal swabs is recommended for pregnant women between 36 and 37 weeks
Carriage	• 20% of general population persistent carriers in nares > perineum, vagina > axillae, toe webs • 30% of population are intermittent carriers • About 2% of adults carry methicillin-resistant *Staphylococcus aureus* (MRSA); a similar rate (2.1%) was found in a small study of pregnant women admitted for delivery	10% of general population carry *S. pyogenes* in the throat
Toxins/proteins produced	• Exfoliative toxin-A (ET-A) • Exfoliative toxin-B (ET-B) • Toxic shock syndrome toxin (TSST-1) • Panton-valentine leukocidin (causes neutrophil lysis)	• Pyrogenic exotoxins, streptolysins, streptokinase, and several other enzymes • Antistreptolysin O (ASO) titer is a marker of previous streptococcal infection. A fourfold rise in titer on paired serum samples 7–14 days apart indicates an acute infection. Antibodies to deoxyribonuclease (DNase) B and to hyaluronidase are more often raised
Penicillin responsiveness	• Produces penicillinase which makes it resistant to penicillin • MRSA is resistant to all beta-lactam antibiotics other than penicillin too	• Uniformly susceptible to penicillin • But reports of resistance are on the rise

TABLE 3: Nonbullous and bullous impetigo.

	Nonbullous impetigo	Bullous impetigo
Etiology	In the past, usually caused by streptococci; now, most cases caused by *Staphylococcus aureus* but sometimes by streptococci or by a combination of both bacteria	Almost always caused by *Staphylococcus aureus*. It can also be regarded as localized staphylococcal scalded skin syndrome (SSSS)
Pathogenesis	• Direct skin infection by the bacteria • Usually develops following bruising, abrasions, minor trauma, insect bites, or maceration • When it is superimposed on lesions of preexisting dermatoses such as eczema, scabies, or pediculosis, it is termed impetiginization	• Toxin-mediated • Exfoliative toxins A and B produced by *S. aureus* are trypsin-like serine proteases and cleave desmoglein-1 in the stratum granulosum. Additionally, the toxins act as superantigens, stimulating B and T cell proliferation • Lesions are localized as production of the toxin is local (unlike in SSSS where it is disseminated hematogenously). Cultured from blister fluid can yield *S. aureus*
Epidemiology	• ¾ of all cases of impetigo • Most common pediatric skin infection; also affects adults including pregnant women, especially those living in crowded circumstances and in occupations involving bruising such as sportspersons and military personnel • Most frequent in late summer • Can cause epidemics • Highly contagious • Spreads by direct contact and through fomites	• ¼ of cases of impetigo • Most common in children between 2 and 5 years old but adult cases are perhaps under-reported • Can affect pregnant women in any trimester • Some authorities recommend human immunodeficiency virus (HIV) screening in adults with bullous impetigo • Neonatal bullous impetigo (earlier pemphigus neonatorum) usually starts after the second week of life. Rarely, it can present at birth, in case of premature rupture of membranes • Not so contagious; more sporadic

Continued

Continued

	Nonbullous impetigo	**Bullous impetigo**
Clinical features: • Morphology • Distribution • Regional lymphadenopathy • Fever	• Transient initial thin walled vesicle on erythematous base • Rapidly ruptures leaving superficial purulent erosion • Dries up forming adherent, honey-colored "glued-on cornflakes" crusts • Lesions are 1–2 cm in size and grow centrifugally; asymptomatic or mildly itchy • Satellite lesions are caused by self-inoculation; scratching can produce linearly distributed lesions • Predominantly involves exposed areas, i.e., the limbs and face, particularly perioral and perinasal areas • Common • Rare	• Vesicles can enlarge up to 1–2 cm in size and remain for 2–3 days • Initially clear blister fluid later turns purulent • As the blister roof ruptures an erythematous moist base, covered with brownish crusts is visible; the remainder of the roof is seen as a peripheral collarette • There is confluence of lesions with peripheral extension resulting in circinate and polycyclic figures • Intertriginous regions, such as the diaper area, axillae, and neck are frequently involved • Face usually spared, but any area can be involved, including palms and soles and even buccal mucosa • Rare • More common

Continued

Continued

	Nonbullous impetigo	Bullous impetigo
Differential diagnosis	• Herpes simplex • Scabies • Pemphigus foliaceus • These conditions can all be impetiginized, thereby further confounding the picture	• Herpes simplex • Bullous tinea • Bullous insect bite hypersensitivity • Pemphigus vulgaris • Linear immunoglobulin A (IgA) dermatosis • In pregnant women, it needs to be distinguished from other blistering dermatoses including impetigo herpetiformis (misnomer, refers to pustular psoriasis of pregnancy), pemphigoid gestationis, other autoimmune blistering disorders, herpes simplex, contact dermatitis, and so on
Complications	• SSSS is a rare complication seen in the staphylococcal form • Cellulitis can occur in the streptococcal from, especially with concomitant malnutrition or underlying systemic disease • Other rare complications include sepsis, arthritis, endocarditis, pneumonia, lymphangitis or lymphadenitis, guttate psoriasis, and toxic shock syndrome • When the "danger area of the face" is involved there is risk of cavernous sinus thrombosis • Acute post-streptococcal glomerulonephritis (PSGN) affects 1–5% of cases of nonbullous impetigo. It depends on the infecting strain and is seen in up to 25% of infections due to *S. pyogenes*, type M-49. For pyoderma, the latent period for development of nephritis is 18–21 days (about 10 days for throat infections). Unfortunately prompt antibiotic treatment of streptococcal impetigo may not prevent this serious complication • Generally rheumatic fever is not a complication of streptococcal impetigo	

Management of Nonbullous and Bullous Impetigo

Investigations

Investigations are not routinely warranted; the diagnosis is mainly clinical. Gram staining can differentiate *Staphylococcus* from *Streptococcus*. Pus culture and sensitivity may be done if methicillin-resistant *Staphylococcus aureus* (MRSA) is suspected or in recurrent or resistant cases.

Treatment

Supportive Care

Daily with soap and warm water cleaning is advised to keep area clean. Regular soap is preferable over the so-called antiseptic soap; soaps containing triclosan or triclocarban are best avoided in pregnancy. Crusts should be removed gently after softening with an emollient and topical medications are best applied after crust removal. Touching the area or picking at scabs should be avoided because it can spread the infection. Strict hygiene helps prevent familial transmission. Any underlying problem such as scabies, pediculosis, or eczema is to be treated so that the impetigo does not recur.

Medication

Topical Therapy

Topical antibiotics are the preferred treatment for localized uncomplicated nonbullous impetigo. Mupirocin, fusidic acid, and retapamulin are effective against *Staphylococcus* as well as *Streptococcus*.

The Infectious Diseases Society of America (IDSA) recommends mupirocin and retapamulin as first-line therapy for impetigo. In pregnant women, the topical agent of choice is mupirocin. Mupirocin (pregnancy category B) has very minimal systemic absorption. However, it should not be used in extensive areas or in burns patients, especially with renal impairment, because absorption of the polyethylene glycol vehicle can cause nephrotoxicity.

Mupirocin resistance in methicillin-susceptible *Staphylococcus aureus* (MSSA) and MRSA is on the rise as a result of injudicious use. Moreover, high-level mupirocin strains are also more likely to be resistant to fusidic acid.

Fusidic acid (pregnancy category C) is not recommended by the IDSA and is not available in USA but is widely used in other countries including India. A 2012 Cochrane review put fusidic acid at par with mupirocin for treatment of impetigo. It is also a favored agent to treat infected eczema in combination preparations containing topical steroids. Fusidic acid may cause kernicterus in neonates by displacing bilirubin from plasma albumin, hence it is preferably avoided during the last month of pregnancy.

Retapamulin (pregnancy category B) is recommended by IDSA as a first-line topical agent to treat impetigo but it is preferably avoided in pregnancy because it is a relatively new agent and adequate data is lacking.

Systemic Therapy

Systemic antibiotics are indicated for all cases of bullous impetigo and cases of nonbullous impetigo having more than five lesions, deep tissue involvement, systemic signs of infection, lymph node enlargement, lesions in the oral cavity, infections on the scalp, and if there is suspicion of infection with a nephritogenic strain of *Streptococcus*.

Antibiotic therapy ideally should be guided by culture and sensitivity results. Antibiotics active against staphylococci and streptococci should be used in case of empirical therapy. The IDSA guidelines recommend a 7-day course of an agent active against *S. aureus* unless cultures yield streptococci alone, in which case oral penicillin is the recommended agent. They recommend dicloxacillin or cephalexin as first-line agents. Other effective agents include cloxacillin and amoxicillin-clavulanate. Dicloxacillin, cloxacillin, cephalexin, amoxicillin-clavulanic acid and penicillin are all safe for use in pregnant women and are all pregnancy category B (see **Table 4** for dosage). Erythromycin, though category B is a bit controversial in the first trimester due to some reports of linkage to cardiovascular malformations and pyloric stenosis. Moreover, the estolate salt has been associated with elevated liver function tests in the second trimester and should not be used.

Management of Difficult/Recurrent Cases and Prevention

For resistant cases, it helps to take skin swabs to confirm that bacteria are sensitive to the prescribed antibiotics. When MRSA is suspected or confirmed, IDSA recommends treatment with doxycycline, clindamycin, or sulfamethoxazole-trimethoprim. For pregnant women, clindamycin (pregnancy category B) is the treatment of choice (see **Table 4** for dosage).

If there are frequent recurrences of impetigo, the patient should be evaluated for the presence of staphylococcal carrier state and decolonized. A systematic review concluded that short-term nasal application of "mupirocin is the most effective treatment for eradicating MRSA or MSSA carriage, having a

TABLE 4: Oral antibiotics for impetigo and ecthyma.*

Agents covering MSSA + streptococci	FDA pregnancy category	Adult dosage
Dicloxacillin	B	250 mg QID
Cloxacillin	B	500 mg QID
Cephalexin	B	250 mg QID
Erythromycin stearate	B	250 mg QID
Clindamycin	B	300–400 mg QID
Amoxicillin-clavulanate	B	625 mg TDS
If MRSA suspected or confirmed		
Clindamycin	B	300–400 mg QID
Cotrimoxazole	C	2 DS tabs BD
Linezolid	C	600 mg BD

*The same agents are also used for predominantly staphylococcal cutaneous infections, viz., folliculitis, furuncles, carbuncles, and abscess.

(FDA: Food and Drug Administration; MSSA: methicillin-susceptible *Staphylococcus aureus*)

success of rate of 90%, after 1 week, and approximately 60% after a longer follow-up". The IDSA guidelines recommend nasal decolonization with mupirocin twice daily to both nares for 5 days. For pregnant women too, this is the treatment of choice to eliminate staphylococcal carriage.

Zinc supplementation during the last two trimesters of pregnancy reduces the frequency and duration of impetigo in infants, particularly in those of low birth weight.

Staphylococcal Scalded Skin Syndrome (Ritter Disease)

Etiopathogenesis

About 5% of *S. aureus* strains produce exfoliative toxins (ETs) which can cause staphylococcal scalded skin syndrome (SSSS). The pathogenesis is similar to that of bullous impetigo (discussed earlier). In SSSS, hematogenous dissemination of the staphylococcal ET is there. Exfoliative toxin-A (ET-A) is more often associated with bullous impetigo, whereas Exfoliative toxin-B (ET-B) is more often associated with SSSS.

Epidemiology

It is most commonly seen in children below 6 years of age and in neonates. Adults including pregnant women may also be affected, particularly in the setting of renal failure and immunosuppression. The immunomodulation occurring in pregnancy is believed to be contributory to development of SSSS.

Clinical Features

Localized staphylococcal infection either in the skin or other sites otitis, conjunctivitis, pneumonia, or urinary tract infection can act as trigger. A few days later, a fever, malaise and skin tenderness develops. Subsequently, faint, erythematous, tender patches develop, which coalesce into a widespread eruption. Fragile bullae develop within the erythematous areas followed by epidermal detachment in large sheets, leaving painful moist, raw, red areas that appear scalded. Nikolsky's sign (skin erosion upon tangential pressure) is positive.

There are two clinical variants, i.e., generalized and localized SSSS. Localized SSSS favors the flexures, especially the axillae, groin, and limb flexures.

Within 24 hours after skin peeling, the involved areas dry up forming thin, shiny crusts, and fissures. There is usually a second period of desquamation during the next 10 days. Within 2 weeks the skin generally heals without scarring.

Complications

When the skin is denuded, complications can ensue, such as fluid and electrolyte imbalances, temperature dysregulation, and secondary infections, which require careful and prompt management. The prognosis of SSSS is usually good in children, but more guarded in infants and poor in adults. The mortality rate is below 5% in treated children; in adults it is much higher, up to 63%, possibly due to the underlying comorbidities.

Diagnosis and Investigations

The diagnosis is usually made on clinical grounds. The important differential is toxic epidermal necrolysis (TEN). In SSSS, there is more superficial skin peeling and lack of mucosal lesions. If in doubt, a skin biopsy may be taken. In SSSS superficial intraepidermal separation beneath the stratum corneum is seen. Both TEN and SSSS lack inflammation, but SSSS does not show the full thickness epidermal necrosis characteristic of TEN.

As the blisters are toxin mediated swabs and cultures of blister fluid do not usually grow the staphylococci unlike bullous impetigo. Original septic site culture may isolate the staphylococci.

Management

Management of SSSS is mentioned in **Box 1**.

ECTHYMA

Ecthyma is a cutaneous bacterial infection that extends into the dermis (deeper than impetigo) and heals with scarring. Ecthyma gangrenosum is a more severe variant of ecthyma which results from bacterial invasion of the blood vessel walls in the skin and subcutaneous tissue. The differences between the two are highlighted in **Table 5**.

BOX 1 Management of staphylococcal scalded skin syndrome (SSSS).

Supportive care:

- Admit the patient preferably to intensive care or burns unit
- Closely monitor temperature, hemodynamics, and electrolytes
- Contact precautions, barrier nursing, and nutritional support
- Paracetamol ± opioids for analgesia; avoid nonsteroidal anti-inflammatory drugs (NSAIDs)

Skin care:

- Liberal application of bland emollients (like petroleum jelly) or wrap the skin with paraffin-coated gauze
- Gentle cleansing. During sponging or bathing, removal of dried skin need not be done when the skin is very tender but should be done gently later on
- Antiseptics? Topical antibiotics?
    - When there are large areas of denuded skin, avoid Betadine and silver sulfadiazine due to risk of systemic toxicity
    - Avoid extensive application of mupirocin due to the risk of nephrotoxicity (see section on impetigo treatment)
- Avoid topical steroids

Medication:

- Early administration of antibiotics improves the prognosis
- Empirical antibiotics include penicillinase-resistant penicillin, first- or second-generation cephalosporins, and macrolides (all pregnancy category B) and adjust according to obtained culture sensitivity reports
- If no improvement, consider methicillin-resistant *Staphylococcus aureus* (MRSA) and switch to vancomycin (pregnancy category C) or clindamycin (pregnancy category B)

TABLE 5: Ecthyma and ecthyma gangrenosum, a comparison.

	Ecthyma	Ecthyma gangrenosum
Etiopathogenesis	Dermal invasion by streptococci and staphylococci, either alone or in combination	• Microbial invasion of blood vessel walls in the skin and subcutaneous tissue • Either invasion from within the vessel in case of septicemia or by direct inoculation through the skin • Classically caused by *Pseudomonas aeruginosa,* but can also be caused by • *Staphylococcus aureus, Streptococcus pyogenes,* fungi such as *Mucor*, *Candida,* and *Aspergillus,* and herpes simplex virus
Epidemiology—risk factors	• Poor hygiene, malnutrition, skin surface breach, and other dermatoses, like scabies • In Europe, mostly in children • In tropical climates, it is more common and occurs at any age	Occurs in the critically ill/immunocompromised/those with hematologic malignancies
Clinical features: • Morphology • Sites of involvement • Associated symptoms	• Initial lesion—erythematous plaque about 2–3 cm size • Develops overlying vesiculation or pustulation • Rapidly ruptures • Ulcer with indurated violaceous margins covered by hard, thick, and adherent crusts • Heals after a few weeks with scarring • Commonly feet, legs, thighs, and buttocks • Fever and lymphadenopathy	• Red patch in the skin, rapidly becomes pustular with perilesional erythema • Hemorrhagic blister forms in the center spreading peripherally • Finally gangrenous ulcer surrounded by red halo • Early lesion can rapidly form necrotic ulcer in under 12 hours • Commonly anogenital area, armpits • Usually critically ill patient
Differential diagnosis	• Arthropod bites • Stasis ulcers • Leishmaniasis • Atypical mycobacterial infection	• Vasculitis • Calciphylaxis • Pyoderma gangrenosum • Septic emboli • Disseminated intravascular coagulation
Investigations	• Clinical diagnosis • If needed, Gram-stain and culture of pus or exudates	Skin biopsy, tissue culture, blood cultures, and septic screen

Continued

Continued

	Ecthyma	Ecthyma gangrenosum
Treatment	• The Infectious Diseases Society of America (IDSA) recommends oral antibiotics effective against both staphylococci and streptococci • For pregnant women, options are dicloxacillin, cloxacillin, cephalexin, amoxicillin-clavulanic acid (all pregnancy category B)	• Send off cultures and start prompt treatment with broad-spectrum antibiotics with antipseudomonal activity • For pregnant women, initial empiric therapy with piperacillin/tazobactam or cephalosporin such as cefepime (both pregnancy category B) • Narrow down or switch antibiotic cover after culture results available

Erysipelas (Saint Anthony's Fire) and Cellulitis (Table 6)

These are diffuse spreading bacterial skin infections involving the dermis and subcutaneous tissues. Some authorities consider erysipelas it to be a superficial subtype of cellulitis while some consider both the terms to be synonymous.

Pregnancy is one of the predisposing factors for cellulitis due to the fact that it often leads to leg edema and also is an immunosuppressed state.

Treatment of Erysipelas and Cellulitis

The IDSA guidelines do not distinguish between erysipelas and nonpurulent cellulitis. A modified version of their guidelines as appropriate for pregnant women is presented in **Table 7**.

First-line therapy for nonpurulent erysipelas/cellulitis is an antimicrobial active against streptococci with/without coverage against MSSA. For mild cases, the recommended treatment duration is 5 days, but it should be extended if the infection has not resolved within this time period. For moderately severe infections with systemic symptoms, hospitalization and intravenous (IV) antibiotics are advisable. Empirical coverage for community-acquired MRSA is recommended in patients who do not respond to β-lactam therapy in 48–72 hours. Other scenarios which warrant MRSA coverage include presence of penetrating trauma, evidence of MRSA infection elsewhere, nasal colonization with MRSA and injection drug use.

In patients who have severe infections (failed oral antibiotic therapy, show severe systemic toxicity, are immunocompromised, or show signs of deeper infection), vancomycin plus either piperacillin-tazobactam or imipenem/meropenem is recommended as a broad-spectrum empirical regimen. In such patients, surgical inspection or debridement should also be seriously considered.

For purulent cellulitis, IDSA guidelines recommend empirical therapy for community-acquired MRSA and pending culture results. Treatment of severe infections is along the same lines as in severe nonpurulent cellulitis and the threshold for surgical intervention should be low.

TABLE 6: Erysipelas and cellulitis, a comparison.

	Erysipelas	**Cellulitis**
Etiology	• Almost always Streptococci • Group A beta-hemolytic *Streptococcus* is the most common etiologic agent	• Majority of cases caused by streptococci • However, *Staphylococcus aureus* can be causative too (purulent cellulitis)—classically in an open wound or postpenetrating trauma, or sites of illicit drug injection • *Haemophilus influenzae* is an important cause of facial cellulitis in children aged < 2 years • In immunocompromised person, other bacteria and fungi maybe the cause
Epidemiology—risk factors	Predisposing factors include wounds, fissured toe-web intertrigo, pressure ulcers, lymphedema, venous insufficiency, chronic edema (including that caused by pregnancy) local surgical operations, subclinical lymphatic dysfunction, obesity, diabetes mellitus, and history of previous cellulitis	
Depth of involvement	Dermis ± upper subcutis	Subcutis
Clinical features	• Single elevated, erythematous, warm, painful plaque, approximately 10–15 cm in its largest dimension • With a well-defined, raised clearly demarcated edge, which advances with disease progression • Skin surface have peau d'orange appearance due to superficial edema surrounding hair follicles which are tightly tethered to the dermis • Blistering is common and superficial hemorrhage in blister of skin may be seen • Commonly affected sites are the leg and the face • In newborns, the periumbilical area is often affected	• Recent onset of diffuse pain, redness, warmth, and swelling of the involved area • With poorly demarcated borders • There may be clear fluid filled blistering; petechiae and ecchymoses may result in hemorrhagic cellulitis • The most commonly affected site is the lower limbs. Upper limbs, trunk, perineum, or head and neck can be involved

Continued

Continued

<table>
<tr><th></th><th>Erysipelas</th><th>Cellulitis</th></tr>
<tr><td>Acute complications</td><td>• Associated lymphangitis and lymphadenopathy are more frequent than in cellulitis
• Systemic symptoms such as fever, malaise, and vomiting can be quite severe</td><td>• Abscesses, necrosis, fasciitis, septicemia are more frequent than in erysipelas
• Periorbital cellulitis can lead to cavernous sinus thrombosis, cerebral abscess, and meningitis
• In purulent cellulitis, there is associated purulent drainage or exudate in the absence of a drainable abscess</td></tr>
<tr><td>Long-term complications</td><td colspan="2">• Recurrent erysipelas/cellulitis in 20%
  ○ Lymphedema, venous insufficiency, tinea pedis, and obesity predispose to recurrences
• Persistent limb edema
• Post-streptococcal glomerulonephritis can also occur following erysipelas or streptococcal cellulitis</td></tr>
<tr><td>Differential diagnoses</td><td>• Cellulitis
• Necrotizing fasciitis
• Contact dermatitis
• Deep vein thrombosis</td><td>• Necrotizing fasciitis—warning signs include purple blisters, necrosis, or ecchymosis, pain out of proportion, wooden hard induration, crepitus, and marked systemic toxicity
• Deep vein thrombosis
• Deep cutaneous abscess in early stage
• Acute lipodermatosclerosis</td></tr>
<tr><td>Investigations</td><td colspan="2">• Diagnosis is mainly clinical
• In immunocompromised patients/those immersion injuries or animal bites/those who fail to improve with empirical antibiotics, blood cultures, cultures and microscopic examination of cutaneous aspirates, biopsies, or swabs are to be done
• Purulent infections should be debrided and cultured
• Plain radiography can reveal gas if necrotizing fasciitis is suspected
• Ultrasonography can detect underlying abscesses
• Doppler ultrasound can help to rule out deep vein thrombosis
• CT and MRI are helpful in imaging the deeper fascial planes, but if necrotizing fasciitis is seriously being considered, imaging should not delay surgical intervention</td></tr>
<tr><td>Treatment—general measures</td><td colspan="2">• Rest
• Elevation of the affected limb
• Treatment of predisposing factors
• Cool sterile saline dressings if there are bullae</td></tr>
<tr><td>Criteria for hospitalization</td><td colspan="2">• Lesions on the face
• Comorbidities such as immunosuppression, heart, or kidney failure
• Signs of local severity such as blisters and necrosis
• General severity such as confusion and hypotension
• Failure of oral antibiotics</td></tr>
</table>

TABLE 7: Guidelines for management of typical erysipelas/cellulitis in pregnant women.

Grade of erysipelas/nonpurulent cellulitis	Treatment setting	Treatment target	Drug and FDA pregnancy category		Dose
Mild—nil signs of systemic infection	• Outpatient treatment • Oral antibiotics	*Streptococcus* cover alone	Penicillin V	B	250–500 mg QID
		Streptococcus + MSSA coverage	Cephalexin	B	250 mg QID
			Dicloxacillin	B	250 mg QID
		If MRSA coverage required*	Clindamycin	B	300–400 mg QID
			Linezolid	C	600 mg BD
			Cotrimoxazole	C	2 DS tablets BD
Moderate—mild signs of systemic infection present	• Hospitalization • IV antibiotics	Strep*tococcus* cover alone	Penicillin	B	2–4 million units every 4–6 hours IV
		Strep*tococcus* + MSSA coverage	Cefazolin	B	1 g TDS IV
			Ceftriaxone	B	1–2 g every 24 hours IV
		If MRSA coverage required*	Clindamycin	B	600–900 mg TDS IV
		If no response to clindamycin*	Vancomycin	C	30 mg/kg/day in two divided doses IV
			Linezolid	C	600 mg BD IV

Continued

Continued

Grade of erysipelas/nonpurulent cellulitis	Treatment setting	Treatment target	Drug and FDA pregnancy category	Dose
• Severe • Severe signs of systemic infection present ○ Temperature > 38°C ○ Pulse > 90 beats/min ○ Respiratory rate > 24 breaths/min ○ WBC count > 12,000 or <4,000 • Immunocompromised	• Empirical broad-spectrum coverage • Surgical inspection/debridement • Culture and sensitivity to guide further Rx	• Vancomycin plus piperacillin/tazobactam* • Vancomycin plus imipenem/meropenem*		
Adjuvant therapy		• For significant edema, compression dressings or stockings, leg elevation, and diuretics when indicated, will help • As per the IDSA guidelines oral corticosteroids (e.g., prednisone 40 mg daily for 7 days) can be considered in nondiabetic adults with cellulitis as an adjuvant to antibiotic therapy		

*The treatment options marked with an asterisk apply to purulent cellulitis as well.

(FDA: Food and Drug Administration; IDSA: Infectious Diseases Society of America; IV: intravenous; MRSA: methicillin-resistant *Staphylococcus aureus*; MSSA: methicillin-susceptible *Staphylococcus aureus*; WBC: white blood cell)

Prevention of Recurrences

Identification and correction of any predisposing factor helps prevent recurrences. Wounds, eczema, or toe-web intertrigo should be treated appropriately and any underlying venous insufficiency or lymphedema should be managed by compression stockings/bandaging or pneumatic pressure pumps.

Despite attempts to control predisposing factors, if patients have three to four episodes of erysipelas/cellulitis per year, prophylactic antibiotics can be considered. Options recommended by IDSA include oral penicillin or erythromycin 250 mg BD for 4–52 weeks, or intramuscular benzathine penicillin every 2–4 weeks, as long as the predisposing factors persist.

CUTANEOUS ABSCESS, FURUNCLE, AND CARBUNCLE (TABLE 8)

Cutaneous abscesses are collections of pus within the dermis and deeper skin tissues.

FOLLICULITIS

It is an inflammatory disorder of the hair follicle, the etiology can be infectious as well as noninfectious. In this chapter we will limit ourselves to bacterial folliculitis. *S. aureus* is most frequent bacterial cause. Other pathogens include *Streptococcus*, *Pseudomonas* (hot tub folliculitis), *Proteus*, and coliform bacteria. The various types of folliculitis caused *by S. aureus* include superficial folliculitis, a special subtype called dermatitis cruris pustulosa et atrophicans and deep folliculitis or sycosis. The latter two types mainly affect men so we will confine the discussion to superficial folliculitis which can affect women including pregnant women.

Superficial Folliculitis (Bockhart's Impetigo)

In superficial folliculitis, the inflammatory changes are confined to the follicular infundibulum.

Epidemiology

Bockhart's impetigo occurs worldwide at all ages; being most common in childhood. Nasal carriage of *S. aureus*, occlusion, maceration, hot and humid temperatures, itchy skin diseases (e.g., scabies and eczemas), diabetes mellitus, obesity, and topical steroids overuse are some risk factors. It is also common in close contact sportspeople (e.g., wrestlers, hockey, and football players).

Clinical Features

Yellow pustules, sometimes with narrow, red areolae develop in crops, followed by crusting and finally heal without scarring within 7–10 days. Lesions are often itchy, especially when crusted but pain is rare. The lesions do not interfere with

TABLE 8: Cutaneous abscess, furuncles, and carbuncles.

	Abscess	Furuncle	Carbuncle
Definition	Pus collection within the dermis and deeper skin tissues	An abscess involving a hair follicle (mostly of the vellus type) and the perifollicular tissue	Deep infection involving multiple contiguous hair follicles and their surrounding tissues
Etiology	• Vast majority caused by *Staphylococcus aureus* including MRSA • Lesions near mucous membranes may be polymicrobial	Almost always *S. aureus*. MRSA is on the rise	
Epidemiology	General risk factors include preexisting dermatoses, minor trauma, and subcutaneous drug use. Specific risk factors for MRSA include MSM, military personnel, athletes, drug users, and hemodialysis	• Common in adolescents and young adults • Recurrent furunculosis risk factors include nasal *Staphylococcus* carriage, especially with PVL positive strains, iron deficiency anemia, malnutrition, diabetes, immune suppression, obesity, and alcoholism	• More often in middle aged or elderly men • Predisposing factors include diabetes, malnutrition, cardiac failure, generalized dermatoses, and prolonged steroid therapy
	Can be seen in pregnancy too		
Clinical features: Morphology	Painful, swollen, red, tender, fluctuant mass, often studded with pustule and surrounded by a rim of erythematous swelling	To begin with a small, follicular erythematous, and firm nodule, which: • Evolves into a tender fluctuant mass, and • Eventually opens to the skin surface	Begins as a dome-shaped painful hard red nodule • Then enlarges to form broad, swollen, erythematous, deep, painful mass of size 3–10 cm or more • Drains pus through multiple follicular orifices
Common sites of involvement	Extremities and trunk	Favors areas exposed to friction and sweating—face, neck, fingers, arms, wrists, buttocks, and anogenital region	Most often on the nape of the neck
Other points of note	Can be associated with surrounding cellulitis and deep abscesses associated with extensive cellulitis may be difficult to diagnose	PVL—toxin carrying strains produce larger, more red, and painful furuncles Clinical course variable from single self-limiting lesion to recurrent crops of multiple lesions	Constitutional symptoms common

Continued

Continued

	Abscess	Furuncle	Carbuncle
Differential diagnoses	• Inflamed epidermal cyst • Skin lesions secondary to systemic infections with atypical organisms—in the immunocompromised	• Folliculitis—more superficial • Disseminated HSV—crops of vesicopustules • Nodulocystic acne—coexistent comedones and papules	• Anthrax—hemorrhagic crust and vesicular margin • Mycetoma—more chronic, sinuses, grains • Kerion—usually scalp
Investigations	• Diagnosis usually clinical • Ultrasound useful to accurately differentiate from cellulitis • Gram-stain and pus culture ± fungal and mycobacterial culture, especially in patients who fail incision and drainage	• Diagnosis usually clinical • Nasal swabs to exclude staphylococcal carriage in recurrent cases	Gram-stain and pus culture recommended by IDSA to confirm diagnosis
Treatment	• Incision and drainage (I&D) is the treatment of choice for cutaneous abscesses. After incision and complete drainage, the wound is left to heal by secondary intention and the cavity is packed loosely with gauze and dressed. Recently, the need to routinely pack a drained abscess has also been questioned • Exception—small lesions < 2 cm in size may be treated by repeated applications of a clean, warm, and humid compress • Antibiotic therapy is not routinely required for abscesses and furuncles. It is used as an adjunct to I&D in patients with multiple lesions, surrounding cellulitis, associated septic phlebitis, carbuncles, systemic symptoms, abscesses in areas that are difficult to drain (i.e., face, hands, and genitalia), extremes of age, lack of response to I&D and immunocompromised • Empirical antibiotic therapy should cover community-associated MRSA and changes can be made if required based on culture-sensitivity results (see **Table 6** for antibiotic classes and dosages relevant to pregnant women)		
Management of recurrent abscesses/recurrent furunculosis	• Staphylococcal carrier state should be looked for and eradicated • If recurrent abscesses at the same site, search for local causes like a pilonidal cyst, hidradenitis suppurativa, or foreign material • Screen for underlying medical conditions, e.g., diabetes mellitus, HIV, and inflammatory bowel disease • If recurrent abscesses began in childhood, neutrophil disorders should be ruled out • Maintain good personal hygiene, avoid sharing personal items, also clean environmental high touch surfaces		

(HIV: human immunodeficiency virus; HSV: herpes simplex virus; IDSA: Infectious Diseases Society of America; MRSA: methicillin-resistant Staphylococcus aureus; MSM: methylsulfonylmethane; PVL: Panton–Valentine leukocidin) hair growth; the hair shaft is frequently seen in the center of the pustule. It can affect any hair-bearing area; in teenage girls and women, the legs are most commonly affected.

Diagnosis

It is usually clinical. Differential diagnoses include acneiform eruption, miliaria pustulosa, subcorneal pustular dermatosis, dermatophytosis, herpetic folliculitis, and pruritic folliculitis of pregnancy.

Pruritic folliculitis of pregnancy is a misnomer and a pregnancy dermatosis where itchy papular and pustular lesions develop on the trunk ± other sites in the second or third trimester. Benzoyl peroxide is helpful.

Investigations

Gram-stain of the pus and pus culture sensitivity can help showing the bacteria and in confirming the diagnosis. A Tzanck smear is useful in case herpetic folliculitis is suspected.

Treatment

Mild staphylococcal folliculitis is often self-limiting, or may respond to cleansing or topical antibacterials. In more severe cases, antibiotics may be required. Topical options include mupirocin (pregnancy category B), fusidic acid (pregnancy category C), erythromycin, (pregnancy category B), clindamycin (pregnancy category B), and benzoyl peroxide (pregnancy category C). Oral agents include dicloxacillin, cephalexin, amoxicillin-clavulanic acid, and clindamycin (for dosage see **Table 4**). The IDSA guidelines do not make any specific recommendations for folliculitis.

Management of Recurrent Infections and Prevention

In recurrent infections, diabetes mellitus should be ruled out. Staphylococcal carriage should be eradicated. This has been covered in the section on impetigo. General measures to prevent folliculitis include avoiding tight-fitting clothes. Patients should be advised to shave the hair in the direction of its growth. Athletic equipment should not be shared among players.

TOXIN-MEDIATED DISEASES

Bullous impetigo and SSSS have been discussed earlier in the chapter. We will also take a brief look at toxic shock syndrome **(Table 9)**.

Pseudomonas Infection

Caused by gram-negative aerobic bacilli, *Pseudomonas aeruginosa* is an opportunistic bacterium, causing various skin and soft tissue infections and can cause severe disease, especially in immunocompromised host. Various diseases caused by *Pseudomonas* in skin and soft tissue include ecthyma gangrenosum, burn wound infections, hot tub folliculitis, nail and paronychial infection (green

TABLE 9: Toxic shock syndrome.

	Staphylococcal toxic shock syndrome	Streptococcal toxic shock-like syndrome
Etiopathogenesis	*Staphylococcus aureus,* mediated by its toxic shock syndrome toxin 1 (TSST-1), a pyrogenic toxin superantigen	Mediated by streptococcal toxins; most common causative agent is group A streptococci
	The tampon-linked disease received great publicity, but it can occur along with staphylococcal infection of any severity, at any site, in any age—group and gender	Occurs only in association with severe invasive group streptococcal infections. Can be seen in association with postpartum sepsis due to group A or group B streptococci
Clinical features	• Acute illness with fever, rash fever, rash, hypotension, multiorgan involvement, and desquamation • Has significant mortality • In the skin, initially widespread macular erythema + mucosal erythema; subsequently, widespread itchy maculopapular rash, and eventually, desquamation, which is either localized to extremities or generalized	
Diagnosis	Supported by the confirmation of the presence of staphylococcal or streptococcal infection	
Treatment	• Hospitalization, intravenous (IV) antibiotics, and intensive supportive care • IV flucloxacillin + clindamycin ± vancomycin and then adjust as per cultures • Intravenous immunoglobulin (IVIG) can be used as an adjuvant to neutralize the toxin	
Prognosis	Overall better prognosis, mortality <10%	Poor prognosis especially if along with necrotizing fasciitis; mortality >40%

nail syndrome), toe web space infections, external otitis, cellulitis, panniculitis, etc. Ecthyma gangrenosum and subcutaneous nodules caused by *Pseudomonas aeruginosa,* necrotizing skin, and soft tissue infections are frequently associated with bloodstream infections, more so in immunocompromised hosts. Management of *Pseudomonas* infection often requires a multidisciplinary team along with surgical support. Antibiotic with antipseudomonal activities include beta-lactams, carbapenems, or fluoroquinolones. The duration of antimicrobial therapy for skin and soft tissue infection is 10–14 days; **Table 10** shows antibiotics used for *Pseudomonas.*

Lyme Disease

Caused by *Borrelia burgdorferi, Borrelia afzelii, Borrelia garinii,* and transmitted by *Ixodes* tick after 1–36 days of incubation period. It initially presents as erythema chronicum migrans (ECM) at the site of tick bite. Erythematous ring formation enlarging at a rate of several cm per week, producing "bull's-eye"

TABLE 10: Antibiotics used for *Pseudomonas* and their pregnancy category (US FDA).

Drug	Pregnancy category
Piperacillin-tazobactam	US FDA pregnancy category: Not assigned
Ticarcillin-clavulanate	B
Ceftazidime	B
Cefepime	B
Cefoperazone	B
Aztreonam	B
Ciprofloxacin	C
Levofloxacin	C
Meropenem	B
Doripenem	B
Imipenem	Not assigned
Ceftazidime	B
Ceftolozane-tazobactam	Not assigned
Tobramycin	Not assigned
Gentamicin	D
Amikacin	D

Note: Although we have mentioned the Food and Drug Administration (FDA) pregnancy category of drugs, it is important to note that FDA has replaced pregnancy risk categories with a new system known as the Pregnancy and Lactation Labeling Rule (PLLR). The PLLR got official nod in 2015 and it aims to provide patients and healthcare providers with relevant information that allows for informed clinical interpretation and medical management. Under PLLR older pregnancy categories are being phased out.

appearance. Moderate burning or itching may be present. This is stage 1, when not treated this may lead to stage 2 with multiple ECM lesions along with constitutional symptoms. The last stage is stage 3 due to persistent infection, may result in acrodermatitis chronica atrophicans (ACA) months or years later. In pregnancy, no adverse outcomes yet reported. Diagnosis is confirmed by enzyme-linked immunosorbent assay (ELISA) followed by a more specific Western blot test. For treatment in pregnancy β-lactam antimicrobial is preferred or for various manifestations of Lyme disease. As doxycycline is contraindicated in pregnancy, oral amoxicillin and cefuroxime can be used. In stage 3, parenteral ceftriaxone should be used.

Rickettsial Diseases

Rickettsial infections are caused by bacteria in the genus *Rickettsia* and transmitted by ticks, body lice, and mites. They cause febrile illness often associated with skin rash. Scrub typhus is the most common rickettsial infection in India. Fever, cough, nausea, headache, and myalgia are the common presenting features. Eschar at the site of chigger bite can be seen as early clinical sign; it can be single or multiple. Skin rash is also commonly seen in other rickettsial disorders like spotted fever and rarely in scrub typhus.

Clinically suspected case of rickettsial disease can be further confirmed by ELISA [immunoglobulin M (IgM) capture assays], polymerase chain reaction (PCR) or indirect immunoperoxidase assay (IPA), and immunofluorescence assay (IFA).

Treatment

The drug of choice for treating rickettsial infections is doxycycline (contraindicated in pregnancy), with the dosing and length of therapy depending on the specific causative organism. In pregnant women, use azithromycin 500 mg in a single dose for 5 days. Patient should be managed through interdisciplinary approach with preferable infectious disease specialist. Complicated cases may need IV antibiotics and other supportive care.

SUGGESTED READINGS

1. Hay RJ, Morris-Jones R. Bacterial infections. In: Griffiths C, Barker J, Bleiker T, Chalmers R, Creamer D (Eds). Rook's Textbook of Dermatology. 9th edition. Chichester: Wiley-Blackwell; 2016. pp. 26.1-26.87.
2. Dotters-Katz SK, Kuller J, Heine RP, Wheeler SM. Group B *Streptococcus* and Pregnancy: Critical Concepts and Management Nuances. Obstet Gynecol Surv. 2022;77(12):753-62.
3. Cohen PR. Bullous impetigo and pregnancy: Case report and review of blistering conditions in pregnancy. Dermatol Online J. 2016;22(4): 13030/qt7533z2m0.
4. Etzel TM, Calafat AM, Ye X, Chen A, Lanphear BP, Savitz DA, et al. Urinary triclosan concentrations during pregnancy and birth outcomes. Environ Res. 2017;156:505-11.
5. Elston CA, Elston DM. Treatment of common skin infections and infestations during pregnancy. Dermatol Ther. 2013;26(4):312-20.
6. Bangert S, Levy M, Hebert AA. Bacterial resistance and impetigo treatment trends: a review. Pediatr Dermatol. 2012;29(3):243-8.
7. Dadashi M, Hajikhani B, Darban-Sarokhalil D, van Belkum A, Goudarzi M. Mupirocin resistance in *Staphylococcus aureus*: A systematic review and meta-analysis. J Glob Antimicrob Resist. 2020;20:238-47.
8. Christiansen KJ. Fusidic Acid. [online] Available from http://www.antimicrobe.org/d29.asp. [Last accessed January, 2025].
9. Kriebs JM. Staphylococcus Infections in Pregnancy: Maternal and Neonatal Risks. J Perinat Neonatal Nurs. 2016;30(2):115-23.
10. Redding KS, Jones EH, Patel T, Skinner RB. Staphylococcal scalded skin syndrome in pregnancy. Cutis. 2015;96(4):E7-9.
11. Sonthalia S, Singal A, Khurana R. Ecthyma. Indian Pediatr. 2014;51(6):510-1.
12. Morgan M. Challenging infections in pregnancy. Obstet Gynaecol Reprod Med. 2020;30(9):289-97.
13. Mohamedahmed AYY, Zaman S, Stonelake S, Ahmad AN, Datta U, Hajibandeh S, et al. Incision and drainage of cutaneous abscess with or without cavity packing: a systematic review, meta-analysis, and trial sequential analysis of randomised controlled trials. Langenbecks Arch Surg. 2021;406(4):981-91.

11.6 Other Viral Infections

Sanjeev Gupta, Anushka Lohariwala, Aditi Dabhra

INTRODUCTION

Cutaneous viral infections during pregnancy present a unique clinical challenge due to their potential impact on both maternal and fetal health. The physiological and immunological changes that occur during pregnancy can alter the course and severity of viral infections, as well as the clinical presentation of skin-related symptoms. While many cutaneous viral infections are generally benign in the nonpregnant population, they can lead to significant complications during pregnancy, including miscarriage, preterm birth, fetal growth restriction, and congenital anomalies **(Fig. 1)**. This chapter explores a few common and clinically relevant cutaneous viral infections in pregnancy and their potential maternal and fetal outcomes. Understanding these infections is critical for optimizing prenatal care and mitigating risks to both mother and child environment at the maternal-fetal interface.

HUMAN PAPILLOMA VIRUS

A family of small, nonenveloped, double-stranded deoxyribonucleic acid (DNA) viruses, *Papillomaviridae* comprises over 200 human papilloma virus (HPV) types. HPV strains have traditionally been classified as low-risk and high-risk HPVs. High-risk HPV cause genital lesions and have been dealt with in another chapter. Low-risk HPV strains such as 1, 2, 3, 4, 27, 57, etc., are causative in verruca vulgaris, plantar warts, and plane warts. On the basis of tropism they

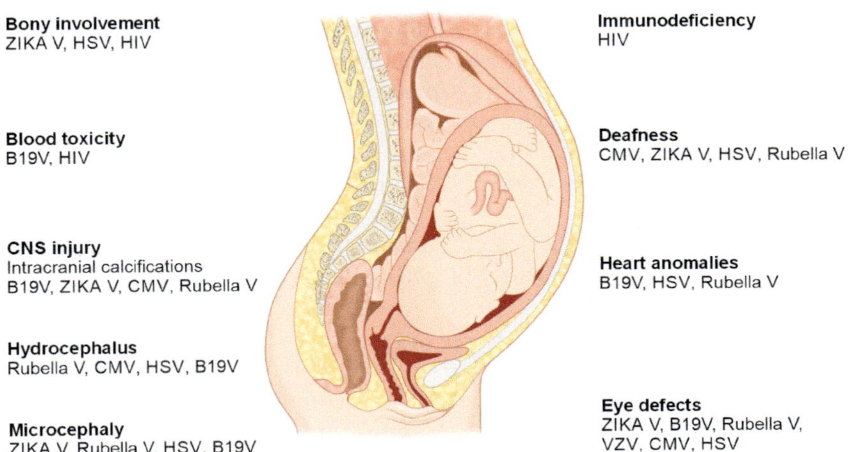

FIG. 1: Various common cutaneous viral infections and organs affected in the fetus.

may lead to cutaneous or to mucosal lesions. Cutaneous HPVs may infect the hair follicle stem cells, thus facilitating persistent infection. These viruses evade the host immune response so there is no viremia.

The altered immunological response in pregnancy may increase the size of already existing warts and lead to the persistence of the infection with a decreased tendency for spontaneous recovery. As there is no viremia so complications in pregnancy and adverse pregnancy outcomes are not associated with verruca vulgaris. Transmission can occur to neonates by inoculation.

Treatment

As warts may be aesthetically unappealing to the patient so various topical treatments can be given:

- *Physical treatment* such as electrocauterization and cryotherapy can be done.
- Various topical treatments which can be used are:
  - 5% KOH—destroys keratin
  - Hydrogen peroxide (1–6%)—oxidizing ability is lethal to virus
  - Trichloroacetic acid (TCA)—causes hydrolysis of cellular protein-inflammation and destruction of tissue
  - Laser ablation—carbon dioxide and neodymium-doped yttrium aluminum garnet (Nd:YAG)
- Treatments which need to be avoided are:
  - *Cantharidin*: Derived from blister beetle *Lytta vesicatoria*. It acts by interfering mitochondria-epidermal cell death, acantholysis, and blister formation.
  - *Imiquimod*: It acts as antiviral agent by inducing secretion of interferon-α (IFN-α).
  - *Quadrivalent vaccine*: Causes immunomodulation. Not effective in adults because of a decrease in vaccine-induced HPV-specific cytotoxic T-cell immune response.
  - Intralesional bleomycin-mutagenic
  - *Salicylic acid (17–40%)*: It is keratolytic. Systemic absorption is 9–25%. Though it can be applied over small areas it cannot be used over large areas. Specifically in the third trimester, it can cause premature closure of ductus arteriosus and oligohydramnios.
  - *Podophyllotoxin*: It is extracted from the Mayapple plant (*Podophyllum peltatum* or *Paeonia emodi*). It is an antimitotic agent. It is mutagenic (category).
  - *Sinecatechins (15%)*: It is a green tea polyphenol extract from *Camellia sinensis*. Induces apoptosis. Not well studied in pregnancy.

MOLLUSCUM CONTAGIOSUM

Molluscum contagiosum (MC) is a benign skin infection characterized by small, pearly, dome-shaped papules with a central umbilication. This condition is caused by the molluscum contagiosum virus (MCV), which is the most common poxvirus affecting humans.

It is of four types, i.e., MCV I, II, III, and IV. MCV I is most prevalent and MCV II is usually seen in sexually transmitted diseases and is more widespread.

Molluscum contagiosum has an incubation period of 2–8 weeks. But it may extend from 6 to 18 months. It evades the host immune system thus discrete papular lesions with central umbilication appear. Later on perilesional erythema appears which is described as the "beginning of the end" (BOTE) sign suggesting regression of lesions. MC usually resolves spontaneously in 6–9 months but occasionally may persist for 3–4 years. MC usually shows only cutaneous involvement but occasionally oral mucosal and cervical involvement have been reported.

Molluscum contagiosum is more commonly seen in children. Disseminated lesions are seen in immunosuppressed patients. Pregnancy as a cause for dissemination has not been reported.

Molluscum contagiosum is transmitted by skin-to-skin contact and fomites. Sexual transmission is also seen. Molluscum has been observed in a newborn and neonatal period. Mollusca lesions are highly contagious so genital lesions can lead to transmission to child during the intrapartum period. Appearance of these lesions within the incubation period duration further supports this mode of transmission. Studies have reported lesions appearing on the scalp or eyes in neonates thus speculating the presence of undiagnosed cervical or vaginal lesions in mothers. Presence of molluscum lesions since birth and on atypical site like shoulder in a newborn suggests vertical transmission of this virus.

During pregnancy MC lesions are usually not disseminated but they persist longer. Multiple lesions may appear in clusters **(Fig. 2)**. Due to associated pruritus, pseudo-kernelization is also seen.

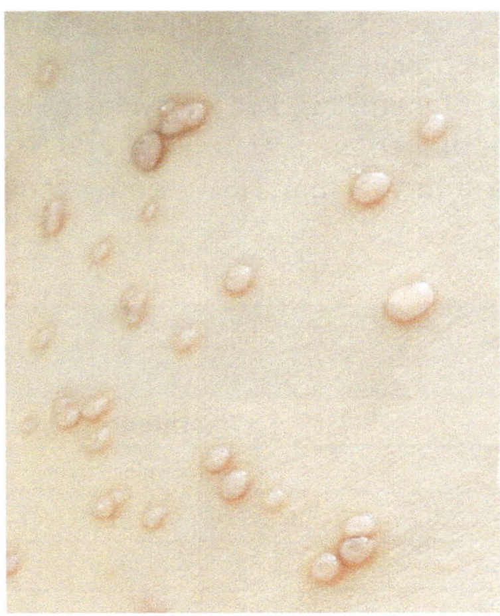

FIG. 2: Grouped lesions of molluscum in pregnant female.

Treatment

- In individuals with a healthy immune system, MC lesions typically resolve on their own within 6 months to 2 years without treatment.
- In those with weakened immune systems, the lesions often persist and can spread indefinitely, making specific treatment more necessary.

Various modalities of treatment which can be used and those which need to be avoided are as mentioned in **Table 1**.

- MC usually involves skin but can also involve mucosa.
- MC genotype MCV 2 has been identified in vaginal lesion samples.
- It is believed that mother-to-child transmission may occur during vaginal delivery.
- Vertical transmission of virus has also been reported.
- Lesions may emerge at various times after birth, from 1 week to 3 months.
- In congenital MC, maternal lesions were documented in many but not all. Undiagnosed cervical/vaginal mucosal lesions could have been the cause.

MONKEYPOX

Monkeypox is a viral zoonosis induced by an enveloped, double-stranded DNA virus belonging to the *Orthopoxvirus* genus of the Poxviridae family. Clinically lesions appear as vesicles after prodrome of constitutional symptoms. There are only a few cases of monkeypox in pregnancy reported. But these cases had moderate and severe disease. Also the rate of abortions and perinatal loss was high.

HERPES LABIALIS

Herpes simplex is a virus from the Herpesviridae family. It is categorized into two types: herpes simplex virus 1 (HSV1) and herpes simplex virus 1 (HSV2), which are distinguished by their specific glycoproteins I and II, respectively. After the initial infection, the virus travels to the sensory ganglia and remains dormant. This results in a lifelong infection marked by cycles of latency and reactivation. Traditionally, HSV1 was linked to oral lesions and HSV2 to genital lesions. However, recent trends indicate that HSV1 now accounts for approximately

TABLE 1: Treatment of molluscum contagiosum: Safe treatment options and treatments to be avoided during pregnancy.

Safe treatments	Treatments to be avoided
Cryotherapy	Podophyllotoxin
Curettage	Imiquimod
Squeezing	Salicylic acid
Cautery	Cantharidin
5% KOH	
Hydrogen peroxide (1–6%)	

80% of genital herpes cases in some populations. Approximately 90% of women will test positive for HSV1 antibodies by the age of 50, and about 53% of pregnant women will show positive for HSV1 immunoglobulin G (IgG), indicating a past infection.

The HSV1 prevalence is higher among individuals:

- Compromised immunity (such as during pregnancy)
- Women under 25 years old
- Those from lower socioeconomic backgrounds
- Women with sexual partners under 20 years of age
- Women whose partners have a history of oral herpes lesions

- HSV1 can be transmitted horizontally through mucosal membranes, broken skin, or sexual contact.
- It is estimated that only 0.5–2% of first-time maternal HSV1 infections occur during pregnancy.
- The risk of transmitting HSV from mother to fetus varies based on the pregnant woman's immune status.
- Diagnosing herpetic skin lesions during pregnancy can be challenging due to the frequent occurrence of nonpathological skin eruptions associated with hormonal changes.

Additionally, individuals with altered immunity tend to experience a shorter latency period and more severe symptoms. Transmission risk is higher in cases of a primary first episode infection (30–60%), compared to 25% for nonprimary first episode infections and 1% for recurrent infections. Approximately 61% of maternal HSV infections occur during the third trimester. Maternal HSV infection may present in various ways, most commonly with cold-like symptoms (such as headaches and chills) and classic vesicular lesions in the affected area. There may be recurrences and recrudescence.

- Recurrence generally refers to any episode where the virus reactivates, whether or not symptoms are present.
- Recrudescence specifically refers to reactivation of the virus that result in visible herpetic signs or symptoms.

During pregnancy there may be recrudescent herpes labialis, recrudescent localized intraoral herpes, or recrudescent intraoral herpes infection mimicking primary herpetic gingivostomatitis **(Fig. 3)**.

Treatment in Pregnancy

- For HSV1 infections at any location, the primary treatment is oral antiviral therapy, with acyclovir being the preferred medication during pregnancy.
- Acyclovir has been shown to be safe in pregnancy, with no evidence linking it to congenital abnormalities, and is also considered safe during breastfeeding, though it may cause transient neonatal neutropenia.
- Acyclovir treatment has been proven to alleviate symptoms, reduce the duration of the infection, and decrease viral shedding in pregnant women.
- A 2008 Cochrane review found that using prophylactic acyclovir in pregnant women with known genital HSV reduced the incidence of active genital

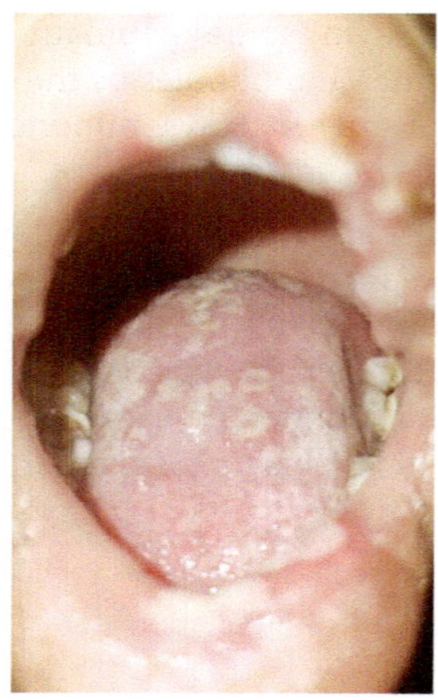

FIG. 3: Herpes infection in pregnant female presenting as gingivostomatitis.

lesions at delivery and decreased the number of cesarean sections. However, there are no guidelines available for prophylactic treatment of nongenital HSV1 during pregnancy.

MEASLES

Measles is an extremely contagious disease caused by the single-stranded, enveloped measles virus, which is part of the genus *Morbillivirus* within the Paramyxoviridae family. It is transmitted through droplet infection. The disease typically begins with general symptoms, followed by a rash within 2–3 days and the appearance of Koplik spots on the mucous membranes.

Maternal Risk

In pregnant women, measles tends to be more severe, with a heightened risk of life-threatening complications such as pneumonia, diarrhea, and subacute sclerosing panencephalitis (SSPE).

Fetal Risk

- *Congenital measles*: Rash appears within 10 days of birth.
- *Postnatal measles*: Rash develops 14–30 days after birth.
- If the mother experiences complications from measles, there is an increased risk of low birth weight, preterm birth, and neonatal death.

RUBELLA

Rubella, also known as German measles, is a contagious viral infection caused by *Rubivirus* of family togavirus. The typical incubation period is 17 days, with a range of 12–23 days.

Rubella is most contagious during the eruption of the rash, but the infectious period spans from 7 days before to 7 days after the rash appears.

Maternal Symptoms

Mild fever, maculopapular rash, arthritis, and lymphadenopathy are the maternal symptoms. Rarely thrombocytopenia or neurological signs may be seen.

While generally mild in children and adults, rubella poses a significant risk during pregnancy due to its potential to cause severe congenital abnormalities.

- *Risk of clinical manifestations of congenital rubella infection (CRI)*:
  - The risk depends on the timing of maternal infection.
  - Highest risk occurs if the maternal infection is acquired during the first 16–17 weeks of gestation.
- *First trimester infections*:
  - Increased prevalence of fetal complications during the first trimester.
  - Specific anomalies include:
    - Cardiac and eye anomalies: Typically result from infections occurring before 8 weeks of gestation.
    - Hearing loss: May result from infections occurring up to 18 weeks of gestation.
- *Second and third trimester infections*:
  - Little to no risk of congenital defects is associated with infections after 18–20 weeks of gestation.
  - Intrauterine growth retardation: May be the primary consequence of infections occurring in the third trimester.

Management in Pregnancy

The approach to managing rubella infection during pregnancy largely depends on the gestational age at the time of infection:

- *Infection before 18 weeks*: There is a high likelihood of fetal damage and major defects. Therefore, termination of pregnancy might be considered in line with local regulations and guidelines.
- *Infection after 18 weeks*: The risk of congenital rubella syndrome is significantly lower, so no specific intervention is usually necessary.

CYTOMEGALOVIRUS

Cytomegalovirus (CMV) is a member of the herpesvirus family. It is a common virus that can infect people of all ages. It can be transmitted by droplet infection, through fomites or sexual route. It is typically asymptomatic or causes mild illness in healthy individuals. CMV infection during pregnancy is a significant concern due to its potential impact on both the mother and the fetus. It can occur first time during pregnancy (primary) or reactivation of latent infection can occur.

Primary infection poses the greatest risk to the fetus. Risk of fetal infection is seen in 30–70% cases.

Congenital Cytomegalovirus Infection

It occurs when a fetus is infected with CMV in utero. This can lead to a range of outcomes, including:

- *Asymptomatic infection*: Many infants with congenital CMV are asymptomatic at birth but may develop symptoms later.
- *Symptomatic infection*: Symptoms at birth can include microcephaly, intrauterine growth restriction, hepatosplenomegaly, jaundice, and petechiae.
- *Long-term complications*: Hearing loss is the most common long-term complication of congenital CMV. Other potential issues include vision loss, intellectual disability, and motor deficits.

  Valaciclovir, ganciclovir, and valganciclovir may be used for treatment.

ZIKA VIRUS

Zika virus is a mosquito-borne *Flavivirus* primarily transmitted by *Aedes* mosquitoes. It can also be transmitted through sexual contact, blood transfusion, and from mother to fetus during pregnancy. The incubation period for the virus is typically between 3 and 7 days.

Zika virus infection is often asymptomatic or causes mild symptoms such as fever, rash, joint pain, conjunctivitis, muscle pain, and headache. Occasionally Guillain-Barré syndrome may be seen.

Fetal Effect

- *Congenital Zika syndrome (CZS)*: The most severe outcome of Zika infection during pregnancy, characterized by a range of birth defects, including:
  - Microcephaly: A condition where a baby is born with a smaller-than-normal head due to abnormal brain development. Even in normocephalic neonates locomotor and other neurological manifestations may be seen.
  - Brain abnormalities: Calcifications, brain atrophy, and other structural brain abnormalities.
  - Eye defects: Such as retinal damage and other vision problems.
  - Hearing defects: Hearing loss is also a common feature.
  - Impaired growth: Restricted growth in utero and low birth weight.
  - Other possible outcomes: Miscarriage, stillbirth, and other neurological conditions have also been associated with Zika virus infection during pregnancy.

Management in Pregnancy

There is no specific treatment available for Zika virus infection. Management involves rest and supportive care, including adequate hydration and the use of acetaminophen to alleviate fever and pain.

PARVOVIRUS B19

Parvovirus B19 is a virus that causes erythema infectiosum, also known as "fifth disease" or "slapped cheek syndrome", which is a common childhood illness. The virus primarily spreads through respiratory droplets. Approximately 50–60% of adults are immune due to previous exposure. The infection often presents with constitutional symptoms followed by maculopapular rash after a week. Rash starts from the face and gradually spreads to extremities. There may be accompanied arthritis.

Parvovirus B19 is a common infection that affects 1–5% of pregnant women, generally with normal pregnancy outcomes. During epidemics, the infection rate can rise to between 3 and 20%, with a seroconversion rate ranging from 3 to 34%. When contracted during pregnancy, the virus can lead to various signs of fetal damage. The risk of adverse outcomes is greater if the infection occurs during the first or second trimester, though it can also affect the fetus in the third trimester. Parvovirus B19 is a notable cause of fetal loss throughout pregnancy, particularly during the second half, when spontaneous fetal loss from other causes is relatively uncommon. Given that parvovirus B19 infection can lead to significant morbidity and mortality, it should be included in the routine evaluation of complicated pregnancies. Assessing the risk of maternal infection is particularly crucial during epidemics, when seroconversion rates are elevated.

Management of Maternal Infection

- Symptomatic therapy is used to manage maternal parvovirus B19 infection.
- There is no specific antiviral treatment available.
- High-dose intravenous immunoglobulin may be used in rare cases to treat persistent aplastic anemia linked to parvovirus B19 infection.
- Complications in mothers are rare, as parvovirus infection generally resolves on its own.

SUGGESTED READINGS

1. Condrat CE, Filip L, Gheorghe M, Cretoiu D, Suciu N. Maternal HPV Infection: Effects on Pregnancy Outcome. Viruses. 2021;13(12):2455.
2. D'Antonio F, Pagani G, Buca D, Khalil A. Monkeypox infection in pregnancy: a systematic review and meta-analysis. Am J Obst Gynecol MFM. 2023;5(1):100747.
3. Neri I, Liberati G, Virdi A, Patrizi A. Congenital molluscum contagiosum. Paediatr Child Health. 2017;22(5):241-2.
4. Luke JD, Silverberg NB. Vertically Transmitted Molluscum Contagiosum Infection. Pediatrics. 2010;125(2):e423-5.
5. Landis MN. Topical and intralesional antiviral agents. In Wolverton SE, Wu JJ (Eds). Comprehensive Dermatologic Drug Therapy, 4th edition Philadelphia: Elsevier; 2021. pp. 494-504.

11.7 Scabies and Other Miscellaneous Infections

Parul Verma, Sucheta Pathania

INTRODUCTION

Pregnancy is a hypermetabolic state which is associated with variable changes in hormonal profile as well as immune status of the patient. Some of these changes are physiological and sometimes there is exacerbation or improvement of the preexisting dermatosis/infections while there are certain conditions which are specific to pregnancy. During pregnancy the cytokine profile is altered, there is elevation in the levels of Th2 cytokines [interleukin (IL)-4, 5, 10, and 13] while in the postpartum period Th1 cytokines [IL-2, tumor necrosis factor (TNF)-alpha, and interferon-gamma] are elevated. The hormonal changes occurring during pregnancy also favors such preferences in the immune status of the antenatal females. In this chapter, we will be discussing miscellaneous skin infections during pregnancy, their presentation, and management.

SCABIES

It is one of the neglected tropical disease caused by the mite, *Sarcoptes scabiei* var. *hominis* and is transmitted by direct skin to skin contact. It is highly contagious. Transmission occurs person-to-person through prolonged direct skin contact, making it common within households, close living quarters, and among sexual partners. Scabies can also spread through infested clothing, bedding, or furniture, though this is less common. Outbreaks are a concern in healthcare and communal settings.

Prevalence

Its global prevalence is estimated at over 200 million cases annually, with higher rates in tropical and subtropical regions due to increased humidity and overcrowding.

The prevalence of scabies in pregnancy is 2–6%.

Clinically it is characterized by papules and nocturnal pruritus with burrows being the pathognomonic sign. Commonly affected areas include the finger webs, wrists, elbows, armpits, waistline, genitals, and buttocks.

Scabies in Pregnancy

Altered immune profile of the pregnant females predisposes them to various infections and scabies is one of them. Poverty and overcrowding are important risk factors. There is disturbance in the sleep cycle due to generalized itching which is more common in the night. Itching is more intense in pregnant patients. It has great psychological impact on a pregnant female. Fear of taking medicines (may cause harm to fetus) and transmission to the newborn further increase the stress. Eczematization and superadded bacterial infections due to scratching are the common complications.

Treatment of Scabies during Pregnancy (Table 1)

Permethrin

Permethrin inhibits sodium channels and is neurotoxic. Due to its better efficacy and safety, permethrin 5% cream (on day 1 and day 7) is the preferred treatment of choice for scabies in pregnancy. Permethrin is a category B drug. Though few studies show resistance to permethrin but others believe that it may be due to errors in application technique. Permethrin 5% cream has been found to be more effective than oral ivermectin, lindane, and crotamiton in a meta-analysis. It may cause itching, burning, stinging, or eczema. Only 2% of the drug can be absorbed systemically.

Benzyl Benzoate 25%

Benzyl benzoate inhibits respiration of mite. It is an emulsion used as second-line treatment in case of nonavailability of permethrin or patient is allergic to first-line drug. It is a category C drug but in a Thai study it was found to have no fetal/maternal toxicity in 444 pregnant females studied.

Camphor (Category C)

It can relieve pruritus due to its local anesthetic effect. Theoretically it can cross placenta and if ingested by fetus/neonate can cause respiratory failure. However, no fetal adverse effects have been observed till date.

TABLE 1: Safety of various topical drugs used for scabies.

Drug	Pregnancy category
First line:	
Permethrin	B
Benzyl benzoate	C
Second line:	
Malathion (0.5%)	B
Spinosad	B
Precipitated sulfur	C
Not used:	
Lindane	C
Supportive therapy:	
• Menthol	N
• Camphor	C
• Crotamiton (10%)	C
• Corticosteroids	C

Precipitated Sulfur (Category C)

No fetal adverse effects have been observed. About 1% of the drug gets systemically absorbed. If first-line drugs fail then limited use of this drug is advised.

Spinosad (Category B)

No systemic absorption and no reported toxicity in animals. Human studies have not been done.

Topical application from head to toe is difficult, especially for pregnant females in tropics may be difficult. Also if skin barrier is disrupted topical application may be difficult.

Ivermectin

Interrupts gamma-aminobutyric acid (GABA)-induced neurotransmission and causes paralysis and death of the mite. Dose is 200 μg/kg/dose and to be repeated after 7–14 days as it is not ovicidal. Ivermectin is reported to be unsafe in children <5 years or in pregnancy.

Ivermectin has been used as part of onchocerciasis mass drug administration programs in sub-Saharan Africa. Nicolas and colleagues did not observe any foetotoxicity after use of ivermectin in pregnant females. Weill et al. suggested that ivermectin can be used safely after first trimester. Normally P-glycoprotein prevents ivermectin crossing the blood–brain barrier. Also this P-glycoprotein is present in the placenta. Hence chances of fetal toxicity are not there. But patients who have mutation of this P-glycoprotein may have fetal adverse effects, but these have not been reported.

Moxidectin

Another compound belonging to macrocyclic lactone group, moxidectin, is under evaluation (phase II) for treatment of scabies during pregnancy.

Scabies during Lactation

Expressed milk feeding should be encouraged in postnatal period as the lesions are predominantly present around the nipples and the chances of transmission to the child can be increased by direct skin contact. In the breast milk, about 1% of oral ivermectin gets secreted. This amount of ivermectin has been found safe during lactation but still it is not Food and Drug Administration (FDA) approved.

Associated pruritus and eczema can be managed with antihistaminic and topical steroids, if required. Other close contacts and family members should also be treated to prevent recurrence of disease. Manage secondary bacterial infections with pregnancy safe antibiotic.

LEISHMANIASIS

Leishmaniasis affects ~12 million people worldwide with an annual incidence of 2 million cases. It is a vector borne disease, caused by a group of protozoan parasites of genus *Leishmania* and is transmitted to humans by the bite of infected sandfly. It is endemic in many countries of the world and India is one among them. In humans, leishmaniasis can present as cutaneous, mucosal or mucocutaneous, or visceral disease. Cutaneous leishmaniasis (CL) is the most common subtype. Clinical manifestation of CL varies from erythematous papules to noduloulcerative lesions, predominantly over exposed parts of the body.

During pregnancy the presentation and evolution of the disease is more severe. Lesions are more exuberant, larger, and have been associated with a higher rate of disseminated lesions, mucosal disease, and recurrent disease compared to nonpregnant patients. Associated lymphadenopathy is more common. The Th2 predominant response which is considered to be beneficial for the maintenance of pregnancy favors the persistence and severity of *Leishmania* infection. Increased neutrophilic infiltration and fibrinoid necrosis is seen on histopathological examination. In spite of exuberant growth no definitive amastigotes of *Leishmania* may be visualized by hematoxylin and eosin (H&E) stain or CD1a immunohistochemistry. It is speculated that an intense inflammatory reaction, similar to what is observed in tuberculoid leprosy, might make it more difficult to detect the parasites in histopathological examinations. Recent evidence indicates that disease severity and relapse risk are influenced by more than just a straightforward type 1 versus type 2 immune response. Instead, they involve a complex interplay of various immune components, including T-helper 17 cells, regulatory T cells, and humoral immunity. Polymerase chain reaction (PCR) may help to confirm diagnosis.

There is increased risk for congenital transmission. Moreover because it causes immune alterations it is associated with increased fetal complications such as preterm delivery, stillbirths, and intrauterine growth retardation.

Standard treatment of choice is antimonial but it is considered to be abortigenic and hence avoided during pregnancy. In patients with limited disease, local treatment with cryotherapy, diathermy, intralesional injections of pentavalent antimonials, as well as topical paromomycin (12%) can be tried. No teratogenic effect was noted with topical administration of these drugs in antenatal females. Topical paromomycin (12%) and methylbenzethonium chloride (15%), a quaternary ammonium salt that exhibits antileishmanial activity, have been used together in combination with good results in Israel and Latin America for >20 years but little is known about its efficacy in case of antenatal females. Amphotericin B, particularly its liposomal derivative, is considered safe and effective in the treatment of visceral leishmaniasis (VL) in pregnancy. However, exact guidelines for the management of CL are still lacking as in most of the studies pregnant females are excluded.

During pregnancy, VL can be transmitted vertically to the fetus. There may be present as severe anemia in the newborn.

CUTANEOUS TUBERCULOSIS

Cutaneous tuberculosis (TB) is a rare entity caused by *Mycobacterium tuberculosis* complex, *M. bovis* and Bacillus Calmette-Guérin (BCG) and constitutes

1–2% of all extrapulmonary TB. Pregnancy is not associated with increased risk of developing pulmonary TB or any site specific TB; however, concomitant immunodeficiency states such as human immunodeficiency virus (HIV) coinfection, chronic kidney disease, and immunosuppression are risk factors for development of cutaneous TB. Its burden among pregnant females is not well known. Taking into consideration incidence of TB among women of reproductive age group and number of births annually Jana et al. calculated that approximately 20,000–40,000 pregnant women annually are likely to suffer from active TB in India. There is no specific data on skin TB in pregnancy.

Depending on the immune status of the host, mode of inoculation and various environmental factors, it can have a varied presentation. The signs and symptoms of TB are masked by pregnancy which is exacerbated in the immediate postpartum period. The clinical spectrum of cutaneous TB in pregnant females remains same as nonpregnant females. Inoculation can occur either by exogenous route, where the direct inoculation of the organism occurs at the site of injury leading to presentations such as TB chancre, TB verrucosa cutis, and by endogenous route. Hematogenous spread as well as contiguous spread from the site of the involvement can give rise to presentations such as lupus vulgaris, scrofuloderma, orificial TB, and miliary TB. Cutaneous TB is also classified as multibacillary and paucibacillary types depending upon the number of acid-fast bacilli (AFB) identified on the smear examination. Since often it is associated with pulmonary TB, so it should always be ruled out. Diagnosis is made by proper history taking, asking all relevant questions such as any history of contact, fever, cough, night sweats, etc., careful physical examination of lesion, doing Mantoux test, sputum for AFB, and skin biopsy of the lesion. Skin tissue and pus should also be sent for culture, cartridge-based nucleic acid amplification test (CB-NAAT), in accordance with the concept of universal drug sensitivity testing.

Impact of Tuberculosis on Pregnancy

Though pulmonary TB during pregnancy may have unfavorable outcomes for both pregnant women and their infants, but this cannot be generalized for exclusive cutaneous TB, where the disease is limited to skin and the disease is paucibacillary.

Treatment

The treatment of cutaneous TB should not be delayed in pregnant females as delay in treatment of active disease is associated with poor maternal and fetal outcome. A 6 months course of a combination of isoniazid (INH), rifampicin (RIF), ethambutol (EMB), and pyrazinamide (PZA) daily for 2 months, followed by INH, RIF, and EMB daily for 4 months (HREZ × 2 + HRE × 4) is recommended by the WHO as safety in pregnancy of these first-line medications have been proven. This regimen is associated with cure rate in 90% of cases with improved perinatal outcomes. Since INH is associated with peripheral neuritis and neonatal seizures, pyridoxine (25–50 mg/day) is recommended in all case as long as treatment is continued.

Multidrug-resistant Tuberculosis in Pregnancy

What is the global burden of multidrug-resistant tuberculosis (MDR-TB) among pregnant females is not well known, but these patients are recognized as a population that is particularly vulnerable to MDR-TB. In a systematic review and meta-analysis of 275 pregnant patients with MDR-TB, the pooled proportion of treatment success was 72.5%, and the pooled proportion of favorable pregnancy outcomes was 73.2%. In this analysis looking into adverse effect, impaired liver function, kidney functions, hearing loss, and hypokalemia were most common, occurring in >50% of the patients. This analysis included pulmonary and extrapulmonary TB, with no specific mention of skin TB.

For treating MDR-TB in pregnancy following points are noteworthy:

- Collaboration between treating physician and obstetrician.
- When the pregnancy is <20 weeks, advice *Mycobacterium tuberculosis* curli pili (MTP) (24 weeks will apply wherever the bill is passed).
- Ethionamide is contraindicated during the first 32 weeks of pregnancy (teratogenicity in first trimester and risk of hypothyroidism in the infant in second trimester).
- Therefore the shorter oral bedaquiline (which contains ethionamide) cannot be administered in pregnant women before 32 weeks.
- Beyond 32 weeks, the choice of regimen needs to be a decision between the obstetrician and physician. Longer oral M/XDR-TB regimen can be designed to prevent known side effects, until better safety profiles are established.

Shorter regimen: 4–6 Bdq (6 months) with Lfx, Cfz, Eto, Hh, Z, E, followed by 5 months of Lfx, Cfz, Z, E. No modifications allowed.

Longer regimen: 18–20 Lfx, Bdq (atleast 6 months or longer) Lzd, Cfz, and Cs. Lzd dose to be tapered to half after 6–8 months based on bacteriological response. Modify regimen if one or more drug cannot be used due to reasons of resistance, tolerability, contraindication, availability, etc.

(H: isoniazid; Hb: high-dose isoniazid; Lfx: levofloxacin; Cfz: clofazimine; Bdq: bedaquiline; Cs: cycloserine; Eto: Ethionamide; Lzd: linezolid; Z: pyrazinamide; E: ethambutol)

NONTUBERCULAR MYCOBACTERIAL INFECTIONS

Nontubercular mycobacteria (NTM), also known as mycobacteria other than TB (MOTT), causes skin and soft tissue infection, lymphadenitis, pulmonary infection, disseminated infection, mainly in susceptible population as, immunocompromised patients, patients with indwelling medical equipment, recent surgery or a penetrating trauma or nonsurgical procedures. Type of disease depends on the mode of inoculation and the susceptibility of the host to infection. Common skin presentations are nodules, abscesses, nonhealing furuncle like lesions, discharging sinuses, etc. In the last decade, there has been steady rise in the cases of NTM infections of skin, especially so after postsurgery and postintervention. In India, skin infections are mostly by the fast growers which include *Mycobacterium fortuitum, M. abscessus,* and *M. chelonae*. Other important skin pathogens are *M. marinum* causing fish tank granuloma and *M. ulcerans* causing painless skin ulcers. **Table 2** shows classification of NTM and **Table 3** shows the diseases caused by them.

The evaluation of skin NTM infections includes tissue culture, AFB staining, histopathology, and PCR for NTM wherever possible. The laboratory should be sensitized regarding the possibility of NTM infection. In patients already on antibiotics culture is often negative; therefore, it is important to send the cultures before starting the patient on antibiotics. Treatment for rapid growers includes

TABLE 2: Classification of nontubercular mycobacteria (NTM).

Slow growing (Weeks to months for growth)	Rapidly growing mycobacteria (7–30 days to grow)
• *Mycobacterium marinum* • *Mycobacterium ulcerans* • *Mycobacterium kansasii* • *Mycobacterium haemophilum* • *Mycobacterium scrofulaceum*	• *Mycobacterium chelonae/abscessus* • *Mycobacterium mucogenicum* • *Mycobacterium smegmatis* • *Mycobacterium fortuitum*

TABLE 3: Diseases caused by nontubercular mycobacteria and its management

Organism	Disease	Treatment
Mycobacterium marinum	Fish tank granuloma, aquarium granuloma, or swimming pool granuloma	Superficial cutaneous infections: • Clarithromycin • Doxycycline • Minocycline • Trimethoprim-sulfamethoxazole Severe infections: Combination of rifampicin and ethambutol
Mycobacterium ulcerans	Buruli ulcer and Bairnsdale ulcer	• 8-week course of rifampicin and streptomycin • Or 4-week course of rifampicin and streptomycin followed by 4 weeks course of rifampicin and clarithromycin
• *Mycobacterium kansasii* • *Mycobacterium haemophilum* • *Mycobacterium avium-intracellulare*	Skin nodules, ulcers, etc., have been reported	Rifampicin, clarithromycin, and ciprofloxacin (in various combination)
• *Mycobacterium fortuitum* • *Mycobacterium abscessus* • *Mycobacterium chelonae*	Subcutaneous nodules, abscesses, cellulitis, ulcers, sporotrichoid nodules, sinus tracts, drainage from chronic wounds, erythema, papules, pustules, and folliculitis	• Clarithromycin, azithromycin, ciprofloxacin, levofloxacin, moxifloxacin, doxycycline, minocycline, linezolid, trimethoprim-sulfamethoxazole • Parental medications: Initially, such as amikacin, cefoxitin, tigecycline, or imipenem

varies oral and injectable antibiotics. There are no guidelines for treating skin infections. Dabas et al. treated *M. fortuitum* skin infection in pregnant female with *linezolid 600 mg twice daily and ofloxacin 400 mg PO daily*. Katayama et al. managed *M. fortuitum* infection in a pregnant female with tetracycline ointment and surgical incision during pregnancy followed by oral minocycline and rifampicin after delivery. The antibiotics should be used in combination (use of single drug is highly discouraged). **Table 4** shows antibiotics uses for NTM and its pregnancy category.

Subcutaneous Fungal Infections

Sporotrichosis, mycetoma, chromoblastomycosis, and phaeohyphomycosis are some of the subcutaneous fungal infections seen; sporotrichosis being the most common among them. There is no difference in the course of these diseases in pregnancy except for the clinical presentation, which can be more florid and extensive during the course of pregnancy. Evaluation of these

TABLE 4: Systemic drugs used in various skin infections and their pregnancy category.

Drug	Pregnancy category (US Food and Drug Administration)
Oral	
Clarithromycin	C
Azithromycin	B
Ciprofloxacin	C
Levofloxacin	C
Moxifloxacin	C
Doxycycline*	D
Minocycline	D
Linezolid	C
Rifampicin*	C
Trimethoprim-sulfamethoxazole*	D
Amoxicillin*	B
Dapsone*	C
Parental medications	
Amikacin*	D
Cefoxitin	B
Tigecycline	D
Imipenem	C
Streptomycin	D
Gentamycin	D
Crystalline penicillin*	B

*Drugs used in actinomycetoma.

diseases remains same; skin biopsy and cultures should be done accordingly. However, the management differs as most of the antifungal drugs are contraindicated during pregnancy except for a few of them such as terbinafine and amphotericin B which are considered to be pregnancy category B.

Sporotrichosis

Sporotrichosis is caused by dimorphic fungi *Sporothrix schenckii*, with women in childbearing age and at-risk population to acquire this mycosis. Presenting as plaques or crusted nodules involving local lymphatics. Treating sporotrichosis in pregnancy is a therapeutic challenge. Treatment modalities such as heat therapy and cryosurgery have been tried in sporotrichosis with good results in antenatal females but studies with larger sample size are still lacking.

- Thermotherapy is the most reported therapeutic option described in pregnant females, daily self-application of heat to the lesions for weeks is needed.
- Cryosurgery is another modality tried and has found to be useful.
- If severe sporotrichosis cases are to be treated during pregnancy, amphotericin B is recommended.

Cryosurgery enhances the immune response by increasing the antigen presenting cells, neutrophils, and macrophages in the subcutaneous tissue. It is considered to be good option in pregnancy; however, it should be avoided in individuals with extensive lesions and those who are sensitive to cold. Fichman et al. successfully treated four pregnant females with sporotrichosis using cryotherapy.

Chromoblastomycosis

Chromoblastomycosis is caused by number of different pigmented fungi, the common of which are *Fonsecaea pedrosoi, Fonsecaea monophora,* and *Cladophialophora carrionii.* It presents as single or multiple verrucous hyperkeratotic infiltrated plaques. Though nothing specific has been mentioned in literature regarding its management in pregnancy, but as it goes with cutaneous sporotrichosis local application of heat, cryotherapy, and surgical reductions may be useful modalities in pregnancy.

Mycetoma

Mycetoma can be either eumycetoma or actinomycetoma. There have been reports of mycetoma following an aggressive course during the pregnancy. Treating eumycetoma is again challenging as except terbinafine and amphotericin B, no other oral antifungals are recommended. For actinomycetoma drugs which are used are listed in **Table 4**. Surgery has been used in pregnancy as a debulking procedure and it may buy some time.

Overall in all these infections, the cases should be managed depending upon the severity; mild disease and long-term single lesion can be treated after delivery, when necessary physical modalities as mentioned may be used. Use of systemic therapy to be used only when benefit outweighs the risk associated.

One can combine the drugs which are safe during the pregnancy, and regimen can be modified according to the response in postpartum period. Collaboration between the treating physician and obstetrician is of utmost importance for better maternal and fetal outcome.

For systemic fungal infections such as histoplasmosis, cryptococcosis, coccidioidomycosis, and blastomycosis, liposomal amphotericin B is preferred in pregnant patients when treatment is necessary.

SUGGESTED READINGS

1. Patel VM, Lambert WC, Schwartz RA. Safety of Topical Medications for Scabies and Lice in Pregnancy. Indian J Dermatol. 2016;61(6):583-7.
2. Weill A, Bernigaud C, Mokni M, Gil S, Elefant E, Chosidow O. Scabies-infested pregnant women: A critical therapeutic challenge. PLoS Negl Trop Dis. 2021;15:e0008929.
3. Morgan DJ, Guimaraes LH, Machado PR, D'Oliveira A Jr, Almeida RP, Lago EL, et al. Cutaneous leishmaniasis during pregnancy: exuberant lesions and potential fetal complications. Clin Infect Dis. 2007;45:478-82.
4. Bitton Y, Diav-Citrin O. Cutaneous Leishmaniasis: Case Series on Pregnancy Outcome. Open Forum Infect Dis. 2020;7:ofaa479.
5. Dutra WO, Barbosa DF, de Souza PEA, Morgan D, Poetker S, Guimarães LH, et al. A Th2-type response is associated with exuberant lesions in pregnant women infected with Leishmania braziliensis. J Infect Dis. 2019;219:480-8.
6. Gould JM, Aronoff SC. TB and pregnancy—maternal, fetal, and neonatal considerations. Microbiol Spectr. 2016;4(6).
7. Miele K, Bamrah Morris S, Tepper NK. Tuberculosis in Pregnancy. Obstet Gynecol. 2020;6:1444-53.
8. Hui SYA, Lao TT. Tuberculosis in pregnancy. Best Pract Res Clin Obstet Gynaecol. 2022;85: 34-44.
9. Esmail A, Sabur NF, Okpechi I, Dheda K. Management of drug-resistant tuberculosis in special sub-populations including those with HIV co-infection, pregnancy, diabetes, organ-specific dysfunction, and in the critically ill. J Thorac Dis. 2018;5:3102-18.
10. Dabas G, Sharma K, Narang T, Sharma M, Chatterjee D, Dogra S. Cutaneous non-tubercular mycobacterial infection in pregnancy and treatment consideration. Eur J Obstet Gynecol Reprod Biol. 2019;237:215-6.
11. Fichman V, Valle AC, de Macedo PM, Freitas DF, Oliveira MM, Almeida-Paes R, et al. Cryosurgery for the treatment of cutaneous sporotrichosis in four pregnant women. PLoS Negl Trop Dis. 2018;12:e0006434.
12. Hay RJ. Mycetoma, mycoses and pregnancy. Acta Term Venereol. 2015;3:259-60.

CHAPTER 12

Specific Dermatological Disorders in Pregnancy

12.1 Atopic Eruption of Pregnancy

Sanjeev Gupta, Neha Rani, Aditi Dabhra

INTRODUCTION

Atopic eruption of pregnancy (AEP) is a pruritic disorder of pregnancy that presents as an eczematous or papular eruption. Atopic dermatitis in pregnancy may occur de novo or may be a recurrence and exacerbation of chronic atopic dermatitis. AEP includes a number of dermatoses that are grouped together due to similar clinical features as given in the **Box 1**.

Atopic dermatitis is characterized by itchy eczematous lesions over skin caused by epidermal barrier impairment and immunological changes in skin. The highest incidence and prevalence of atopic dermatitis in early childhood, but can reoccur during adolescence or adulthood, especially in geriatric population and pregnancy. In atopic dermatitis, due to impairment of skin barrier there is reduced diversity in skin microbiome with a predominance of *Staphylococcus aureus*. There is also subclinical inflammation in skin that is characterized by increased number of inflammatory dendritic cells and T helper 2 (Th2) cells.

During disease flares, predominantly Th2 cells increase along with Th1, Th17, and Th22, whereas the number of Th1 cells increase during chronic phase. However, some variations are possible in this general trend depending on the

BOX 1 Synonyms.

- Early onset prurigo of pregnancy
- Prurigo of pregnancy
- Prurigo gestations
- Pruritic folliculitis of pregnancy
- Eczema of pregnancy

phenotype. Th22 and Th17 cells are seen more in Asian patients and almost absent in black patients with atopic dermatitis. In this chapter, we will be discussing at pathogenesis and clinical features and management of atopic dermatitis during pregnancy.

EPIDEMIOLOGY OF ATOPIC ERUPTION OF PREGNANCY

Atopic eruption of pregnancy is one of the most common dermatological conditions that occur during pregnancy, affecting approximately 5–20% of pregnant women. AEP accounts for nearly 50% of all pregnancy-specific skin disorders, making it a significant cause of pruritus (itching) in pregnant women. It is more common in those with a preexisting history of atopy.

Geographic and ethnic variation: AEP is more common in areas where atopic conditions are more frequent. It is more common in Caucasians.

Age: Women of reproductive age with a preexisting history of atopy, particularly those in their late 20s to early 30s, are at increased risk of developing AEP. Younger women (under 30 years) are generally more likely to be affected.

Parity: Primigravida are more likely to develop AEP.

SKIN AND HORMONES

- Various hormones such as glucocorticoids are both synthesized and metabolized in the skin. Therefore, skin can be considered as an extra-adrenal organ which connects endocrine, nervous and skin immune system with reciprocal interactions and influence on each other. Even the steroid hormone precursors can also be synthesized in the skin.
- In the skin, estrogen receptors are expressed in the epidermis and dermis mainly by fibroblasts, hair follicles, blood vessels, and sebaceous glands. Whereas androgen receptors are expressed by hair follicles and sebaceous glands.
- Estrogen and progesterone regulate the collagen content and water-binding capacity of skin and there by affect skin structure and elasticity. Estrogen improves skin barrier function and increases the water binding capacity and fluid retention in the skin. Estrogen also decreases the cellular immune response and downregulates sebum production.
- Progesterone and androgens have negative effects on skin barrier function. Androgens also lead to increase in sebum production.
- Physiological changes are seen in the levels of estrogen and progesterone during menstrual cycle, which correlates with the higher occurrence of certain skin diseases such as atopic dermatitis during the luteal phase with improvement during menstruation. This can lead to cyclical improvement and worsening of symptoms in atopic dermatitis patients.
- There are studies which have reported variations in reactivity in epicutaneous contact allergen testing during menstrual cycle. This skin test reactivity has been described to increases during luteal phase and decreased during the

TABLE 1: Changes in the skin and skin immunity with different hormones.

	Estrogen	Progestogen	Androgen
Skin barrier	↑	↓	↓
Water binding capacity	↑	↓	↑
Sebum production	↓	?	↑
Th1	↓	↓	↑
Th2	↑	↑	↓
Th17	↓	↓	↓
Treg	↑	↑	↑

follicular phase. It is hypothesized that during ovulation, estradiol suppresses the late phase immune response.

- Cyclical changes in skin barrier functions, sensitivity, dryness, and transepidermal water loss demonstrates the marked effects of these hormones on these skin changes **(Table 1)**.

PATHOPHYSIOLOGY OF ATOPIC ERUPTION OF PREGNANCY (TABLE 1)

The pathophysiology of AEP is complex and primarily driven by the unique hormonal and immunological changes that occur during pregnancy.

- Estrogen improves skin barrier function and water holding capacity.
- Progesterone and androgens have a negative effect on skin barrier.
- Estrogen decreases sebum production while progesterone and androgen increases it.
- Estrogen suppresses cell-mediated immune response.
- Skin is dry, sensitive, and have increased transepidermal loss during luteal phase and increases during menstruation.

ATOPIC DERMATITIS AND HORMONES

- There are several differences in innate and adaptive immune responses seen in males and females. One of the differences is higher expression of toll-like receptor 7 on human plasmacytoid dendritic cells with consecutively higher induction of type 1 interferons after stimulation in females. CD4+ cell counts and the CD4+/CD8+ ratio are also higher in females as well as the number of activated T cells, proliferation of T cells, cytotoxic activity, and Th2 immune responses. The number of B cells and different antibody production is also more in females.
- Another example is the higher toll-like receptor 9 expression on peripheral blood mononuclear cells (PBMCs), as well as toll-like receptor 4 expression of neutrophils and macrophages in the males. These differences are present from puberty, adulthood, and older age.

- Some of these differ due to the influence of estrogen on immune system. These include the support of Th2 immune response, increased release of Th2 cytokines by innate lymphoid cells as well as dendritic cell differentiation, responsiveness and cytokine release, and increased mast cell activity.
- Estrogen and progesterone stimulate Th2 immune response and regulatory T-cell function and down regulate Th1 and Th17 immune response. Whereas androgen support Th1 immune response and regulatory T cells while down regulate Th2 and Th17 responses. These effects of estrogen and progesterone are responsible for increased Th2 inflammation and susceptibility to allergic reactions that occur in the course of menstrual cycle or pregnancy.
- Studies have also demonstrated that Th2 immune response is overall more pronounced in females than in males which in parts is also caused by immunosuppressive effects of testosterone. Although there is slightly higher incidence of atopic dermatitis in boys in infancy, during childhood incidence is similar in boys and girls. Some studies suggest female predominance whereas male patients predominate among those older than 65 years of age.

PREGNANCY AND Th2 IMMUNITY

- Pregnancy is considered to be a Th2 driven event. But the nature of cytokines and type of immune response change in every trimester.
- Human chorionic gonadotropin is essential for the pregnancy from its very early stage and therefore its levels increase rapidly and reach a peak in the middle of first trimester. It is an important amplifier for production of progesterone. Progesterone in turn is regarded as an important driver of Th2 cells.
- During implantation and placentation, an inflammatory cytokines milieu predominates to increase the receptivity of the uterus and to increase reorganization of adhesion molecules during attachment of blastocyst.
- The second trimester of pregnancy is dominated by anti-inflammatory Th2 milieu which supports the rapid fetal growth and is considered to be important for the survival of the fetus.
- Toward the full development of fetus, immune status shifts from Th2 to Th1 type immune response. This Th1 type immune state is necessary for the delivery.
- Progesterone and estrogen levels are associated with a stronger Th2 immune response in the first and second trimester, which might be the reason for the occurrence of atopic dermatitis in these trimesters.
- During pregnancy, atopic eczema (AEP) is often seen in women with a history of worsening atopic dermatitis during menstruation, highlighting the influence of estrogen and progesterone.
- AEP frequently presents with normal total immunoglobulin E (IgE) levels and no prior allergic or atopic conditions, complicating its diagnosis. Traditional atopic dermatitis diagnostic criteria, such as those from Hanifin and Rajka, are not always applicable, as they rely on features like high IgE levels or a history of atopy, which are often absent in AEP.

- Consequently, the diagnosis of AEP remains difficult due to the lack of specific criteria, necessitating a comprehensive understanding of pregnancy-related skin conditions to differentiate AEP from other dermatoses during pregnancy.

PATHOPHYSIOLOGY OF ATOPIC ERUPTION OF PREGNANCY

Atopic eruption of pregnancy is thought to be triggered by pregnancy specific immunological changes such as reduced cellular immunity and reduced production of Th1 cytokines [interleukin-12 (IL-2), interferon gamma, and IL-12], dominant humoral immunity, and increased secretion of Th2 cytokines (IL-4 and IL-10). Thus, dominant Th2 immune response which is typical for pregnancy to prevent fetal rejection causes exacerbation of preexisting atopic eczema or may cause first manifestation of atopic skin changes in pregnancy.

Several key factors contribute to the development of AEP:
- Hormonal changes
- Immunological shift to Th2 predominance
- Altered skin barrier function
- Genetic predisposition
- Environmental triggers

CLINICAL FEATURES OF ATOPIC ERUPTION OF PREGNANCY

- It usually presents in first trimester. In 75% of the patients, present before the third trimester. It has a tendency to recur in subsequent pregnancy.
- All of the different phenotypes of atopic dermatitis occurring during pregnancy are referred to as atopic eruptions of pregnancy.
- Despite a similar clinical presentation, different endotypes, and phenotypes of atopic dermatitis have been identified, i.e., classic extrinsic phenotype and intrinsic phenotype. The classic extrinsic phenotype is seen in about 80% patients of atopic dermatitis and is characterized by high total serum IgE levels, eosinophilia, personal and family history of atopic dermatitis, and skin barrier impairment. The other 20% of patients with atopic dermatitis have intrinsic phenotype with normal total serum IgE levels and have delayed onset of disease with a female predominance.
- It needs to be distinguished from other diseases during gestation associated with pruritus or eczema. AEP is associated with severe itching, usually presents in first or second trimester of pregnancy.
- About 20% of patients presents with an exacerbation of preexisting atopic eczema with a typical clinical picture. The remaining 80% of patients develop atopic skin changes for the first time in pregnancy or after a long period of remission (e.g., since childhood).
- The skin eruptions are of either E-type or P-type. Two-thirds of these patients presents with wide spread eczematous lesions called as E-type AEP, affecting

typical atopic sites such as face, neck, décolleté, and flexural surfaces of limbs. The remaining one-third of patients present with papular lesions, called as P-type AEP, which is characterized by small erythematous papules disseminated on the trunk and limbs as well as typical prurigo nodules mostly over shins and arms.

- AEP may occasionally present as follicular and papulopustular eruption (formerly known as pruritic folliculitis of pregnancy). Lesions first appear on the abdomen but may spread to the trunk and extremities. It is only mildly pruritic.
- A key feature is severe dryness of the skin and frequent atopic minor features according to Hanifin and Rajka criteria of atopic eczema. Patients may have a personal or family history of atopy or asthma.
- Symptoms usually improve within 2 weeks of delivery.

Clinical features of AEP:
- Onset in first or second trimester, improves within 2 weeks postpartum.
- Usually arises de novo in pregnancy but there may be exacerbation of preexisting atopic dermatitis.
- Depending on clinical feature AEP is of two major types; E type and P type.
- Depending on immunological factor it is of two types: Extrinsic and intrinsic.

DIFFERENCES FROM OTHER PREGNANCY DERMATOSIS

- Polymorphic eruptions of pregnancy can also occur on limbs and trunk but the skin lesions have an urticarial or papulovesicular component which is not seen in atopic eruptions of pregnancy. In these cases, clinical history and typical localization bullae that can be easily distinguished from atopic eruptions of pregnancy.
- In intrahepatic cholestasis of pregnancy, pruritus can be present without any skin lesion.
- Acute urticaria or exacerbation of chronic spontaneous urticaria can be seen in pregnancy.
- Other dermatosis like scabies or contact dermatitis may also occur during pregnancy. In these cases, clinical history and typical localization of lesion helps in diagnosis of these conditions.

Clinical mimics of AEP:
- Polymorphic eruption of pregnancy
- Intrahepatic cholestasis of pregnancy
- Acute urticaria/exacerbation of chronic urticaria
- Scabies
- Contact dermatitis

DISEASE COURSE AND PROGNOSIS

In pregnancy, about 30–40% of women with preexisting atopic dermatitis experience worsening of their condition, while 20% may see improvement or remission, and 40–50% have stable symptoms.

Maternal prognosis is good even in severe cases as lesions respond quickly to the therapy, but recurrence in subsequent pregnancies is common. Fetal prognosis is unaffected, but infant may be at risk of developing atopic skin changes later in life.

INVESTIGATIONS

- AEP is diagnosed clinically which is confirmed by ruling out other diagnosis.
- Laboratory tests may reveal elevated serum IgE levels in 20–70% of the patients (especially in E type AEP).
- Histopathology of skin lesions is nonspecific and varies with clinical type and stage of the disease and shows subepidermal pustules and perifollicular neutrophilic infiltration. There may be epidermal hyperplasia, spongiosis, and parakeratosis on histopathological examination.
- Both direct and indirect immunofluorescences are negative. There are no reliable diagnostic criteria for AEP.

MANAGEMENT (FLOWCHART 1)

General Considerations

Treating pregnant women presents unique challenges, primarily because treatments must be safe for the fetus. Many women prefer to avoid medication during pregnancy due to concerns about potential harm to the baby, as highlighted by a UK survey where over 70% of women expressed such fears. However, untreated conditions like atopic dermatitis can lead to complications such as eczema herpeticum or staphylococcal infections, and significant maternal distress, which may impact the unborn child and increase the risk of atopic diseases in the offspring. Therefore, a careful evaluation of risks and benefits is essential **(Table 2)**.

Topical Treatment

- *Moisturizers*: Moisturizers are the fundamental treatment for AEP. Topical therapies to relieve itching and dryness are initial treatment recommendations, such as pramoxine and 1–2% menthol. These should be chosen on an individual basis and should be used at least once daily. These emollients can also be used by wet wrap technique as well if necessary. Adequate skin hydration is as important as fundamental treatment. Antihistamines can be used to relieve itching, e.g., chlorpheniramine, cetirizine, and loratadine.
- *Topical corticosteroids (TCS)*: TCS are the first-line treatment of atopic dermatitis. There is higher level of evidence for safety of TCS use during pregnancy. Therefore, medium to high potency TCS are recommended both as proactive and reactive therapy during pregnancy. The amount of 200 mg/month is considered safe for use during pregnancy. If a larger dose of TCS is required for treatment it indicates a poorly controlled disease, which requires

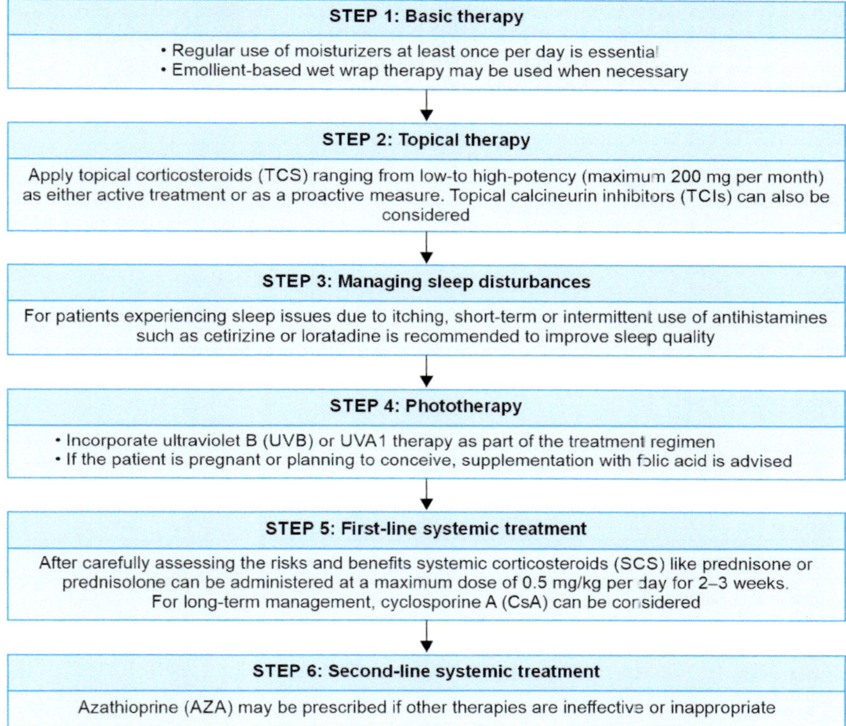

FLOWCHART 1: Stepwise approach to atopic eczema of pregnancy.

therapy escalation. Ultra high doses of TCS can be used for shorter duration as a rescue treatment or at localized areas. Only TCS that should not be used during pregnancy is fluticasone propionate, because it is not metabolized by the placenta and thus can reach the fetus in high concentrations.

- *Topical calcineurin inhibitors*: There are no studies available on the use of topical calcineurin inhibitors during pregnancy; however, oral tacrolimus has been used extensively in pregnant women following solid organ transplantation. No teratogenic or mutagenic effects have been observed in these patients. But an increased risk of prematurity has been demonstrated, it may be associated with maternal disease. Furthermore, due to larger molecular size of tacrolimus and pimecrolimus, systemic absorption is considered to be very low. Although, the use of these topical calcineurin inhibitors is not approved in pregnancy, these can be used for face, intertriginous areas, and thighs where the use of TCS is not favorable due to the risk of striae formation.
- *Ultraviolet (UV) therapy*: If the topical therapy is insufficient in controlling disease, next step in atopic dermatitis treatment is UV therapy. Broadband UVB, narrowband UVB, and UVA1 can be used as therapy in atopic dermatitis and are considered safe during pregnancy. But it can increase pregnancy-

TABLE 2: Treatment modalities for atopic dermatitis and their safety in pregnancy.

Substance	Recommended washout time before conception	Preconceptive	Pregnancy
Topical therapy:			
Moisturizers	Safe	[+++]	[+++]
Mild-to-medium-potency TCS	Safe	[+++]	[+++]
High-to-ultra-high-potency TCS	Safe	‡	‡
TCI	Safe	‡	‡
Crisaborole	NA	++	++
UV therapy:			
Broad- or narrowband UVB	Safe	[+++]	[+++]
UVA1	Safe	[+++]	[+++]
PUVA	3 months	–	–
Systemic therapy:			
Systemic corticosteroid	Safe	[+++]	[+++]
Cyclosporine	Safe	++	++
Methotrexate	3–6 months	–	–
Azathioprine	Safe	++	++
Mycophenolate mofetil	3 months	–	–
Dupilumab	Safe	‡	‡
Tralokinumab	Safe	‡	‡
Baricitinib	1 week	‡	‡
Upadacitinib	4 weeks	‡	‡

Note: [+++]: Best evidence, [++]: Possible if necessary, [+/–]: Limited evidence, [–]: Contraindicated (PUVA: psoralen plus ultraviolet A; TCI: topical calcineurin inhibitor; TCS: topical corticosteroids; UV: ultraviolet; UVA1: ultraviolet A1; UVB: ultraviolet B);

induced hyperpigmentation. Some studies show that UVB therapy decreases serum folic acid levels, and this should be compensated for with folic acid supplements before conception and during the course of pregnancy. Although, there are no specific recommendations on folate supplementation in pregnant women undergoing UV therapy. Therefore it is recommended that women who are trying to conceive while undergoing UV therapy receive folic acid at the doses that are normally recommended preconception. In addition, pregnant women undergoing UV therapy should receive a standard dose of folate daily regardless of trimester and serum folate levels should be measured at least once in a trimester while using UV therapy during pregnancy. Psoralenes are not recommended in pregnancy because of potential mutagenic effects.

Systemic Therapy

If the disease cannot be controlled with moisturizers, TCS, and UV therapy, next step in the treatment escalation is systemic therapy. Different amounts of evidence are available on the use of systemic anti-inflammatory drugs during pregnancy.

- *Oral antihistamines*: Sufficient evidence of safety of second-generation oral antihistamines such as cetirizine and loratadine is available for use in pregnancy. There is also some evidence for the safe use of third-generation antihistamines during pregnancy, but more clinical studies are required to support this. There is insufficient evidence to use oral antihistamines as treatment of atopic dermatitis and these are not a replacement for topical therapies. However, short term or intermittent use of oral antihistamines can be given in addition to primary treatment to improve pruritus and sleep quality due to sedative effect. Oral antihistamines should be used in a standard dose, up dosing of these is not recommended in pregnancy. Also, the patient should be counseled about the side effects such as sedation and impaired cognitive functions.
- *Systemic corticosteroids*: These can be used for atopic diseases in pregnancy as a rescue therapy for acute flare ups of the disease. However, their long-term safety profile is unfavorable due to many side effects such as osteoporosis, osteopenia, hypertension, glaucoma, and type 2 diabetes mellitus. During pregnancy, it may also increase the risk of gestational diabetes, preeclampsia, preterm delivery, and membrane rupture. Systemic corticosteroids have also been linked to fetal malformations like oral clefts; however, this association is not confirmed by a large cohort study on pregnant patients who used oral or inhalation steroids in first trimester. Therefore, based on this evidence of safety, use of systemic corticosteroids can be used as a short-term rescue therapy only if the topical or UV therapy is unable to control the disease. Maximum recommended dose is 0.5 mg/kg/day, prednisone or prednisolone can be used but not dexamethasone.
- *Cyclosporine A (CsA)*: There is large body of evidence on safety of CsA use in pregnancy, which is formed by the studies on patients of solid organ transplantation or patients with systemic autoimmune diseases. But there is slight tendency for preterm or low birth weight in newborns; however, this can be attributed to maternal underlying disease. No teratogenic or mutagenic effects have been reported. Common side effects of CsA include renal function impairment or development of arterial hypertension. Therefore close monitoring is required for these parameters in pregnant women. Thus, based on data, CsA can be used in pregnancy in special cases when the benefits for mother justify the potential risk to the fetus. The European task force on atopic dermatitis categorizes CsA as a first-line systemic treatment during pregnancy when long-term systemic therapy is required for disease control.
- *Azathioprine*: It can be used as off-label for AEP when topical and UV therapy are ineffective and CsA cannot be given or ineffective. No teratogenic or mutagenic effects have seen but there is an increased risk of preterm delivery.
- *Methotrexate*: Is contraindicated for use in pregnancy and before conception. Methotrexate causes embryopathy and skeletal abnormalities in the fetus

even after a low dose. Women of childbearing age are strongly recommended to use effective contraception if receiving methotrexate. The European league against rheumatism task force recommends that methotrexate should be stopped 1–3 months before planning a pregnancy. The European task force on atopic dermatitis recommends to stop methotrexate at least 6 months before conception.

- *Mycophenolate mofetil*: It is an antimetabolite drug, is known to be teratogenic and associated with specific abnormalities including embryonal malformation (microtia, aural atresia, cleft palate and lip, polydactyly, and hypertelorism) play and abnormalities of renal, cardiovascular, and central nervous systems. Women of childbearing potential are recommended to use an effective contraception at least 3 months before conception.

Treatment:
- Emollients are first line of treatment
- TCS (mid potency) can be added
- Topical steroids may be used
- Narrowband UVB, broadband UVB, or UVA1 phototherapy can be given in AEP.
- Oral corticosteroids are given when topical treatment is not beneficial. Oral prednisolone can be given at a maximum dose of 0.5 mg/kg/day for 2–3 weeks.
- Immunosuppressants such as azathioprine and CsA may be used in pregnancy when benefits outweigh any potential risk to the fetus.

Novel Treatment for Atopic Dermatitis in Pregnancy

- *JAK inhibitors*: The first US Food and Drug Administration (FDA) approved JAK inhibitor for atopic dermatitis in adults is baricitinib. But, a very limited data is available on its safe use in pregnancy. Because JAK/STAT pathway is involved in cell adhesion and polarity, its inhibition may affect embryonic development. However, in rats and rabbits, reduction in fetal growth and weight, skeletal malformations have been observed at exposures 10–39 times the human exposure. Therefore its use is contraindicated in pregnancy and women of childbearing ages are strongly recommended to use effective contraceptive methods during and at least for 1 week after the treatment.
- Upadacitinib and abrocitinib are other US FDA approved JAK inhibitors for atopic dermatitis and are also contraindicated in pregnancy. They have shown to be teratogenic in rats and rabbits. Therefore women of childbearing ages are recommended to use effective contraceptive methods during treatment and at least 4 weeks after stopping the treatment.
- *IL-13/-4Ra chain inhibitors*: Dupilumab is the first monoclonal antibody approved for moderate to severe atopic dermatitis in adult patients. Currently available clinical studies about dupilumab exposure in pregnant women show no teratogenic or mutagenic potential. Therefore, product information states that the use of dupilumab in pregnancy is allowed only if the benefits justify the potential risk to fetus. Dupilumab is an immunoglobulin G (IgG) antibody; therefore, it is expected to cross placenta thus cannot be recommended to use unconditionally.

- Tralokinumab is another novel anti-IL-13 antibody, which was approved by the FDA and European Medicine Agency in 2021. There is no published data on the use of tralokinumab in pregnant women. However, based on studies product information does not list pregnancy as a contraindication for its use but recommends avoiding its use during pregnancy.
- *PDE4 inhibitor*: A novel PDE4 inhibitor is crisaborole which is the FDA approved for use in atopic dermatitis. There is no available data about crisaborole in pregnant women, but it advised not to use crisaborole ointment preconceptionally and during pregnancy.

CONCLUSION

The complexity of the hormonal and immunological changes during pregnancy leads to the exacerbation of atopic dermatitis or development of de novo disease, collectively known as atopic eruptions of pregnancy. The diagnosis of atopic eruptions of pregnancy is challenging as it does not meet the standard criteria of atopic dermatitis. It also needs to be distinguished from other pruritic or eczematous skin diseases occurring during gestation. The treatment of atopic eruptions of pregnancy should be escalated gradually depending upon the diseases severity and maternal quality of life. First-line therapeutic therapy includes TCS and topical calcineurin inhibitors. UV therapy and systemic therapy can be added if initial treatment shows poor response. Systemic treatment includes oral antihistamines, oral prednisone, cyclosporine, etc. Cessation of nicotine and alcohol consumption, avoidance of severe stress, and vaginal mode of delivery may reduce the risk of atopic dermatitis in children.

SUGGESTED READINGS

1. Balakirski G, Novak N. Atopic dermatitis and pregnancy. J Allergy Clin Immunol. 2022;149(4):1185-94.
2. Kroumpouzos G, Cohen LM. Specific dermatoses of pregnancy: an evidence-based systematic review. Am J Obstet Gynecol. 2003;188(4):1083-92.
3. Ambros-Rudolph CM, Müllegger RR, Vaughan-Jones SA, Kerl H, Black MM. The specific dermatoses of pregnancy revisited and reclassified: results of a retrospective two-center study on 505 pregnant patients. J Am Acad Dermatol. 2006;54:395-404.
4. Roth MM, Cristodor P, Kroumpouzos G. Prurigo, pruritic folliculitis, and atopic eruption of pregnancy: Facts and controversies. Clin Dermatol. 2016;34:392-400.

12.2 Polymorphic Eruption of Pregnancy

Resham Vasani

INTRODUCTION

Polymorphic eruption of pregnancy (PEP) is a benign inflammatory skin disorder that usually affects primiparous women in the last few weeks of pregnancy or immediately postpartum. It was described in 1979 by Lawley et al. It is also called as pruritic urticarial papules and plaques of pregnancy (PUPPP) but the term PEP has begun to supplant PUPPP. Historical terminologies for the same entity which now stand abandoned include toxemic erythema of pregnancy, Nurse's late-onset prurigo of pregnancy, Bourne's toxemic rash of pregnancy, and linear immunoglobulin M (IgM) dermatosis of pregnancy.

EPIDEMIOLOGY

Incidence:
- PEP is one of the most common specific disorders of pregnancy. It occurs approximately 1 in 160–300 pregnancies.
- It appears in late pregnancy (during third trimester) but can also present postpartum.
- It is most common in primigravida or in females who have never given birth, with the first pregnancy resulting in a spontaneous abortion.

ETIOPATHOGENESIS

Exact etiology is unknown and there are multiple theories:
- The degree of stretching of the abdominal skin is thought to play a role since PEP is seen more commonly with multiple gestation. It is hypothesized that stretching causes damage to the connective tissue that exposes the dermal antigens and triggers an inflammatory response. Supporting this theory is that PEP is usually seen at 35–37 weeks when the abdominal stretching is maximum.
- Several studies have reported the preponderance of male fetuses in women with PEP. One study also demonstrated the presence of fetal DNA in maternal skin lesions, possibly because of blood chimerism. Though the hypothesis is not confirmed, a graft versus host disease like immunological response to the circulating fetal antigens could result in PEP.
- The immunohistology profile of the patients with PEP strongly expresses the HLA-DR genotype suggestive of an antigenically driven immune hyperactivation to an unknown antigen.
- Uncertain pathogenetic theories include the possible role of reproductive hormones, medications like tocolytic drugs and prolonged progesterone therapy, paternity, atopy and autoimmunity.

RISK FACTORS

- *Multiple pregnancy*:
  - Twin pregnancy (2.9–16%)
  - Higher risk in triplets
- Hydramnios
- Macrosomic fetus

Risk factors implied but relation to PEP not established:
- Male fetus
- Rh negative maternal blood

- Maternal weight gain during pregnancy
- Familial tendency

CLINICAL FEATURES

- Usually occurs in nulliparous women.
- There is an abrupt onset in third trimester. The onset of the condition is usually around 35 weeks gestation. Rarely the condition can manifest in the second trimester. In 15–16% cases present postpartum (usually after 2 days to 2 weeks).
- Lesions start as intense pruritic papules 1–2 mm in size within abdominal striae **(Figs. 1A and B)**. Inspite of the disabling pruritus, excorations are uncommon.
- Abdominal lesions along the striae sparing the periumbilical area are the most common initial manifestations **(Fig. 2)** and it may be the only site involved.

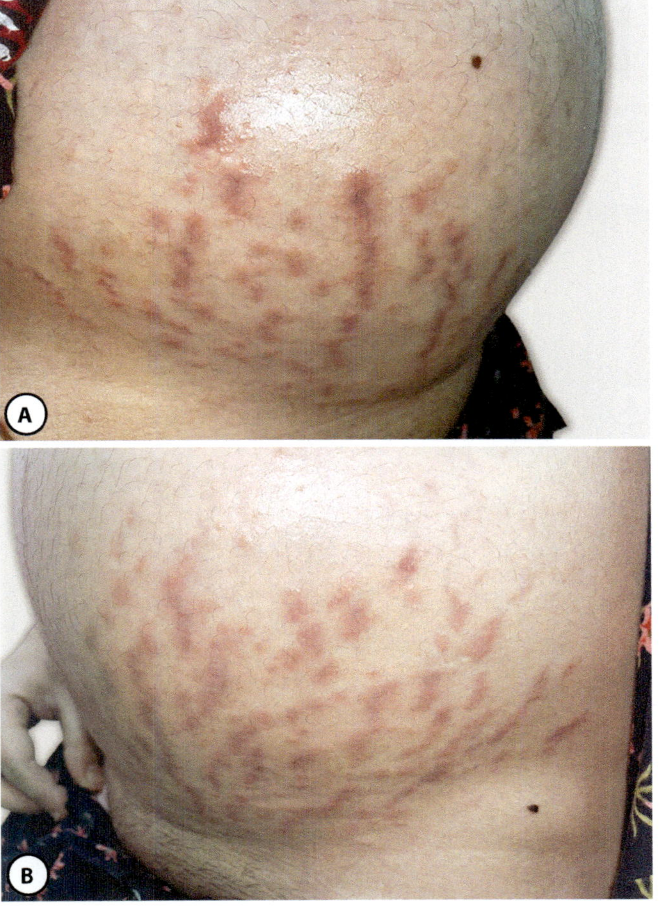

FIGS. 1A AND B: Erythematous papules that begin within the abdominal striae.

The papules then spread to the other parts of the body—on upper/lower limbs **(Figs. 3A and B)**, chest, back **(Fig. 4)**, and coalesce to form urticarial plaques **(Figs. 5A and B)**. The face, palms, and soles are usually spared.

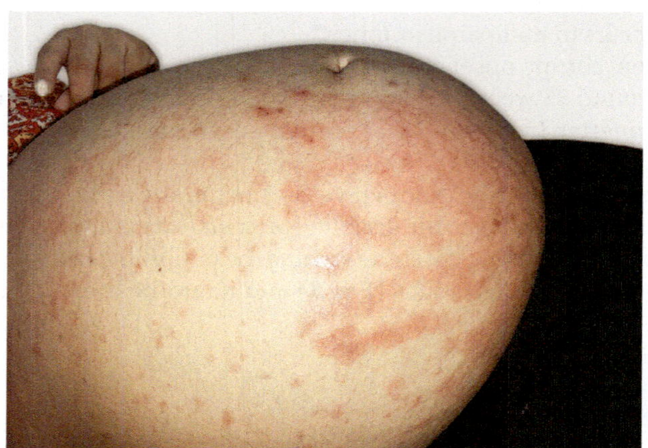

FIG. 2: Erythematous urticated papules that start within the abdominal striae further involve the adjacent abdominal skin.

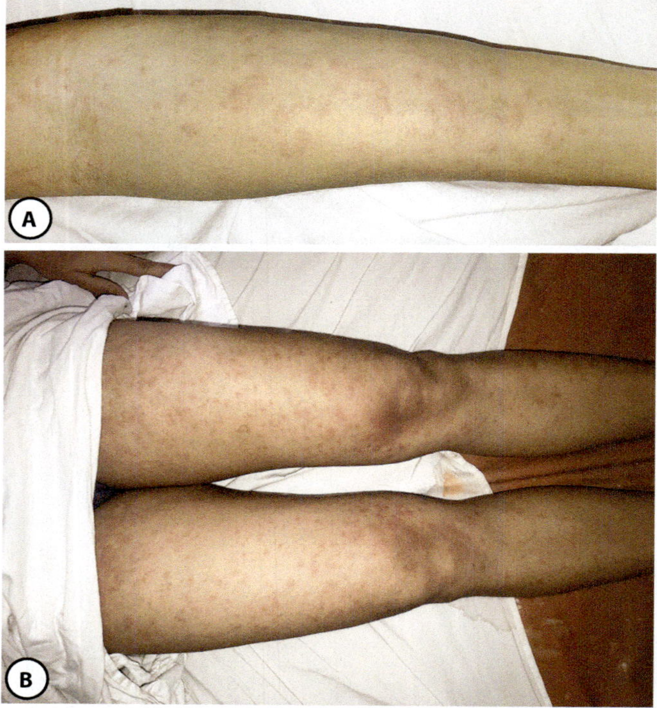

FIGS. 3A AND B: Erythematous edematous papules over the upper and lower extremities.

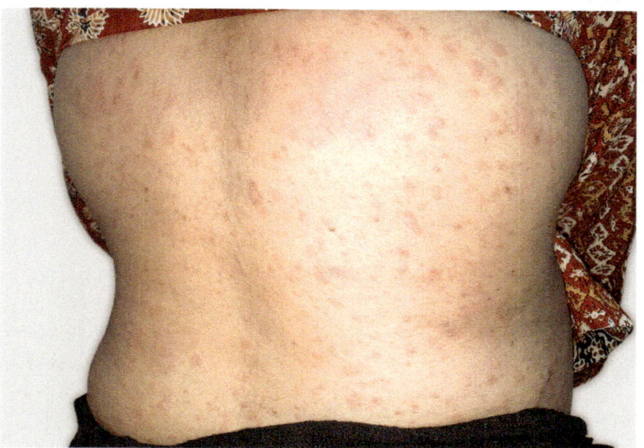

FIG. 4: Erythematous edematous papules on the back.

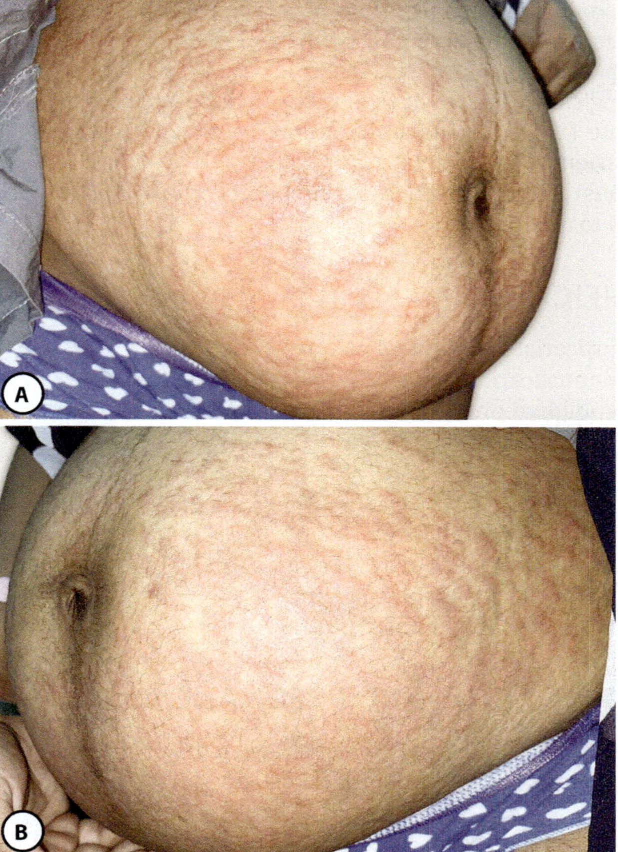

FIGS. 5A AND B: Erythematous papules coalesce to form urticarial plaques on the abdomen.

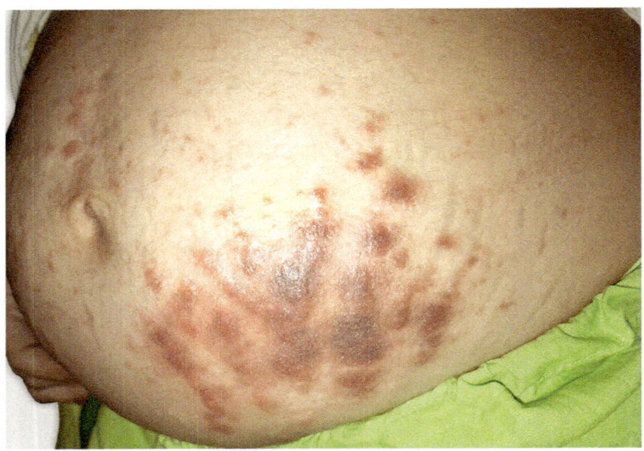

FIG. 6: Eczematous variant of polymorphic eruption of pregnancy (PEP) along the abdominal striae.

- There are occasional reports of localization of PEP only on the extremities or on the face with involvement of palms and soles. Photosensitive distribution is also reported.
- Morphological variations in the lesions include—papulovesicular, erythema multiforme (EM)-like/target-like lesions, eczematous lesions **(Fig. 6)**, and bullous lesions.
- The lesions are associated with intense pruritus—that can be extremely refractory to treatment.

CLASSIFICATION

- Type 1—urticarial papules and plaques
- Type 2—nonurticarial erythema papules and vesicles
- Type 3—combination of the two forms

RESOLUTION

- Intrapartum or prior to delivery
- 60% resolve within 1 week of delivery
- <1% resolve several weeks postpartum
- Mean clearance—3 weeks postpartum

EFFECT ON FETUS AND PREGNANCY

- Maternal and fetal outcomes are not altered if the patient has PEP.
- One case report where similar lesions on the infant born with mother diagnosed PEP.
- Preterm delivery prior to 37 weeks of gestation was seen in 18.4% of PEP patients compared to 5.8% in the control group. Early onset of symptoms before 35 weeks of pregnancy.

- Rate of cesarean section in patients with PEP (40% vs. 13.1%) in control.
- Higher rate of induction of labor
- Recurrences in subsequent pregnancies—infrequent and mild

DIAGNOSIS

- PEP is primarily a clinical diagnosis based of history and clinical examination.
- PEP has a broad clinical spectrum + diverse clinical features. Hence, investigations are done in doubtful cases to rule out other entities that can particularly have an unfavorable maternal or fetal prognosis.
- As a part of diagnosis, two biopsies are suggested; one from lesional skin for histopathology and one from nonlesional skin for direct immunofluorescence (DIF).
- Histopathology is expected to show superficial and deep perivascular and interstitial lymphocytic infiltrate with eosinophils. Epidermal changes show mild epidermal hyperplasia, spongiosis, and parakeratosis. Some cases show lymphohistiocytic vasculitis.
- DIF in lesional skin is usually negative or can show IgM, C3, IgA deposition in nonspecific granular pattern around blood vessels. Findings are not diagnostic and not consistent. This is important to differentiate PEP from pemphigoid gestationis (PG) which shows linear deposition along the dermoepidermal junction.
- Indirect immunofluorescence is always negative.

DIFFERENTIAL DIAGNOSIS

- *Other pregnancy-specific dermatosis*: PG, autoimmune progesterone dermatitis (APD), and atopic eczema of pregnancy (AEP) need to be differentiated from PEP **(Table 1)**.
- *Other differentials*: EM, drug eruptions, viral exanthem, pityriasis rosea, urticaria, and contact dermatitis

TREATMENT

- Goal of treatment is relieving the symptoms.
- Symptomatic treatment consists of cooling baths, frequent application of emollients, menthol or pramoxine containing topical medications, and light cotton clothing.
- Antihistamines such as first-generation chlorpheniramine or second-generation nonsedating antihistamines such as loratadine and cetirizine may be helpful to control pruritus.
- Topical mid potency to high potency topical corticosteroids are the initial treatment. Topical mid potent and high potent topical corticosteroids are generally safe during pregnancy as supported by multiple observational studies and meta-analysis. However, the use of potent or superpotent topical corticosteroids exceeding 300 g during whole pregnancy may be associated with an chances of increased low birth weight.

TABLE 1: Difference between PEP and other pregnancy specific dermatosis.

Feature	PEP	PG	APD	AEP
Parity	Primi	No relation	No relation	No relation
Timing	Typically third trimester, often in first pregnancy	Second or third trimester, but can occur anytime	During pregnancy or in response to menstrual cycle	Anytime during pregnancy, often early
Presentation	Red, itchy bumps, starting in stretch marks on the abdomen, spreading to thighs, buttocks, and arms	Red, itchy papules and plaques progressing to tense blisters (bullae), often starting around the belly button	Varies from eczema-like rashes to hives, mimicking PEP or PG	Exacerbation of preexisting eczema or new onset, red, itchy inflamed patches, typically on face, neck, and flexural areas
Site of involvement	Primarily abdomen, often within stretch marks; can spread to thighs, buttocks, and arms	Starts around the belly button, spreading to the trunk, back, and limbs; face typically spared	Varies, may involve any skin area, commonly affects areas exposed to progesterone fluctuations	Face, neck, flexural areas; may affect hands and feet
Cause	Unknown, possibly related to skin stretching, and male fetus	Autoimmune disorder where antibodies attack the skin	Immune response to the body's own progesterone	Immune changes during pregnancy, often in women with a history of atopic conditions (e.g., asthma and hay fever)
Recurrence in subsequent pregnancy	Rare recurrence; typically a one-time occurrence	High recurrence rate in subsequent pregnancies	Can recur with subsequent pregnancies or hormonal fluctuations	May recur, especially in women with a history of atopic conditions
Histopathology	Nonspecific findings: Spongiosis, perivascular lymphocytic infiltrate, and eosinophils may be present	Subepidermal blister formation with a dense infiltrate of eosinophils	Varies; spongiotic dermatitis, perivascular lymphocytic infiltrate, eosinophils, or leukocytoclastic vasculitis	Spongiosis, acanthosis, perivascular lymphocytic infiltrate, occasionally eosinophils

Continued

Continued

Feature	PEP	PG	APD	AEP
Immunohistochemistry	Negative or nonspecific	Positive direct immunofluorescence (DIF) showing linear C3 and IgG deposition along the basement membrane	Variable; may show perivascular IgE or immune complexes	Negative or nonspecific; may show features consistent with atopic dermatitis
Prognosis	Resolves after delivery, no long-term effects	Can worsen postpartum, may recur in future pregnancies, small risk of preterm delivery and low birth weight	Resolves after delivery or with hormonal regulation	Generally improves postpartum, but some women may experience ongoing symptoms
Treatment	Topical corticosteroids, antihistamines for itching; and symptoms resolve postpartum	Systemic corticosteroids, immunosuppressants for severe cases; may require treatment postpartum	Hormonal modulation, corticosteroids, antihistamines; avoid progesterone triggers	Topical corticosteroids, emollients, antihistamines; manage as typical eczema, with focus on symptom control

(AEP: atopic eczema of pregnancy; APD: autoimmune progesterone dermatitis; IgE: immunoglobulin E; PEP: polymorphic eruption of pregnancy; PG: pemphigoid gestationis)

- In severe cases, a short course of oral corticosteroids such as prednisolone 0.5 mg/kg/day for 1 week tapered over 1–2 weeks may be given for rapid resolution of symptoms. It is favored over betamethasone given the lower risk of fetal hypothalamic–pituitary–adrenal axis suppression.
- Narrowband ultraviolet B (NB-UVB) is rarely given as a treatment considering the relatively short duration of PEP but has been found to be effective. It can cause degradation of folate and hence additional folate supplementation during pregnancy is recommended.
- Autologous hemotherapy has an immunomodulatory effect.
- Early delivery to end symptoms is rarely necessary.

CONCLUSION

- PEP also known as PUPPP is a common benign, self-limiting, and pregnancy-specific dermatoses.
- Onset is usually in primigravida, toward the end of pregnancy and distribution is within or adjacent to the abdominal striae.
- Diagnosis is clinical. In doubtful cases, PG should be ruled out by DIF.
- Treatment is mainly symptomatic, with focus on relieving the pruritus.

SUGGESTED READINGS

1. Taylor D, Pappo E, Aronson IK. Polymorphic eruption of pregnancy. Clin Dermatol. 2016; 34(3):383-91.
2. Brandão P, Sousa-Faria B, Marinho C, Vieira-Enes P, Melo A, Mota L. Polymorphic eruption of pregnancy: Review of literature. J Obstet Gynaecol. 2017;37(2):137-40.

12.3 Pemphigoid Gestationis (Herpes Gestationis)

Sivasankari M, Biju Vasudevan, Debdeep Mitra, Aakansha Sharma

INTRODUCTION

Pemphigoid gestationis (PG) is rare among the various autoimmune bullous disorders. As the name suggests, it is a disorder occurring specifically in pregnancy and has clinicopathological resemblance with bullous pemphigoid. It was earlier called as herpes gestationis due to the morphological similarity of the vesicles to that of herpes. However, it has been studied that there is no association with old or active herpes virus infection. The lesions usually manifest in the third trimester in the form of intensely pruritic polymorphic skin lesions. It has a tendency to recur earlier in subsequent pregnancies with more severity.

INCIDENCE AND PREVALENCE

An incidence of 1 in 50,000–60,000 pregnancies has been reported. No ethnic predominance has been noted so far. The age of onset varies from 26 to 32 years.

Pemphigoid gestationis occurs commonly in multiparous women. The onset is earlier in multigravidae compared to that in primigravida. It usually manifests in the second or third trimester of pregnancy. However, onset has been reported in the first trimester or puerperium also.

ETIOPATHOGENESIS

BPAg1 and BPAg2, also known as BP230 and BP180 respectively, are key components of the basement membrane zone (BMZ) and play crucial roles in the structural integrity of the skin. While BPAg 230 (BPAg1) is found in hemidesmosome, BPAg 180 (BPAg 2) is transmembranous spans the plasma membrane of basal keratinocytes, extending into the extracellular matrix and interacts with other proteins in the basement membrane, such as laminin-332, to help anchor the epidermis to the dermis. The pathogenesis of PG is similar to that of bullous pemphigoid. There is deposition of autoreactive antibodies which are directed against BP180 antigen. Major antigen target is noncollagenous 16A (NC16A), though other sites on BP180 may also be targeted. The BP180 antigen is expressed on the basement membranes of skin and of the amniotic epithelium of both the placenta and the umbilical cord. The primary immune response is due to an abnormal expression of major histocompatibility complex (MHC) class II antigens by the placental trophoblasts and amniochorionic stromal cells. This presents the BP180 antigen to the maternal immune system. As a result, the placental BP180 antigen proteins are considered as foreign proteins and anti-placental immunoglobulin G (IgG) antibodies are produced against them. The risk is further increased in egg donated in vitro fertilization pregnancy as in these cases 100% of foetal DNA is foreign to the mother (Renata Heck, Katerina Patsatsi, Dedee Murrell 2024). There is cross reaction of the antibodies with similar antigen present in the skin as well. The autoimmune response thus triggered leads to formation of bullae and also tissue destruction **(Flowchart 1)**. Through epitope spreading BPAg 230 ma also get involved.

Immunological factors also have a role in the pathogenesis of PG as the maternal MHC class II haplotypes HLA-DR3 and HLA-DR4 have been found to have strong association with PG.

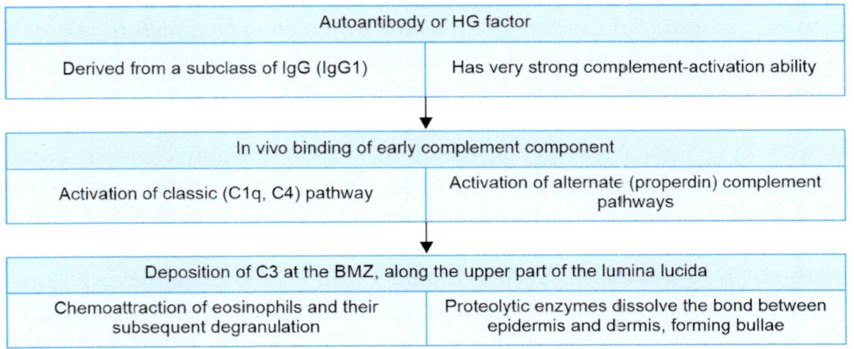

FLOWCHART 1: Mechanism of blister formation.

ASSOCIATED DISEASES

Pemphigoid gestationis has been reported to have association with other autoimmune diseases such as autoimmune thyroid disease (Graves' disease) and pernicious anemia. Rare association with hydatidiform mole and choriocarcinoma has also been reported.

HORMONES

The role of sex hormones has been proposed in the pathogenesis of PG. Progesterone has an inhibitory effect on antibody production. Fall in progesterone levels in postpartum and in premenstrual period leads to flare of PG activity. Estrogen increases the B cell response hence increasing risk and severity of PG. Flares are also observed after oral contraceptive pills.

CLINICAL FEATURES

Symptoms

Pruritus is usually the presenting symptom. They often precede the onset of bullous lesions. The intensity of pruritus is very severe in some patients to the extent that it can cause an emotional impact on the patient. Some patients report with inflammatory skin lesions as the initial symptom. It typically starts between the 12th and 24th weeks of pregnancy, with the average onset around 21 weeks. Although determining the exact prevalence at the onset is challenging, it is estimated that 18% of cases occur in the first trimester, 34% in the second trimester, and another 34% in the third trimester. However, PG can arise anytime from 9 weeks of gestation to 1 week postpartum.

Signs

Skin lesions are polymorphic. They manifest as erythematous urticarial papules or plaques or as erythema multiforme like lesions which later form into vesicles and bullae. The bullae are tense with an erythematous background. They heal without scarring **(Figs. 1 and 2)**. The lesions typically start in the periumbilical region in a majority of cases **(Figs. 3A and B)**. Later they spread to rest of the abdomen, thighs, and acral areas. There is sparing of the face and mucosae.

The interval between the onset of eruption and the development of bullous lesions was found to be usually within 2–4 weeks. The duration of individual lesions is in general 1–3 weeks. The bullous eruption usually clears in 4 weeks postpartum, and the urticarial lesions may persist up to 60 weeks. Breastfeeding may shorten this duration to 5 weeks for bullous lesions and 24 weeks for urticarial lesions.

Around 5–10% of infants born to mothers with PG have cutaneous lesions in the form of transient urticarial or vesicular lesions which resolve spontaneously within around 3 weeks. It is hypothesized that by that time the maternal antibodies are catabolized.

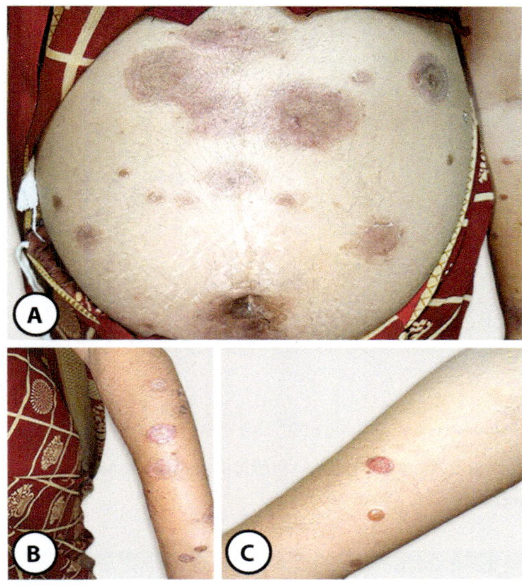

FIGS. 1A TO C: Erythema multiforme (EM) like erythematous plaques which later become bullae; resolving without scarring.

Courtesy: Dr Sriram CK, Velammal Medical College, Madurai.

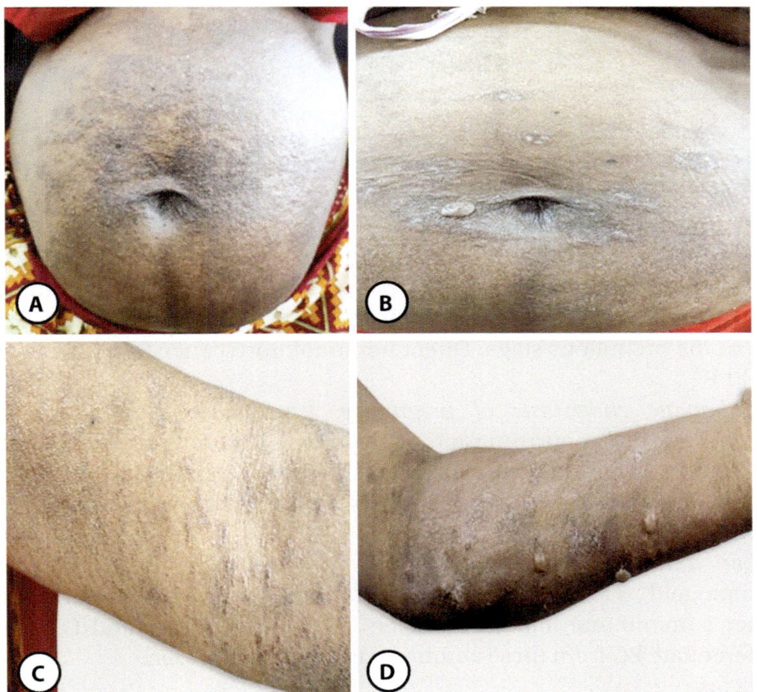

FIGS. 2A TO D: Pemphigoid gestationis. (A and C) Prebullous stage; (B and D) Bullous stage.

Courtesy: Dr Mangaiyarkarasi, Madurai Medical College.

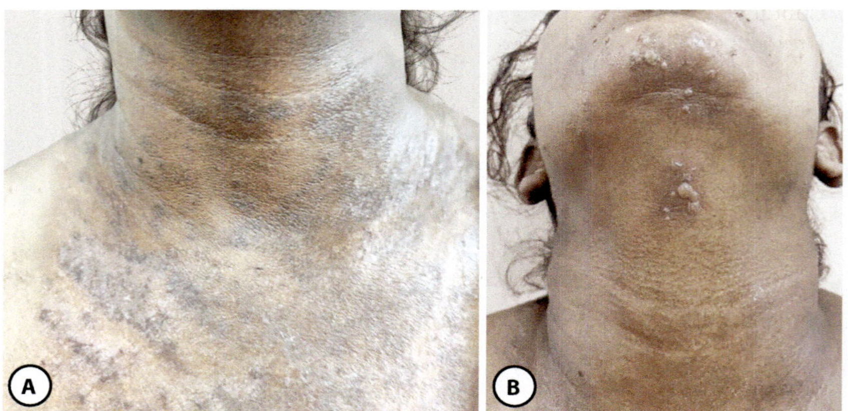

FIGS. 3A AND B: Pemphigoid gestationis. (A) Prebullous stage; and (B) Bullous stage.
Courtesy: Dr Mangaiyarkarasi, Madurai Medical College.

TABLE 1: Difference between presentation of pemphigoid gestationis depending on gestational period.

During second trimester	Postpartum presentation
• Less explosive • Often a period of relative remission in the last few weeks of pregnancy (33–40th week) • Abrupt relapse postpartum	• "Explosive" and "within hours of delivery" • More likely to recur in next pregnancy with earlier onset and florid expression

On the basis of time of presentation, features as shown in **Table 1** are seen.

DIFFERENTIAL DIAGNOSIS

- *Polymorphic urticarial papules and plaques of pregnancy (PUPPP)*: The lesions develop in the third trimester of pregnancy. They have clinical similarity to PG in the prebullous stage. Direct immunofluorescence (DIF) is negative in PUPPP.
- *Intrahepatic cholestasis of pregnancy*: Pruritus is the main symptom manifesting in the late trimesters of pregnancy. Excoriations due to scratching and icterus are common. Serum bile acid levels are elevated.
- *Atopic eruption of pregnancy*: Occurs in the first or second trimester of pregnancy.
- *Other autoimmune bullous disorders*: Linear IgA dermatosis, bullous pemphigoid, cicatricial pemphigoid, and dermatitis herpetiformis are other autoimmune bullous disorders. A detailed history and DIF helps to differentiate PG from these autoimmune bullous disorders
- Urticaria

- Contact dermatitis
- Drug hypersensitivity reactions
- Pityriasis rosea
- Scabies

INVESTIGATIONS

- Histopathology **(Table 2)**
- *DIF of perilesional tissue*: The most sensitive and specific test for diagnosis of PG. There is a linear deposition of C3 (complement 3) at the dermoepidermal junction in all cases while IgG deposition is seen in 25-50% of cases. DIF remains positive for 6 months to 4 years after remission.
- *Indirect immunofluorescence (IIF)*: It detects IgG autoantibodies targeting the basement membrane of the skin. It is also known as "HG factor".
- Enzyme-linked immunosorbent assay (ELISA) of the anti-BP180 IgG autoantibodies. The assay has specificity of 94–98% and helps to differentiate from other pregnancy related pruriginous dermatoses. It is used to monitor the disease activity.
- *Immunochemistry*: It reveals deposition of C4d immunoreactant in a linear fashion along the basement membrane.
- In conjunction with these findings, the following findings have also been observed:
  - Increased incidence of antigastric parietal cell antibodies has been reported and increased antithyroid antibody titers
  - Peripheral leukocytosis with eosinophilia (marker of severity)

TABLE 2: Difference in histopathology of an urticated and blister in pemphigoid gestationis.

Early stage: Urticarial and nonblistered areas	Late stage: Bullous stage
• Nonspecific findings • Superficial and deep, dense, and perivascular infiltrate: Lymphocytes, histiocytes, and eosinophils • "Reactive perivasculitis" • Spongiosis and vacuolization of epidermal cells • Intraepidermal microvesicles • Marked dermal edema, spongiosis, and necrosis of basal cells at tip of dermal papillae • Dermal infiltrate may be of two types: Completely lymphocytic with few eosinophils or predominantly eosinophilic with nuclear fragmentation (nuclear dust)	• Damage to basal cell plasma membrane, resulting in destruction of basal cells with blister formation • Basement membrane remains on the floor of the bulla initially, with time gets disrupted • Necrosis: Not only basal cells but also squamous cells • Level of split: Lamina lucida

TREATMENT

Pemphigoid gestationis is a self-limiting disease which usually wanes off after delivery. Treatment of PG mainly depends on the severity and the stage of the lesions.

The main aim of treatment is to provide relief from itching and to arrest the progress of the disease by stopping the blister formation. This in turn helps in improvement of the emotional and physical impact of the disease on the patient. Dressings and topical antibiotics application on the erosion will help to prevent secondary infection. The large intact bullae need to be drained without deroofing. Topical emollients containing pramoxine or menthol and oatmeal baths can help to alleviate the pruritus.

- *In mild cases with localized skin lesions*: Oral antihistamines help to alleviate the itching. First-generation oral antihistamine like chlorpheniramine or second-generation antihistamines such as loratadine and cetirizine are preferable due to their relative safety. Mild to moderate potent topical corticosteroids are used for localized disease with less blistering.
- *In moderate to severe skin lesions*: In patients who show poor or less response to topical corticosteroids in mild cases and those with lesions exceeding 10% of the body surface area, systemic corticosteroids are the drug of choice. Systemic corticosteroids in the dose of 0.3–0.5 mg/kg help to control the disease. Prednisolone and prednisone are nonfluorinated systemic steroids which are preferred in the treatment of PG as they are easily inactivated by the placental 11 beta-hydroxylase and hence the concentration crossing the placental barrier is less. Prednisolone concentration in the breast milk is about 0.1% of the ingested dose and hence it is relatively safe in lactating mothers. Breastfeeding of the baby after 3–4 hours after the oral corticosteroids is optimum. Though there is not much effect of corticosteroids on the pregnancy outcome, features of adrenal insufficiency have to be ruled out in the mother and newborn.
- *Cases less responsive/resistant to systemic corticosteroids or in case of progressive skin lesions*: The following second- or third-line drugs can be given as adjuvants to the systemic corticosteroids:
    - Intravenous immunoglobulin (IVIG): It is a second-line therapy for management of PG as it is a steroid-sparing agent. It is useful in severe and refractory cases. It is also used in patients with risk factors such as immunosuppression and uncontrolled diabetes. The recommended dose of IVIG ranges from 0.4 to 0.5 g/kg/day for 2–5 days. IVIG is an effective and safe treatment both in pregnancy and the postpartum period. The common adverse effects are fatigue, headache, flushing, and fall in blood pressure.
    - Plasmapheresis: It can be used in combination with corticosteroids or IVIG in the treatment of corticosteroid resistant cases. It causes a rapid response with clearance of lesions. The side effects are less on the mother but its effect on the placental microcirculation needs to be considered as it can affect the growth of fetus.
    - Immunoadsorption: It is a process in which the IgG are selectively removes from the plasma with the help of substances with high affinity adsorption.

The use of immunoadsorption as a treatment modality in PG has been reported in few cases with success.

- Third-line therapy:
  - Rituximab: This anti-CD20 receptor chimeric monoclonal antibody directed has been used in few cases of PG with complete remission and no side effects. However, it is not recommended to use rituximab during pregnancy because of insufficient data on the effect on fetus
  - Cyclosporine: It is a third-line drug in the management of PG. It is effective and nontoxic in pregnancy. In spite of it crossing the placental barrier, it gets rapidly cleared. Hence it does not have teratogenic effects on the fetus. However, cyclosporine has been reported to cause preterm deliveries and also growth retardation in the fetus. Other known adverse effects include hypertrichosis, bone marrow suppression, preeclampsia, and gestational hypertension.
  - Azathioprine: It has been used in persistent and sever cases of PG as an adjunct to systemic corticosteroids. The known side effects are bone marrow suppression, liver impairment, and hypersensitivity reactions. It can cause preterm, low birth weight, and birth defects. But it can be given in lactating women.
  - Dapsone: It is used as an adjuvant to corticosteroids in patients with severe and persistent PG. It has an anti-inflammatory effect. Hemolytic anemia is a known adverse effect in pregnant women who are deficient in glucose-6-phosphate dehydrogenase.
  - Methotrexate: It is effective for controlling disease activity in autoimmune bullous disorders but it is contraindicated in pregnant women because of its teratogenicity. It is also contraindicated in lactating women as it is present in the breast milk.

Other Treatments

- Goserelin and ritodrine have been tried in few cases of PG.
- Doxycycline/minocycline and nicotinamide
  Dupilumab, antibody against interleukin-4 receptor, has been recently tried.

PROGNOSIS

The lesions of PG are self-limiting soon after the pregnancy. However, they have a tendency to recur with more severe effects in the subsequent pregnancies. Onset in early trimesters of pregnancy is associated with adverse outcomes. Prognosis in the fetus is generally good. But PG can cause small for gestation and preterm birth. Neonatal pemphigoid can occasionally occur in about 10% cases due to the passive transfer of the maternal autoimmune antibodies. These babies develop fluid filled lesions or urticaria like lesions which are self-limiting. There is no increased risk of abortion or still birth.

Approach to patient of PG is as shown in **Flowchart 2**.

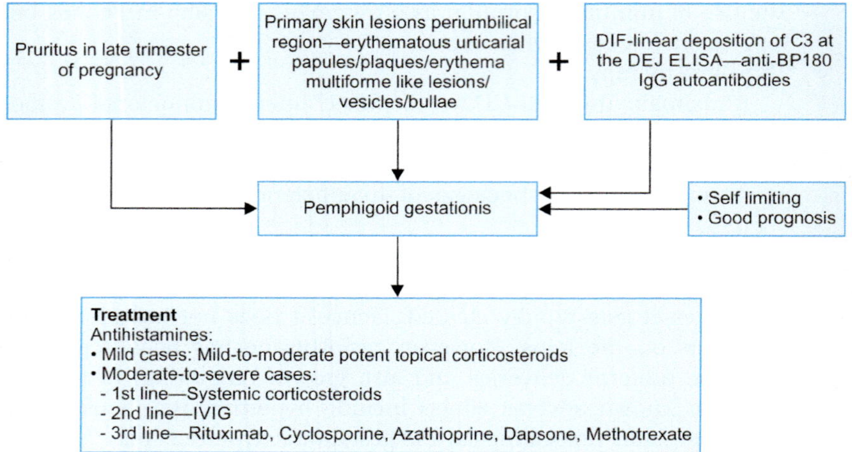

FLOWCHART 2: Approach to patient of pemphigoid gestationis.

(DIF: direct immunofluorescence; ELISA: enzyme-linked immunosorbent assay; IVIG: intravenous immunoglobulin)

KEY POINTS

- Rare autoimmune bullous disorder of pregnancy.
- Common in third trimester.
- Autoantibodies against BP180.
- DIF and ELISA for autoantibodies are specific to diagnosis.
- Self-limiting disease with resolution in the puerperium.
- Corticosteroids is usually effective in disease clearance.
- Prognosis is good.

SUGGESTED READINGS

1. Wojnarovska F, Venning VA. Immunobullous diseases. In: Burns T, Breatnach S, Cox N, Griffiths C (Eds). Rook's Textbook of Dermatology, 8th edition. Oxford, UK: Wiley-Blackwell Publishing; 2010. pp. 40.1-40.62.
2. Al-Fouzan AS, Galadari I, Oumeish OY. Herpes gestationis (pemphigoid gestationis). Clin Dermatol. 2006;24:109-12.
3. Radia C, Salim G, Kawtar I, Zahra MF, Taoufiq H. Pemphigoid gestationis: a Moroccan study. Our Dermatol Online. 2017;8(2):128-32.
4. Engineer L, Bhol K, Ahmed AR. Pemphigoid gestationis: a review. Am J Obstet Gynecol. 2000;183(2):483-91.
5. Huilaja L, Mäkikallio K, Sormunen R, Lohi J, Hurskainen T, Tasanen K. Gestational pemphigoid: placental morphology and function. Acta Derm Venereol. 2013;93:33-8.
6. Kelly SE, Bhogal BS, Wojnarowska F, Black MM. Expression of a pemphigoid gestationis–related antigen by human placenta. Br J Dermatol. 1988;118:605-11.
7. Semkova K, Black M. Pemphigoid gestationis: current insights into pathogenesis and treatment. Eur J Obstet Gynecol Reprod Biol. 2009;145(2):138-44.

8. Shornick JK, Stastny P, Gilliam JN. High frequency of histocompatibility antigens HLA-DR3 and DR4 in herpes gestations. J Clin Invest. 1981;68:553-5.
9. Shornick JK, Black MM. Secondary autoimmune diseases in herpes gestationis. J Am Acad Dermatol. 1992;26:563-6.
10. Matsumoto N, Osada M, Kaneko K, Ohara K, Noguchi D, Udagawa H, et al. Pemphigoid gestationis after spontaneous expulsion of a massive complete hydatidiform mole. Case Rep Obstet Gynecol. 2013;2013:267268.
11. Intong LR, Murrell DF. Pemphigoid gestationis: pathogenesis and clinical features. Dermatol Clin. 2011;29(3):447-52.
12. Sävervall C, Sand FL, Thomsen SF. Pemphigoid gestationis: current perspectives. Clin Cosmet Investig Dermatol. 2017;10:441-9.
13. Sävervall C, Thomsen SF. Managing Pemphigoid Gestationis. Eur Med J. 2020;5(2):125-35.
14. Butler DC, Heller MM, Murase JE. Safety of dermatologic medications in pregnancy and lactation: Part II. Lactation. J Am Acad Dermatol. 2014;70(3):417.e1-10.
15. Elliott AB, Chakravarty EF. Immunosuppressive medications during pregnancy and lactation in women with autoimmune diseases. Womens Health (Lond). 2010;6(3):431-40.
16. Shornick JK, Black MM. Fetal risks in herpes gestationis. J Am Acad Dermatol. 1992;26:63-8.

12.4 Pruritus Gravidarum (Intrahepatic Cholestasis of Pregnancy)

Resham Vasani

INTRODUCTION

Intrahepatic cholestasis of pregnancy (ICP) is also called pruritus gravidarum, obstetric cholestasis, recurrent jaundice of pregnancy, icterus gravidarum, and idiopathic jaundice of pregnancy. This entity is characterized by generalized pruritus with an elevation of the serum bile acid levels in developing the late second trimester and/or third trimester of pregnancy.

EPIDEMIOLOGY

- Intrahepatic cholestasis of pregnancy is the most common liver disease occurring in pregnancy. It occurs in <1–27.6% globally. In Indian population, the incidence is 0.5–1.5%.
- Seasonal variation in the form of increased incidence in the winter months has been seen in certain geographic locations for no definite reasons.

RISK FACTORS

- A history of ICP is a strong risk factor for recurrence in subsequent pregnancies.
- Advanced maternal age, personal or family history of cholestatic disorders, chronic hepatitis C, and multiple gestation are other risk factors.

ETIOLOGY

Genetic Susceptibility

A genetic susceptibility to develop ICP is thought to be possible on account of familial clustering of cases, presence of the condition in first-degree relatives of patients with ICP, and increased risk in some ethnic groups. Heterozygous mutation in the gene ABCB4 (adenosine triphosphate binding cassette, subfamily B, member 4) which encodes MDR3 (multidrug resistance 3) has been found in multiple cases of ICP. This gene mutation is primarily involved in a subtype of progressive familial intrahepatic cholestasis. MDR3 is canalicular transport translocator and other genes related to the same function like *ABCB11, ATP8B1, ABCC2, NR1H4* can also be involved.

Hormonal Factors

Role of estrogen in the pathogenesis is suggested by:

- Intrahepatic cholestasis of pregnancy occurs in the late second or the third trimester when the serum concentrations of estrogen are at their peak.
- A higher incidence is seen in twin pregnancies where the levels of circulating estrogen are high.
- Ovarian hyperstimulation can induce ICP in early pregnancies when the levels of estrogen are significantly high.
- Intrahepatic cholestasis of pregnancy resolves following delivery of placenta which is a major source of estrogen.
- Estrogen-progesterone containing contraceptive pills can cause cholestasis.

Role of progesterone in pathogenesis: The hepatic transport system is responsible for the biliary excretion of the progesterone metabolites that are synthesized in large amounts in genetically predisposed pregnant females. A saturation of the transport system causes increased sulfated progesterone metabolites causing activation of TGR5 causing the sensation of pruritus.

Environmental Factors

Seasonal, geographic variability and high incidence of ICP in places where there are low selenium levels in the diet, low vitamin D levels are the possible environmental factors that have been implied in the pathogenesis of ICP. Serum selenium levels decrease with advancing pregnancy. Glutathione peroxidase action depends on selenium. Increased oxidative stress caused by estrogen thus cannot be handled.

Underlying Liver Disease

Underlying liver conditions which may be preexisting or may be revealed by pregnancy have an association with ICP. Hepatitis C, nonalcoholic cirrhosis, and progressive fibrosis increase the chances of prolonged and recurrent intrahepatic cholestasis.

CLINICAL FEATURES

- The presentation is in the late second trimester or third trimester. Ovarian hyperstimulation syndrome after in vitro fertilization (IVF) can also give rise to transient first trimester symptoms.
- Generalized pruritus is the most prominent clinical symptom. Pruritus first begins on the abdomen and spreads to involve the palms and soles. The intensity varies from being mild to intolerable. There is nocturnal aggravation of pruritus. The itching may be disabling causing sleep deprivation with severe affliction of quality of life at times inducing suicidal thoughts.

  The cause of pruritus is believed to be the accumulation of bile acids in the cutaneous interstitial fluid. However, this may not be the sole explanation in ICP, as pruritus often occurs before bile acid levels increase. Other contributing factors include sulfated progesterone metabolites and serotonin.

  There are no primary lesions. Secondary excoriations and pruriginous lesions may be seen.
- Infrequent symptoms include right upper quadrant pain, nausea, poor appetite, and steatorrhea. Jaundice occurs in 14–25% of the patients, 1–4 weeks after the onset of itching. Jaundice without pruritus is rare and, if present, investigations should be done to rule out other causes. Liver failure or encephalopathy should initiate screening for other causes of liver disease.
- Though pruritus normally increases with gestation, jaundice may not change much. Also rise in bilirubin is mild.
- Presence of steatorrhea is a sign of poor maternal outcome, e.g., postpartum bleeding.
- Symptoms resolve in 2–8 weeks.

Laboratory Findings

Bile Acids

Oxidation of cholesterol occurs in liver leading to formation of primary bile acids [cholic acid (CA) and chenodeoxycholic acid (CDCA)] which are secreted in bile. These bile acids are converted into secondary bile acids [deoxycholic acid (DCA) and lithocholic acid] by deconjugation and dihydroxylation by microbes in ileum and colon. Tertiary bile acid ursodeoxycholic acid (UDCA) is formed by bacterial modification and hepatic metabolism. About 95% bile acids enter the enterohepatic circulation **(Fig. 1)**.

- In normal pregnancy, there is minimal rise in bile acids maximum 10 and 14 µmol/L especially CDCA. Rest may be same as prepregnant level.
- Asymptomatic hypercholanemia of pregnancy (AHP) is defined as raised serum bile acids which is asymptomatic with no other biochemical markers of ICP. AHP is seen in 10% (or even more) of total pregnant patients, of these only 2–3% have ICP.
- In ICP, bile acids are elevated in >90% of affected pregnancies. The rise may be 10–100 times the normal upper cut off limit.
  - Biliary bile acid profile is also altered in ICP: Although both primary and secondary bile acids are increased but increase in CA remains the

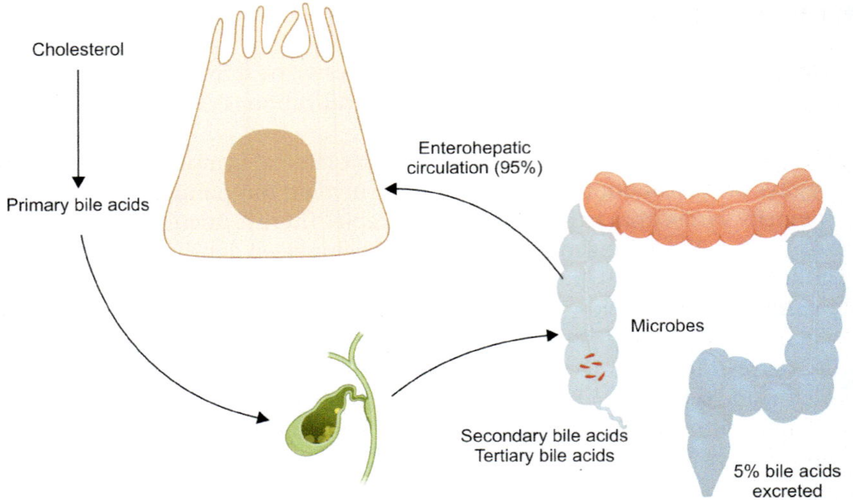

FIG. 1: Conversion of cholesterol to bile acids and its subsequent entry into circulation.

predominant. CA:CDCA ratio is increased (most sensitive marker). DCA is also increased but to a less significant level suggesting impaired enterohepatic circulation. Ratio of CA to DCA increases (normal 1:3).

- In ICP, consumption of a standard test meal causes a more dramatic and prolonged postprandial rise in serum bile acids.

Other Liver Function Tests in Intrahepatic Cholestasis of Pregnancy

- Serum aminotransferases are increased in 60% of cases. The raise in the value is usually two times the normal values but can be increased up to 1,000 units/L. In cases where the transaminases are very highly elevated, it is necessary to rule out viral hepatitis.
- Up to fourfold increase in alkaline phosphatase levels is seen but the increase is not specific for ICP because of the natural elevation of the placental isoenzyme in pregnant state.
- Total and direct bilirubin levels are increased suggesting cholestasis. The usual elevation of the total bilirubin is up to 6 g/dL.
- Serum gamma-glutamyl transpeptidase levels are usually normal but can be modestly elevated in up to 30% of the cases.
- Glutathione S-transferase alpha (GSTA) is a more sensitive and specific marker of hepatic integrity than standard liver function tests (LFTs).

Clotting Factors

Serum prothrombin time is usually normal but can be increased due to vitamin K deficiency. The deficiency in vitamin K is unlikely due to a hepatic cause and is rather due to fat malabsorption due to steatorrhea and can also happen on account of drugs administered in the treatment of cholestasis such as cholestyramine.

Ultrasound abdomen is usually shows a normal hepatic parenchyma and nondilated biliary ducts. In ICP, the fasting and ejection volumes of the gallbladder are increased, which may make these women more susceptible to developing gallstones.

Liver Histopathology

It is not required for diagnosis. It is characterized by the presence of bile plugs within the hepatocytes and canaliculi without significant inflammation.

DIAGNOSIS

The diagnosis of ICP is based on—(1) pruritus of cholestasis, (2) elevated fasting serum bile acids >10 μmol/L (and elevated serum transaminases), (3) spontaneous relief of signs and symptoms within 2–3 weeks after delivery, and (4) absence of other diseases that cause pruritus and jaundice.

Differential Diagnosis

- All specific dermatoses of pregnancy should be ruled out.
- Causes of generalized pruritus without associated primary lesions such as drug-induced pruritus, renal pruritus, hematological disorders such as Hodgkin's disease and polycythemia rubra vera
- Other causes of ICP with elevation of serum liver tests:
    - *In the late first trimester*: Hyperemesis gravidarum
    - *In the third trimester*: Acute fatty liver of pregnancy, HELLP (hemolysis, elevated liver enzyme levels, and a low platelet count) syndrome, preeclampsia, and eclampsia
    - *In all trimesters*: Viral hepatitis, alcoholic hepatitis, drug-induced hepatitis, biliary obstruction, hyperbilirubinemic states, primary biliary cirrhosis, and primary sclerosing cholangitis

FETAL EFFECTS OF INTRAHEPATIC CHOLESTASIS OF PREGNANCY

Elevation of maternal bile acids causes increase in the fetal and amniotic levels of bile acids. This elevation of the bile acids can lead meconium-stained amniotic fluid, fetal demise and stillbirth, fetal arrhythmias, neonatal respiratory distress syndrome, and preterm labor.

- *Meconium-stained amniotic fluid*: Bile acids are known to cause an increase in colonic motility or may cause fetal distress.
- *Fetal arrhythmias*: Increased taurocholic acid may cause abnormal calcium dynamics leading to arrhythmias.
- *Neonatal respiratory distress syndrome*: Increased bile acid levels in the fetal circulation can reverse the action of phospholipase A2, leading to the breakdown of phosphatidylcholine and a deficiency in surfactant.

- *Intrauterine death*: Increased syncytial knot formation and villous edema, which are suggestive of hypoxic insults. Meconium penetrates placenta within 3 hours causing vasoconstriction of umbilical and placental vessels and hence fetal hypoxia and death. A peptide or prostaglandin is suggested to be responsible for this.
- *Preterm labor*: The elevation in the bile acids causes increased expression of the myometrial oxytocin receptors. This increases the chances of preterm labor and spontaneous preterm birth.

TREATMENT

Flowchart 1 outlines the approach to diagnosis and treatment of ICP.

- Clinical decision making in ICP is based on the highest total bile acid level at any point during pregnancy, maternal obstetric history, and symptoms. If the symptoms are suggestive of ICP but the serum bile acid levels are normal, the serum bile acid levels can be estimated weekly, since there is a significantly increased risk of stillbirth if the levels increase to 100 µmol/L. This situation will favor early delivery. Treatment for ICP is generally not started unless there is biochemical evidence of ICP. If UDCA is started empirically, elevated bile acid levels and serum transaminase levels may never be elevated.
- Itching in ICP is initially treated with UDCA. It works by increasing hepatobiliary secretion. It has no fetal or neonatal toxicity. The dose of UDCA is 10–15 mg/kg daily. UDCA enhances biliary secretion through post-transcriptional regulation of the exporters MRP4 and MRP3. Additionally, it has antiapoptotic properties, as it decreases mitochondrial membrane permeability to ions and reduces cytochrome c expression. Furthermore, UDCA lowers serum levels of ethinylestradiol 17β-glucuronide, a key cholestatic estrogen metabolite. It normalizes CA:DCA ratio and decreases harmful effects of bile acids on cardiocytes. Nausea and dizziness can be possible side effects in 25% of the cases. This treatment not only decreases pruritus but has also shown to reduce stillbirth and preterm birth rates. A decrease in pruritus is usually seen within 1–2 weeks and biochemical improvement is seen within 3–4 weeks. In case no improvement is observed, the dose can be titrated every 1–2 weeks up to 21 mg/kg/day. It is not necessary to increase the dose of UDCA to reduce the elevated laboratory results if pruritus is relieved.

In cases where the maximum dose of UDCA does not cause symptomatic relief, the following drugs can be considered.

- *S-adenosyl methionine*: This drug influences the composition of the hepatocyte plasma membrane and increased methylation and biliary excretion of the hormone metabolites. Oral S-adenosylmethionine (1,600 mg/day) is administered to nonpregnant patients. Intravenous therapy is preferred for pregnant patients but prolonged therapy may be required. It has been demonstrated to be less effective than UDCA.
- Cholestyramine acts by decreasing the ileal production of bile salts and increasing the fecal excretion. It is given orally in divided doses starting from 2–4 g per day and gradually increased to 16 g per day. The symptomatic control of pruritus is limited. The side effects include constipation, abdominal pain, fat malabsorption, and that of fat-soluble vitamins.

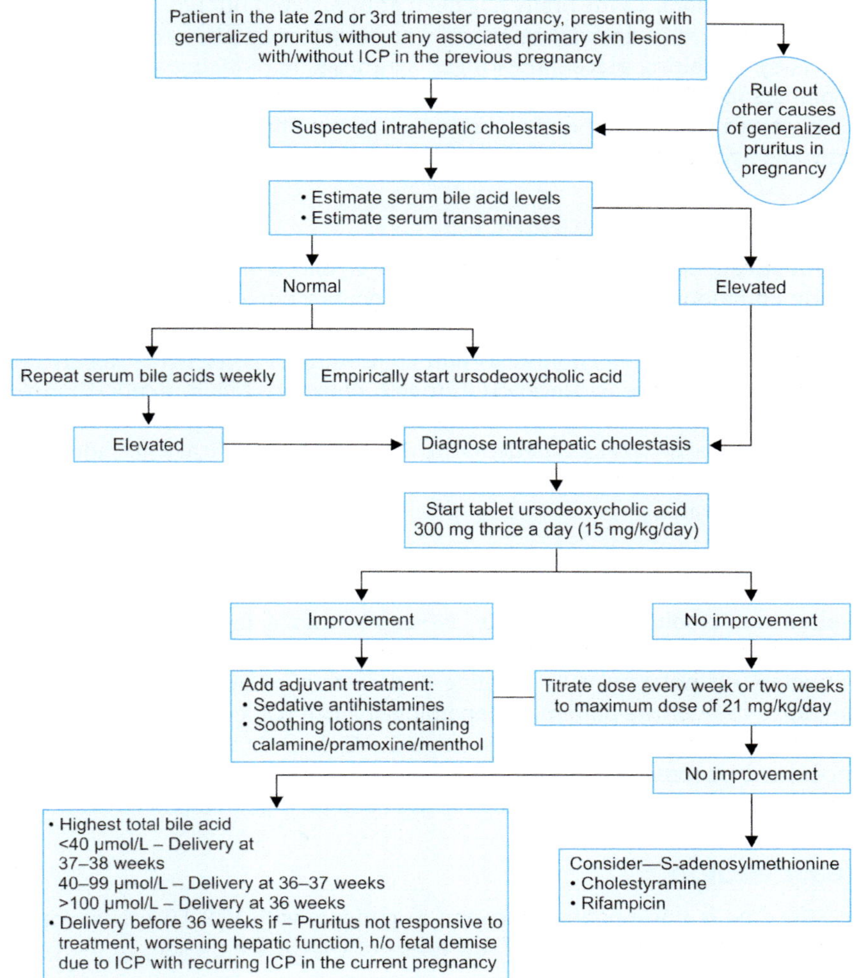

FLOWCHART 1: Approach to diagnosis and treatment.

- *Rifampin/rifampicin*: This drug is a potent agonist of the pregnane X receptor which improves detoxification and hepatobiliary processes. It has been used in nonpregnant cholestasis patients. It can be combined with UDCA in pregnant patients in the dose ranging from 300 to 1,200 mg administered in divided doses.

Other drugs that have been used as adjunctive therapy include:

- Hydroxyzine 25 mg every 6–8 hours orally or chlorpheniramine 4 mg every 4–6 hours orally has been used for their sedative value. The antihistamine efficacy in reducing pruritus is minimal.
- Calamine lotion with 2% menthol or pramoxine has been used as soothing lotions to temporarily alleviate symptoms.

- Dexamethasone 12 mg orally has been administered but has not been found to be effective in decreasing pruritus or normalizing laboratory values. This acts by inhibiting placental estrogen synthesis by reducing secretion of the precursor, dehydroepiandrosterone sulfate, from the fetal adrenal glands.

Other treatments have demonstrated uncertain efficacy, including charcoal, ultraviolet light, phenobarbital, and herbal remedies.

Management of Pregnancy

The American College of Obstetricians and Gynecologists (ACOG) has made recommendations to reduce the adverse pregnancy outcome. They recommend antenatal surveillance with fetal nonstress tests after viability and beginning at the time of diagnosis of cholestasis and continuing once or twice weekly until delivery. For a total bile acid level <100 µmol/L, delivery is recommended between 36 and 39 weeks of gestation. For a total bile acid level >100 µmol/L, delivery is recommended at 36 weeks. If patients are diagnosed with ICP at a gestational age later than recommended gestation for delivery, delivery is recommended at the times of diagnosis.

Maternal Outcome

Spontaneous resolution of pruritus is seen within a few days post delivery along with the normalization of the biochemical parameters. In case the liver parameters do not return to baseline and remain persistently elevated, it is imperative to refer the patient to hepatologist since ICP can be associated with subsequent diagnosis of gallstones, hepatitis C, hepatic fibrosis, hepatobiliary cancer, and pancreatic diseases. Higher incidence of thyroid disease, cardiovascular diseases, and diabetes mellitus has been demonstrated in few studies.

Breastfeeding

Breastfeeding is not a contraindication in patients with ICP. UDCA is stopped when the labor starts and even if low levels of UDCA are present in the breast milk, it is not harmful to the fetus.

Recurrence

60–70% recurrence with variable intensity is seen in subsequent pregnancies.

Contraception

Any nonhormonal contraceptive can be used in these patients. Though combined oral contraceptives can be given after the LFTs are normal, the patients should be warned about the possible recurrence of cholestatic pruritus and the pills need to be discontinued. Progestin only pills can be an acceptable choice.

Flowchart 1 outlines the approach to the diagnosis and management of a case of intrahepatic cholestasis.

SUGGESTED READINGS

1. Pusl T, Beuers U. Intrahepatic cholestasis of pregnancy. Orphanet J Rare Dis. 2007;2:26.
2. Ovadia C, Williamson C. Intrahepatic cholestasis of pregnancy: Recent advances. Clin Dermatol. 2016;34(3):327-34.
3. Geenes V, Williamson C. Intrahepatic cholestasis of pregnancy. World J Gastroenterol. 2009;15(17):2049-66.

12.5 Impetigo Herpetiformis

Senkadhir Vendhan, Biju Vasudevan, Santanu Banerjee

INTRODUCTION

Impetigo herpetiformis (IH), a rare and severe variant of pustular psoriasis, is primarily associated with pregnancy. This condition, first described by von Hebra in 1872, manifests as an acute and potentially life-threatening dermatological emergency, typically occurring in the third trimester. Characterized by pustular eruptions on erythematous and edematous skin, IH necessitates prompt recognition and management due to the significant risks it poses to both the mother and the fetus. Von Hebra's initial description of IH highlighted its distinct clinical presentation in pregnant women. Over time, this condition has been better understood and is now considered a form of generalized pustular psoriasis (GPP), triggered by the unique physiological changes of pregnancy.

Impetigo herpetiformis presents in two forms. The classic form occurs only during pregnancy, usually resolving on its own after delivery, but it can reappear in subsequent pregnancies. This form is not linked to a history of psoriasis and is characterized by widespread pustulosis, resembling pustular psoriasis of von Zumbusch type. The other form involves a flare-up of existing psoriasis during pregnancy, which may continue even after childbirth.

PATHOPHYSIOLOGY

The pathophysiology of IH involves a complex interplay of hormonal changes, genetic predisposition, and immunological factors, with contributions from environmental and lifestyle influences.

Hormonal Factors

Hormonal fluctuations during pregnancy, particularly elevated levels of estrogen and progesterone, are thought to play a pivotal role in the pathogenesis of IH. These hormones can modulate immune responses and skin barrier functions, potentially triggering the disease.

Estrogen and Progesterone

Estrogen and progesterone levels increase significantly during pregnancy. Estrogen influences inflammatory processes and immune cell functions, enhancing the production of proinflammatory cytokines such as interleukin-1 (IL-1), IL-6, and tumor necrosis factor-α (TNF-α), which contribute to the development of pustular lesions. Progesterone, primarily known for maintaining pregnancy, also exerts immunosuppressive effects, altering immune homeostasis and potentially exacerbating inflammatory conditions. In IH, estrogen is less and progesterone more than in a pregnant patient without IH. Estrogen is known to suppresses neutrophil migration, whereas progesterone increases it. Hence, in IH, increased neutrophil migration is seen.

Genetic Predisposition

Genetic susceptibility plays a significant role in the development of IH. Mutations in genes associated with pustular psoriasis, particularly the *IL36RN* gene, have been implicated.

IL36RN Gene

The *IL36RN* gene encodes the IL-36 receptor antagonist, which regulates inflammation in the skin. Mutations in this gene result in a defective receptor antagonist, leading to unregulated activation of the IL-36 signaling pathway. IL-36 is a member of the IL-1 cytokine family and is known for its proinflammatory properties. In IH, IL-36 is believed to contribute to the inflammatory response by activating keratinocytes and immune cells, such as neutrophils and T cells. This activation leads to the release of additional proinflammatory cytokines and chemokines, resulting in the recruitment and activation of immune cells at the site of inflammation. The heightened inflammatory environment driven by IL-36 promotes keratinocyte proliferation and epidermal hyperplasia, which are characteristic features of IH. Thus, IL-36 is thought to play a crucial role in amplifying the inflammatory cascade and sustaining the pathology of this condition.

Immunological Factors

A complex interplay between keratinocytes, neutrophils, skin-resident dendritic cells (DCs), infiltrating macrophages, T cells, and other immune cells contributes to unchecked keratinocyte proliferation, dedifferentiation, and angiogenesis. In individuals with a genetic predisposition, activation of TLR9 on DCs by triggers the release of IL-36 (α, β, and γ), IL-12, and IL-23. These cytokines drive the polarization of effector T cells, which secrete TNF-α, interferon-γ (IFN-γ), IL-17, IL-22, and other inflammatory mediators. Cytokines released in response to IL-36 (α, β, and γ) synergize to stimulate epithelial cells, leading to the production of various growth factors and inflammatory mediators, thereby perpetuating and intensifying a vicious cycle in this skin condition.

Cytokine Imbalance

Pregnancy is associated with a shift in the cytokine profile, favoring a Th2-dominated immune response to prevent fetal rejection. This shift can disrupt the balance of proinflammatory and anti-inflammatory cytokines in the skin. Increased levels of proinflammatory cytokines such as IL-1, IL-6, and TNF-α have been observed in patients with IH. This cytokine imbalance promotes inflammation and the formation of pustular lesions.

Neutrophil Activation

Neutrophils are central to the formation of pustules in IH. The increased levels of proinflammatory cytokines lead to the activation and recruitment of neutrophils to the skin. These neutrophils accumulate in the epidermis, forming subcorneal pustules characteristic of the condition. The excessive neutrophilic infiltration and activity contribute to the intense inflammation and pustule formation observed in IH.

Antimicrobial Peptides

In IH, the upregulation of LL-37, β-defensins, and other antimicrobial peptides due to IL-36γ and IL-36β suggests a robust inflammatory and antimicrobial response.

Environmental and Lifestyle Factors

Environmental and lifestyle factors may also influence the development of IH. While hormonal, genetic, and immunological factors are primary contributors, external factors can act as triggers or exacerbating agents.

Stress

Stress has been shown to exacerbate inflammatory skin conditions by affecting the hypothalamic-pituitary-adrenal (HPA) axis. Stress-induced activation of the HPA axis leads to increased production of glucocorticoids, which can alter immune function and exacerbate inflammatory responses. The impact of stress on the immune system can contribute to the onset or worsening of IH, particularly in susceptible individuals.

Infections

Infections, both bacterial and viral, can act as triggers for IH. The immune response to infections can lead to increased production of inflammatory cytokines, which may exacerbate skin inflammation and pustule formation. Patients with a history of recurrent infections may be at higher risk for developing IH.

Medications

Certain medications **(Table 1)** used to treat other conditions can influence the immune system and potentially trigger or worsen IH. Understanding the

TABLE 1: Various medications involved in triggering impetigo herpetiformis.

Category	Medications
Systemic corticosteroids	Prednisone, methylprednisolone
Biologics	• TNF-α inhibitors: Infliximab, adalimumab, etanercept • IL-17 inhibitors: Secukinumab • IL-23 inhibitors: Ustekinumab
Antibiotics and antivirals	• Antibiotics: Amoxicillin, ciprofloxacin • Antiviral agents: Acyclovir
Miscellaneous	• Calcium channel blockers: Nifedipine • Lithium • NSAIDs: Ibuprofen, naproxen

(IL: interleukin; NSAID: nonsteroidal anti-inflammatory drug; TNF: tumor necrosis factor)

medication history of patients is crucial for identifying potential triggers and managing the condition effectively.

CLINICAL SYMPTOMS AND SIGNS OF IMPETIGO HERPETIFORMIS

Cutaneous Manifestations

Pustular Eruptions

Impetigo herpetiformis is characterized by the acute onset of pustular eruptions **(Figs. 1 to 4)**. These pustules are sterile and filled with neutrophils **(Fig. 5)**, emerging on an erythematous and edematous base. The pustules predominantly initiate in intertriginous areas such as the groin, axillae, and inframammary regions, with potential dissemination to other body parts. The pustules often coalesce to form extensive areas of exudative lesions that may subsequently crust and erode.

Erythema and Edema

The affected dermal regions exhibit pronounced erythema and edema, providing a vivid inflammatory background for the pustular lesions. This erythema is typically intense and sharply demarcated, indicative of significant underlying inflammation. Edema contributes to the swelling and tenderness of the lesions, exacerbating patient discomfort.

Desquamation

As the pustules desiccate and crust, desquamation ensues, leading to the formation of scaly plaques. This shedding of the outer epidermal layer adds to the discomfort and poses cosmetic concerns for the patient.

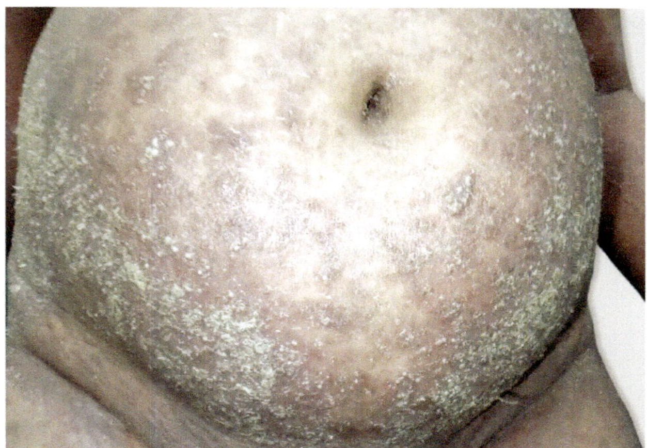

FIG. 1: Clinical image showing multiple pustules over abdomen coalescing to form diffuse plaque.

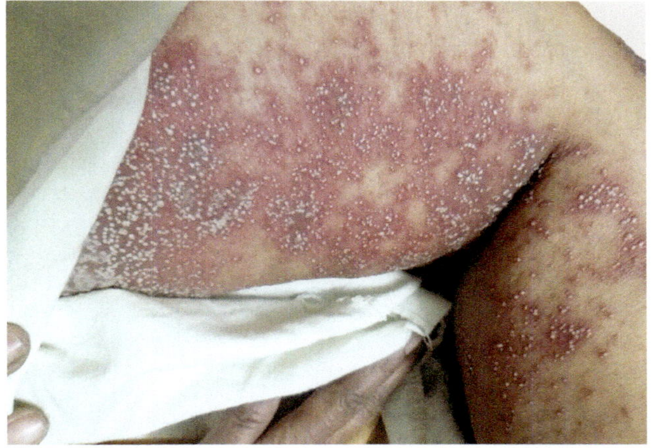

FIG. 2: Clinical image showing multiple pustules in an erythematous background.

Systemic Symptoms

Pyrexia and Malaise

Patients frequently experience systemic symptoms such as fever and malaise. The fever is typically low-grade yet persistent, reflecting the systemic inflammatory response. Malaise significantly impacts the patient's quality of life.

Gastrointestinal Disturbances

Gastrointestinal symptoms, including nausea, vomiting, and diarrhea, are common in IH. These symptoms can be severe, leading to dehydration and electrolyte imbalances, necessitating vigilant monitoring and intervention.

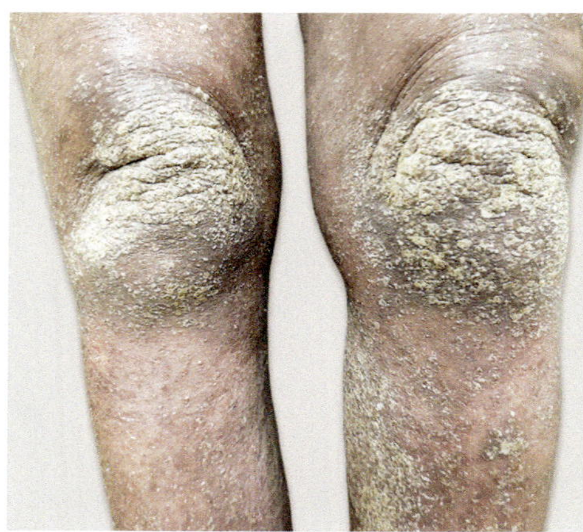

FIG. 3: Clinical image showing pustules over extensors of both the knees.

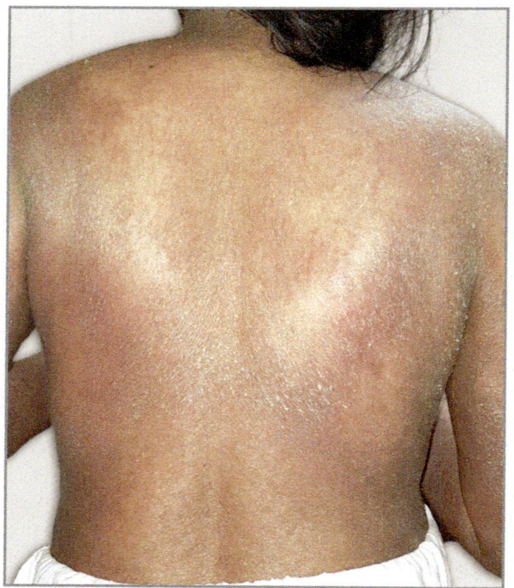

FIG. 4: Clinical image showing diffuse scaling and erythema over back.

Mucosal Involvement

Oral Lesions

Mucosal involvement is a notable feature of IH. Painful erosions and ulcers can appear on the oral mucosa, including the tongue, buccal mucosa, and lips, causing difficulty in alimentation and deglutition. Esophagus may also be involved.

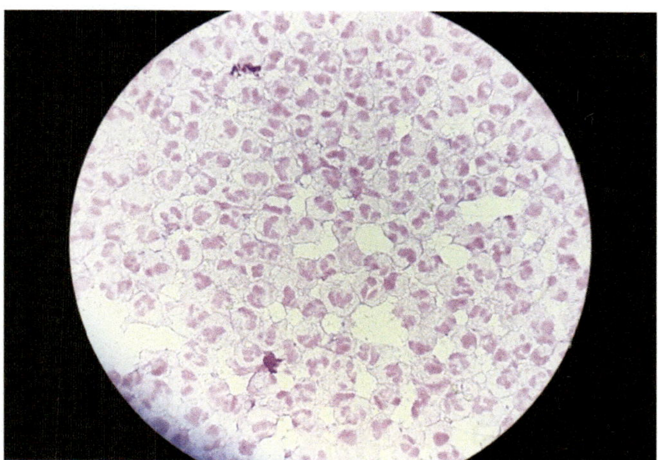

FIG. 5: Tzanck smear from the pustule showing numerous neutrophils.

Genital and Perianal Lesions

Lesions may also manifest in the genital and perianal regions, resulting in significant pain and discomfort. These areas are susceptible to secondary infections, leading to complications such as cellulitis and abscess formation.

Ocular Involvement

In some cases, conjunctival involvement occurs, leading to conjunctivitis and other ocular symptoms. This can result in redness, swelling, and irritation of the eyes.

Nails

Nails are less frequently involved in IH.

DIAGNOSIS

Histopathological features: A skin biopsy is essential for confirming the diagnosis. The biopsy typically reveals subcorneal pustules filled with neutrophils, along with spongiosis, acanthosis, and parakeratosis **(Fig. 6)**. The presence of Munro microabscesses (neutrophil collections within the stratum corneum) and Kogoj pustules (intraepidermal collections of neutrophils) is characteristic.

Laboratory Investigations

Complete Blood Count

- Leukocytosis: An elevated white blood cell count is commonly observed, indicating a systemic inflammatory response. Leukocytosis supports the clinical suspicion of an inflammatory or infectious etiology.

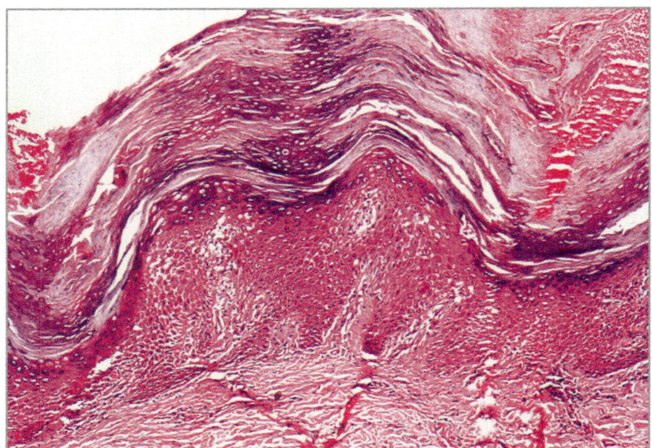

FIG. 6: Histopathological examination in 400× showing parakeratosis, hyperkeratosis, subcorneal pustules, and Munro's microabscesses.

Inflammatory Markers

- *Erythrocyte sedimentation rate (ESR)*: Elevated ESR is a nonspecific marker of inflammation. It is typically increased in IH, reflecting the systemic inflammatory state .
- *C-reactive protein (CRP)*: Similar to ESR, elevated CRP levels indicate an acute inflammatory response. CRP levels can help monitor disease activity and response to treatment.

Serum Calcium Levels

- *Hypocalcemia*: Low serum calcium levels are frequently observed in patients with IH. This is due to the extensive inflammatory process and calcium consumption by the inflamed skin. Monitoring and correcting hypocalcemia is crucial to prevent complications such as tetany and seizures. Hypoalbuminemia and lowered vitamin D further increase hypocalcemia.

Liver Function Tests

- *Hepatic involvement*: Abnormal liver function tests (LFTs) may indicate liver involvement or stress due to systemic inflammation. Elevated liver enzymes can also result from drug toxicity if the patient is receiving multiple medications.

Renal Function Tests

- *Renal function*: Monitoring renal function is important, particularly if immunosuppressive agents like cyclosporine are used, as these drugs can impact renal function. Serum creatinine and blood urea nitrogen (BUN) levels should be regularly assessed.

Serological Tests

- *Autoimmune markers*: In cases where the diagnosis is unclear, serological tests for autoimmune markers can help rule out other conditions such as autoimmune blistering diseases. Tests may include antinuclear antibodies (ANAs) and specific autoantibodies associated with pemphigus and pemphigoid.

Microbiological Tests

- *Culture and sensitivity*: Although the pustules are sterile, cultures may be performed to rule out secondary bacterial infections, which can complicate the clinical picture. Swabs from pustules and erosions should be sent for bacterial, fungal, and viral cultures.

Differential Diagnosis

Generalized pustular psoriasis: Similar pustular lesions but not necessarily associated with pregnancy. The presence of systemic symptoms and the typical histopathological findings help differentiate IH.

Acute generalized exanthematous pustulosis (AGEP): Often drug-induced with a rapid onset and resolution upon withdrawal of the offending agent. Histopathology and patient history of drug intake are crucial for differentiation.

Autoimmune blistering diseases: Conditions like pemphigus and pemphigoid have distinct histopathological features. Immunofluorescence studies can aid in differentiation.

Infectious causes: Bacterial, fungal, and viral infections can present with pustular or vesicular lesions. Negative culture results and characteristic histopathological findings help rule out these conditions.

MANAGEMENT OF IMPETIGO HERPETIFORMIS

The management of IH, a rare and severe variant of pustular psoriasis, necessitates a multidisciplinary approach to ensure the safety and well-being of both the mother and the fetus. Effective management involves pharmacological treatment, supportive care, and close monitoring. This section outlines the key strategies for managing IH, supported by citations and references.

Pharmacological Treatment

Systemic corticosteroids are the cornerstone of treatment for IH due to their potent anti-inflammatory effects.

Prednisolone is commonly used and preferred because of its established safety profile during pregnancy. The dosage is adjusted based on the severity of the disease and the patient's response. Initial high doses are often required to control the acute phase, followed by a gradual tapering.

Immunosuppressive Agents

Immunosuppressive agents are considered in cases refractory to corticosteroid therapy.

- *Cyclosporine*: Cyclosporine is effective due to its ability to suppress T-cell-mediated inflammation. It is often used when corticosteroids alone are insufficient. The dose is tailored to achieve therapeutic levels while minimizing adverse effects.
- *Methotrexate*: Use is limited due to potential teratogenic effects and is typically reserved for postpartum management.

Biologics

Biologics have emerged as a transformative option in the treatment of various dermatological conditions, including severe forms of psoriasis. Their use in IH, although not extensively documented, represents a potential avenue for patients who are refractory to conventional therapies.

Mechanism of Action

Biologics are targeted therapies that modulate specific components of the immune system, offering a more precise treatment approach compared to traditional systemic immunosuppressants. They act on cytokines and cellular pathways implicated in the pathogenesis of pustular psoriasis and related conditions.

Tumor Necrosis Factor-α Inhibitors

Infliximab, adalimumab, and etanercept: TNF-α inhibitors block the activity of TNF-α, a proinflammatory cytokine involved in the inflammatory cascade. By inhibiting TNF-α, these agents reduce inflammation and the formation of pustules.

Interleukin Inhibitors

- *Interleukin-17 inhibitors*:
    - *Secukinumab and ixekizumab*: These biologics target IL-17A, a cytokine that plays a crucial role in the pathogenesis of psoriasis. By neutralizing IL-17A, they help reduce the inflammatory response and clinical symptoms **(Figs. 7 and 8)**.
- *Interleukin-12/-23 inhibitors*:
    - *Ustekinumab*: This agent targets the p40 subunit shared by IL-12 and IL-23, inhibiting the downstream inflammatory pathways. It has shown efficacy in managing plaque psoriasis and is being explored for pustular variants.
- *Interleukin-23 inhibitors*:
    - *Guselkumab and tildrakizumab*: These biologics specifically target IL-23, a key cytokine in the differentiation and activation of Th17 cells, which are implicated in psoriasis. **Flowchart 1** shows the diagnosis and management of IH.

Clinical Evidence and Case Studies

Efficacy in pustular psoriasis: While specific studies on IH are limited, the efficacy of biologics in managing GPP provides valuable insights. GPP shares pathophysiological mechanisms with IH, suggesting that biologics could be similarly beneficial.

Case Reports and Series

- Several case reports have documented the successful use of biologics in patients with severe pustular psoriasis unresponsive to conventional therapies. For instance, infliximab has been reported to induce rapid clinical improvement in severe cases of GPP.

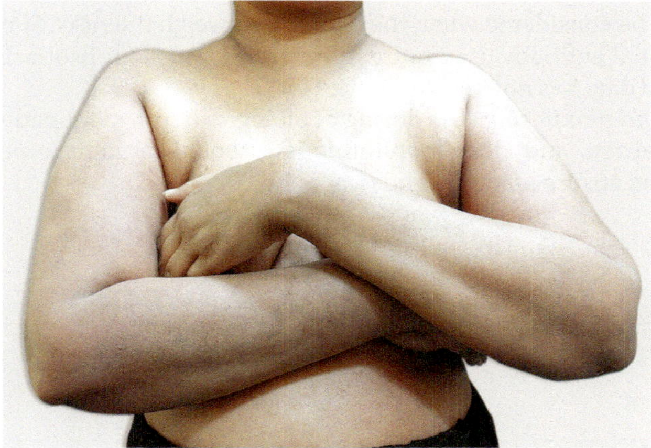

FIG. 7: Clinical image of the trunk and abdomen showing improvement in the erythema and scaling after 3 months of injection secukinumab.

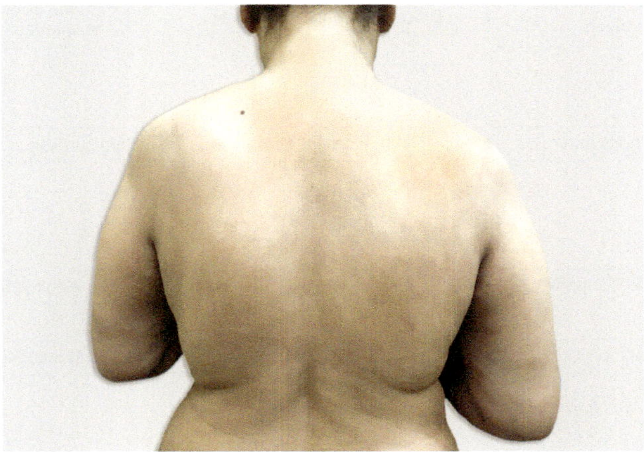

FIG. 8: Clinical image of the back showing improvement in the erythema and scaling after 3 months of injection secukinumab.

- A case series highlighted the use of secukinumab in patients with refractory pustular psoriasis, demonstrating significant clinical improvement and disease control.

Potential Use in Impetigo Herpetiformis

Given the similarities between GPP and IH, biologics offer a promising therapeutic option for patients with IH, particularly those who are refractory to corticosteroids and other immunosuppressants.

Considerations for Use

- *Safety in pregnancy*: The use of biologics during pregnancy requires careful consideration due to potential risks to the fetus. TNF-α inhibitors, such as infliximab and adalimumab, have the most extensive safety data in pregnancy and may be considered when the benefits outweigh the risks. Spesolimab is a monoclonal antibody used to treat generalized pustular psoriasis (GPP) due to limited data has not been approved for IH as yet.
- *Dosing and monitoring*: The dosing of biologics in pregnant patients must be individualized, and close monitoring is essential to manage potential side effects and ensure maternal and fetal safety.

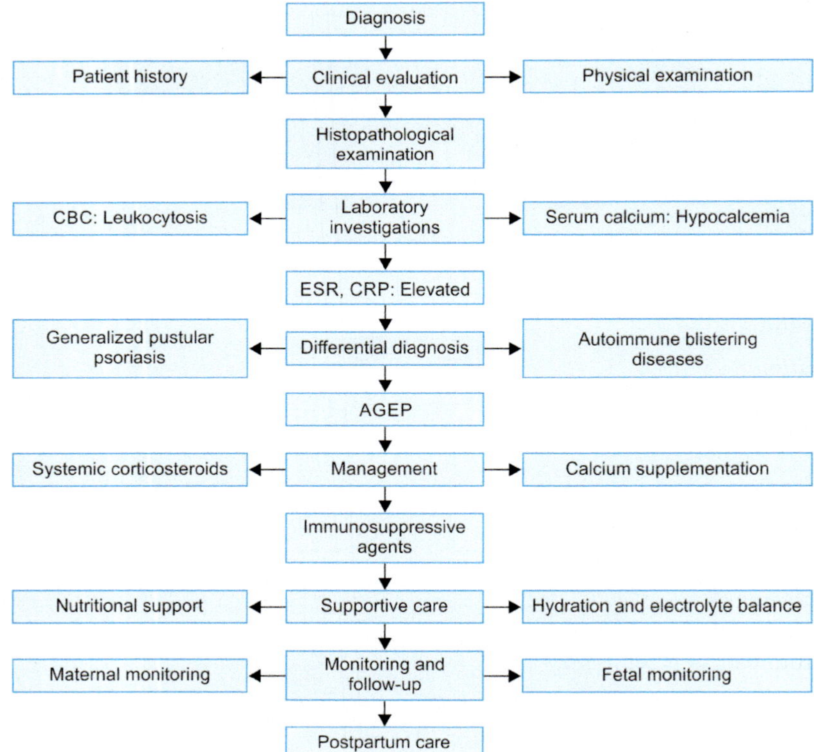

FLOWCHART 1: Diagnosis and management of impetigo herpetiformis.

(AGEP: acute generalized exanthematous pustulosis; CBC: complete blood count; CRP: C-reactive protein; ESR: erythrocyte sedimentation rate)

Safety and Monitoring

Risk of infections: Biologics can increase the risk of infections due to their immunosuppressive effects. It is crucial to screen patients for latent infections, such as tuberculosis, before initiating therapy. Continuous monitoring for signs of infection during treatment is also necessary.

Food and Drug Administration (FDA) category: Most biologics fall under FDA category B or C for pregnancy, indicating that they should be used with caution and only when the potential benefits justify the potential risks.

Calcium Supplementation

Hypocalcemia is a common complication in IH, necessitating calcium supplementation.

Oral calcium supplements: Oral calcium supplements are administered to maintain normal serum calcium levels and prevent complications such as tetany and seizures. Monitoring serum calcium levels is crucial during treatment.

Antibiotics

While the pustules in IH are sterile, secondary bacterial infections can complicate the clinical picture.

Broad-spectrum antibiotics: Broad-spectrum antibiotics are used to treat secondary bacterial infections. The choice of antibiotic is guided by culture and sensitivity results to ensure effective coverage.

Supportive Care

Nutritional Support

Adequate nutrition is essential, especially in patients with significant systemic symptoms.

Nutritional assessment and support: Nutritional assessment and support are provided to ensure adequate caloric and nutrient intake. Enteral or parenteral nutrition may be necessary in severe cases.

Hydration and Electrolyte Balance

Maintaining hydration and correcting electrolyte imbalances are critical components of supportive care.

Intravenous fluids: Intravenous fluids are administered to prevent dehydration and correct electrolyte imbalances, particularly in patients with severe gastrointestinal symptoms such as vomiting and diarrhea.

Monitoring and Follow-up

Regular Monitoring

Close monitoring of maternal and fetal well-being is essential throughout the treatment course.

Maternal monitoring: Regular follow-ups are necessary to adjust treatment and monitor for potential side effects. This includes frequent assessment of skin lesions, systemic symptoms, and laboratory parameters.

Fetal monitoring: Fetal well-being is monitored through regular ultrasound examinations and fetal heart rate monitoring. This ensures early detection of any complications that may arise due to maternal illness or treatment.

Postpartum Care

The condition typically resolves postpartum, but careful postpartum follow-up is important.

Postpartum monitoring: Monitoring for potential recurrence in subsequent pregnancies is crucial. Patients should receive counseling about the risk of recurrence and the importance of early prenatal care in future pregnancies.

Psychosocial Support

The psychological impact of IH on pregnant women can be significant.

Psychosocial support: Providing psychosocial support, including counseling and support groups, can help address the emotional and psychological challenges faced by patients. This holistic approach is vital for overall well-being.

CONCLUSION

The management of IH requires a comprehensive approach involving pharmacological treatment, supportive care, and close monitoring. Early intervention and a multidisciplinary approach can significantly improve outcomes for both the mother and the fetus. Recognizing and addressing the complex needs of patients with this rare condition is essential for effective management.

SUGGESTED READINGS

1. Namazi N, Dadkhahfar S. Impetigo Herpetiformis: Review of Pathogenesis, Complication, and Treatment. Dermatol Res Pract. 2018;2018:5801280.
2. Kinoshita M, Ogawa Y, Takeichi T, Okamoto T, Osada A, Shimada S, et al. Impetigo herpetiformis with IL-36RN mutation successfully treated with secukinumab. Eur J Dermatol. 2018;28; 381-2.
3. Ennouri M, Bahloul E, Sellami K, Marrakchi S, Fakhfakh F, Turki H, et al. Pustular psoriasis of pregnancy: Clinical and genetic characteristics in a series of eight patients and review of the literature. Dermatol Ther. 2022;35(8):e15593.
4. Murrieta-Coxca JM, Rodríguez-Martínez S, Cancino-Diaz ME, Markert UR, Favaro RR, Morales-Prieto DM. IL-36 Cytokines: Regulators of Inflammatory Responses and Their Emerging Role in Immunology of Reproduction. Int J Mol Sci. 2019;20(7):1649.
5. Wan Y, Zhang L, Xie B, Wu J, Zhao M, Guo J, et al. Impetigo herpetiformis in the second trimester: a case report and review of the literature. J Int Med Res. 2023;51(12): 3000605231217950.
6. Oumeish OY, Parish JL. Impetigo herpetiformis. Clin Dermatol. 2006;24:101-4.
7. Genovese G, Moltrasio C, Cassano N, Maronese CA, Vena GA, Marzano AV. Pustular Psoriasis: From Pathophysiology to Treatment. Biomedicines. 2021;9:1746.

12.6 Autoimmune Progesterone Dermatitis

Mudita Gupta, Sanjeev Gupta

INTRODUCTION

Autoimmune progesterone dermatitis (APD) is an immune-mediated catamenial skin condition that occurs cyclically in response to endogenous or exogenous progesterone. Progesterone, a steroid hormone, is crucial for regulating the menstrual cycle, maintaining pregnancy, and supporting embryogenesis. In nonpregnant women, progesterone is secreted by the corpus luteum, which forms from the follicle after ovulation and releases the hormone during the luteal phase of the menstrual cycle. During pregnancy, the placenta begins producing progesterone at 8–10 weeks, with levels continuing to rise until just before term.

Exogenous progesterone is extensively used in various medical contexts to support reproductive health and treat gynecological disorders. In hormone replacement therapy (HRT), it is combined with estrogen to alleviate menopausal symptoms and prevent endometrial hyperplasia. For individuals with polycystic ovary syndrome (PCOS), it helps regulate menstrual cycles. Progesterone-only contraceptives, including emergency contraception, are employed for birth control. Additionally, progesterone is used to manage premenstrual syndrome (PMS), premenstrual dysphoric disorder (PMDD), and to induce menstruation in cases of amenorrhea. In assisted reproductive technology (ART), progesterone supports the luteal phase in early pregnancy, reducing the risk of preterm birth. It is also prescribed for recurrent pregnancy loss and threatened miscarriage. Furthermore, progesterone is used in hormone therapy for transgender individuals and in treating hormone-sensitive cancers, such as certain types of endometrial cancer.

Autoimmune progesterone dermatitis was first described by Geber in 1921. The initial description involved a woman who experienced cyclical skin eruptions that coincided with her menstrual cycle. This pioneering observation laid the foundation for recognizing the relationship between hormonal fluctuations, particularly progesterone, and certain dermatological conditions. APD is a rare condition, and its exact prevalence is not well-documented. As of 2021, approximately 200 cases had been reported. APD occurring during pregnancy is even rarer, accounting for only about 14% of these cases.

- APD is an allergic and inflammatory response to increased progesterone levels (endogenous/exogenous).
- Endogenous progesterone increase in premenstrual period and in pregnancy.
- Exogenously progesterone can be given controlling menopausal symptoms, dysfunctional uterine bleeding, treatment of hormone sensitive malignancies, etc.
- During pregnancy it can be given to prevent abortion and preterm labor.
- It is coprescribed in ART.
- It is less reported entity.

ETIOPATHOGENESIS (FIG. 1)

As discussed in earlier chapters, sex hormones play a pivotal role in the homeostasis of both adaptive and innate immunity. Sudden increases in these hormones can alter immune responses, potentially triggering or alleviating various immune-mediated diseases. Conditions such as psoriasis, Behçet's syndrome, atopic dermatitis, other forms of eczema, hereditary angioedema, and persistent postpartum impetigo herpetiformis often show increased disease activity during menstrual cycles. Similarly, APD and autoimmune estrogen dermatitis (AED) are catamenial diseases, with symptoms influenced by hormonal fluctuations.

Increase in endogenous progesterone (luteal phase/pregnancy) or exogenous progesterone may lead to following changes:

- *Delayed type IV hypersensitivity response*: T cells recognize progesterone or progesterone-bound proteins (synthetic progesterone) as antigens. Activated T cells release cytokines such as interferon-gamma (IFN-γ) and tumor necrosis factor-alpha (TNF-α), leading to local inflammation and tissue damage.
- *High expression of progesterone receptors*:
    - G protein coupled receptor modulation of T helper 2 (Th2)
    - Activation of progesterone membrane receptor α (PHR α) on CD8+ cells.
- *Cross sensitivity to other steroids*:
    - Increase in progesterone specific immunoglobulin E (IgE) → mast cell/basophil degranulation → type I hypersensitivity response
    - Immune complex mediated: In some cases, autoantibodies against progesterone or progesterone-receptor complexes may be present, suggesting an autoimmune component.
    - Also progesterone prevents B cell apoptosis and increase autoreactive cell survival.

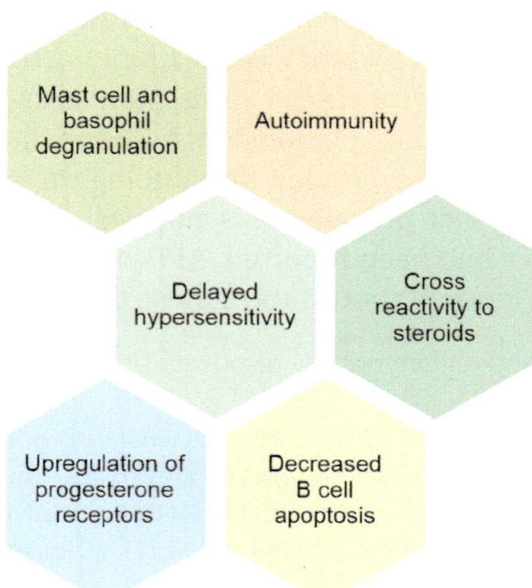

FIG. 1: Etiopathogenic mechanisms of autoimmune progesterone dermatitis.

Various progesterone preparations which can be given during pregnancy are 17-α-hydroxyprogesterone caproate, progesterone given vaginally or orally for prevention of preterm birth. However, mifepristone, a competitive antagonist of progesterone, can lead to a compensatory exaggerated production of progesterone after medical abortion, potentially precipitating APD.

CLINICAL FEATURES

The clinical features of APD are diverse, affecting both the skin and mucous membranes. Dermatological lesions commonly include urticaria, erythema multiforme, and eczema. Other reported manifestations are vesiculobullous eruptions, annular erythema, angioedema, papulopustular eruptions, purpura, fixed drug eruptions, Steven-Johnson-like eruptions, dermatitis herpetiformis-like lesions, and erythema annulare centrifugum-like lesions. These lesions are typically symmetrical and can involve the face, trunk, or extremities.

Mucosal involvement may present as stomatitis, oral ulcers, conjunctivitis, and vulvovaginitis. Systemic symptoms can include generalized pruritus and, in rare cases, systemic reactions such as fever, malaise, joint pain, shortness of breath, and even anaphylaxis. These clinical manifestations usually appear about 3–10 days before menstruation. Recognizing the cyclical nature of these symptoms in relation to progesterone levels is crucial for diagnosing this rare condition.

During pregnancy, there may be worsening of mucocutaneous manifestations or complications such as abortion or preterm delivery may occur. Occasionally there may be onset of APD during gestation. Bierman was the first to observe APD in pregnant patient in two successive pregnancies. However, occasional improvement in symptoms has also been reported. Though pregnancy is associated with increase in progesterone levels but also simultaneous increased in endogenous cortisol may at times lead to blunting of allergic response. Desensitization to hormone occurring as a result of gradual increase in progesterone level may also dampen the immunological response.

- Common clinical features of APD are urticaria, eczema, and erythema multiforme.
- Mucocutaneous manifestations are variable and may range from mild to life-threatening conditions.
- Pregnancy is usually associated with worsening of symptoms.
- Improvement of APD may occur during pregnancy due to desensitization and endogenous cortisol.

INVESTIGATIONS

Various techniques have been used to diagnose APD **(Fig. 2)**.

Hormone Challenge Test

- Intramuscular progesterone challenge-cutaneous lesions appear after 24–48 hours

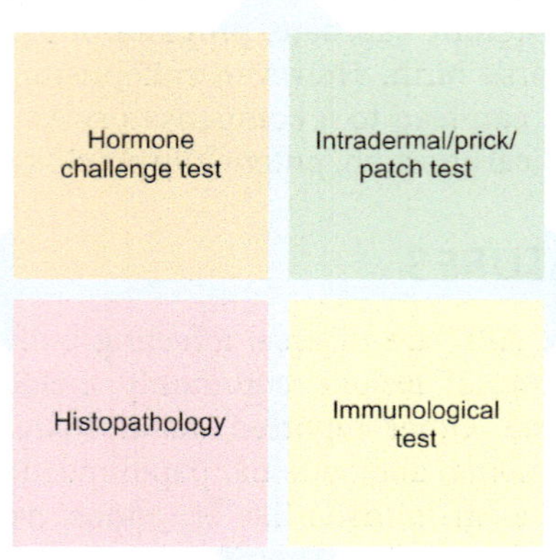

FIG. 2: Techniques for the diagnosis of autoimmune progesterone dermatitis (APD).

- Oral progesterone challenge
- Exogenous progesterone withdrawal

Intradermal Skin Testing

The commonly used concentration of progesterone for intradermal testing is between 0.1 mg/mL and 1 mg/mL. Preferably aqueous base is used but if not available oil ones can be used. There are more chances of false positive with oil preparations. Rehman et al. injected 1% in oil base. Reading is taken within 30 minutes for observing immediate (wheal and flare) and after 48 hours for delayed hypersensitivity reaction (erythema and induration). Saline is used as a control.

Patch Test

In this, 10% progesterone in petrolatum base is used.

Prick Test

A concentration of 50 mg/mL (5%) progesterone in saline is often used for the prick test presence of a wheal and flare at site of prick within 30 minutes is considered as positive test.

Histopathology

Similar to variability seen in morphological features of APD histopathology is also not specific. In the dermis, along with perivascular infiltrate comprising of lymphocytes eosinophils and mast cells are also predominantly seen.

Immunologic Assessments

- *Serum progesterone-specific IgE*: Measure specific IgE antibodies to progesterone to identify an allergic response, although this is not always present in APD.
- *Lymphocyte transformation test (LTT)*: LTT has limitations, including the risk of false positives or negatives and the need for specialized laboratory techniques and expertise. The test measures the proliferation of lymphocytes in response to progesterone, with increased proliferation indicating a hypersensitivity reaction. The lymphocyte response to progesterone is compared with responses to other nonspecific stimulants and a control sample to ensure specificity.
- *Basophil granulation test/leukocyte histamine test*: In the basophil degranulation test, basophils from a blood sample are exposed to progesterone, and their degranulation is measured, with significant degranulation indicating a positive reaction. The leukocyte histamine release test measures histamine release from leukocytes upon exposure to progesterone, with significant release also indicating a hypersensitivity reaction. Both tests require specialized laboratory equipment.
- *Direct and indirect immunofluorescent staining of luteinizing cells in the corpus luteum*: Fluorescently labeled primary antibodies specific to the target antigen (e.g., luteinizing hormone receptors and specific proteins expressed in luteinizing cells) are applied directly to the tissue sections.
- *Detection of circulating antibodies*: Antibodies can be detected to 17-α-hydroxyprogesterone.

DIFFERENTIAL DIAGNOSIS

The dermatological and systemic manifestations of APD are nonspecific, requiring differentiation from other common diseases. The cyclical nature of APD in nonpregnant patients, a high index of suspicion during pregnancy, and targeted investigations are crucial for diagnosis. Warin proposed criteria for diagnosing APD, which include cyclical dermatitis with luteal flare, a positive reaction to intradermal progesterone, and amelioration of symptoms by inhibiting ovulation.

- APD needs to be differentiated from different diseases depending on the morphology.
- Cyclical nature of disease in prepregnant state helps in diagnosis.
- Targeted investigations may be required to suggest diagnosis.
- Response to drugs inhibiting ovulation confirms diagnosis.

TREATMENT

Management of APD aims to control symptoms and inhibit ovulation:

- *First-line treatment*:
  - Avoidance of exogenous progesterone in medications and treatments
  - Use of topical corticosteroids and antihistamines

- *Second-line treatment*:
  - Oral corticosteroids
  - Gonadotropin-releasing hormone (GnRH) analogs (buserelin and triptorelin)
  - Steroid-sparing drugs like azathioprine

Other therapies which have been tried are:

- *Danazol:* An antiestrogen that inhibits ovulation but may affect skeletal mineralization with long-term use
- *Tamoxifen*: Increases progesterone clearance and can alleviate menopausal symptoms
- *Suppressive progestins* (low-dose progestin pills) *or combined oral contraceptives*: May also be successful in suppressing symptoms
- *Lymphatic pumps*: Enhance lymphatic drainage and venous return, reducing inflammation
- *Omalizumab*: An anti-IgE monoclonal antibody, approved for severe allergic asthma and severe chronic spontaneous urticaria, has been tried by Heffler et al. in APD.
- In resistant cases, salpingo-oophorectomy has to be done.

Management during Pregnancy

Managing APD during pregnancy is particularly challenging, as most of the earlier-mentioned medications cannot be prescribed. Stopping systemic progesterone therapy may be detrimental for sustaining pregnancy, but it might still need to be discontinued after counseling the patient. Depending on the gestation and severity of APD, topical or oral corticosteroids and antihistamines can be prescribed.

CONSIDERATIONS FOR KNOWN APD CASES AND PREGNANCY

For known APD cases desiring pregnancy, progesterone supplementation should be avoided. If progesterone treatment is necessary, desensitization should be done prior to planning the pregnancy. Suppression of ovulation is a key target of therapy. With the increasing use of progesterone and its metabolites during pregnancy clinicians need to be vigilant about APD.

- There are various drugs which have been tried in nonpregnant APD.
- During pregnancy only symptomatic treatment is advised.
- In patients who have prepregnant APD in nonpregnant state and wish to become pregnant should be desensitized with progesterone.
- Progesterone supplementation should be started after ruling out APD.

AUTOIMMUNE ESTROGEN DERMATITIS

Autoimmune estrogen dermatitis was first recognized by Zondek and Bromberg. Like APD, AED also shows cyclical dermatological changes in nonpregnant patients. Clinical features are similar to APD. Localization of lesions to face, neck, upper trunk, and arms is seen as more estrogen receptors on face. Urticaria is the most common presentation. Challenging with estrogens provokes this entity. Shelley et al. diluted pure estrone in aqueous suspensions (0.1 mL in a 1:1,000 dilution) for intradermal testing. Result is considered positive if a papule persists for >24 hours.

Like progesterone, estrogen skews Th1 predominant immune response to Th2. This Th2 predominance leads to increased allergic diseases. Also there is increased production of antibodies (IgG, IgE, etc.) from immunoglobulin producing B cells. Type 1 hypersensitivity responses are increased because of degranulation of mast cells, basophils, and upregulation of endometrial nitric oxide synthetase and nitric oxide production. Alteration of dendritic cells also predispose to inflammatory response.

Treatment involves a combination of hormonal regulation, immunosuppressive therapies, and supportive measures. Hormonal regulation can be achieved with oral contraceptives to stabilize hormone levels, GnRH agonists like leuprolide to suppress ovarian function or aromatase inhibitors such as anastrozole to reduce estrogen synthesis. Immunosuppressive and anti-inflammatory therapies include topical and systemic corticosteroids, immunosuppressants like azathioprine or methotrexate, and oral antihistamines for itching. Dapsone and ciclosporin have also been tried. Supportive measures involve gentle skin care with hypoallergenic products, moisturizers, and stress management techniques.

During pregnancy AED also behaves similar to APD with peak in second and third trimester **(Table 1)**. Management involves symptomatic measures only.

TABLE 1: Difference between autoimmune progesterone and autoimmune estrogen dermatitis.

Feature	Autoimmune progesterone dermatitis (APD)	Autoimmune estrogen dermatitis (AED)
Hormone involved	Progesterone	Estrogen
Timing of symptoms	Luteal phase (postovulation)	Follicular phase or around ovulation
Common symptoms	Urticaria, eczema, erythema multiforme, and respiratory symptoms (e.g., wheezing and rhinitis)	Eczema, urticaria, erythema, and other forms of dermatitis
Diagnosis	Clinical history, skin testing with progesterone (skin prick and intradermal), and lymphocyte transformation test	Clinical history, skin testing with estrogen, and immunologic tests
Treatment	Hormonal therapies [oral contraceptives and gonadotropin-releasing hormone (GnRH) agonists], corticosteroids, and immunosuppressive agents	Hormonal regulation (oral contraceptives, aromatase inhibitors, and GnRH agonists), corticosteroids, and immunosuppressants
Management of hormonal fluctuations	Suppress ovulation and reduce progesterone levels using continuous oral contraceptives or GnRH agonists	Stabilize estrogen levels using aromatase inhibitors or combined oral contraceptives
Supportive care	Patient education, stress management, and supportive care	Patient education, stress management, and supportive care

SUGGESTED READINGS

1. Apurwa A, Patil S, Chaudhari P, Nadkarni NJ. Autoimmune Progesterone Dermatitis. Indian J Dermatol. 2018;63(2):188-90.
2. Huang Y, Ye S, Bao X, Yang R, Huang J. Whole course of treatment of autoimmune progesterone dermatitis that had spontaneously resolved during pregnancy: A case report and review of the literature. Front Immunol. 2022;13:939083.
3. Mbonile L. Autoimmune progesterone dermatitis: Case report with history of urticaria, petechiae and palpable pinpoint purpura triggered by medical abortion. S Afr Med J. 2016;106(4):48-50.
4. Kanninen TT, Moretti ML, Lakhi NA. Autoimmune progesterone dermatitis following vaginal progesterone exposure in pregnancy. Obstet Med. 2019;12(2):100-2.
5. DeRosa A, Adams S, Fee EK. Progressively Worsening Cyclic Rash: Diagnosis and Approach to Care. J Am Osteopath Assoc. 2015;115(12):738-44.

CHAPTER 13

Neutrophilic Dermatoses during Pregnancy

Debdeep Mitra

INTRODUCTION

Neutrophilic dermatoses (NDs) are a diverse group of conditions characterized by a noninfectious infiltration of primarily mature neutrophilic leukocytes, found at different levels within the skin. The cutaneous manifestations of NDs are diverse, including pustules, bullae, abscesses, papules, nodules, plaques, and ulcers. Neutrophilic inflammation can affect nearly any organ system, leading to the term "neutrophilic disease."

These conditions present unique challenges when occurring during pregnancy, as they not only impact maternal health but also raise concerns about potential effects on fetal development. Understanding the management of ND in pregnancy is crucial for dermatologists, obstetricians, and other healthcare providers involved in the care of pregnant women. This chapter provides an overview of the clinical manifestations, pathophysiology, and management considerations of ND during pregnancy, highlighting the importance of individualized care and multidisciplinary collaboration.

These conditions can be classified based on the primary depth and type of skin involvement. **Table 1** is an organized classification that includes various forms of NDs.

Hypodermal:

- *Neutrophilic panniculitis*: Involves the deeper layers of the skin and subcutaneous fat
- *Aseptic abscess syndrome*: Characterized by sterile abscesses primarily in the deep layers
- *Rheumatoid neutrophilic dermatosis*: Associated with rheumatoid arthritis, affecting the deep dermis and hypodermis
- *Sweet's syndrome*: Presents with painful, red plaques, and nodules with involvement extending into the hypodermis
- *Pyoderma gangrenosum (PG)*: A rapidly progressing ulcerative condition affecting the dermis and hypodermis

TABLE 1: Classification of neutrophilic dermatoses.

Category	Condition
Primarily epidermal	Transient neonatal pustular melanosis
	Subcorneal pustular dermatosis
	Amicrobial pustulosis of the folds associated with autoimmune disease
	Intraepidermal neutrophilic IgA dermatosis
	Infantile acropustulosis
	Neutrophilic spongiosis
	Acute generalized exanthematous pustulosis
Primarily dermal	
"Classical" neutrophilic dermatoses	Pyoderma gangrenosum
	Sweet's syndrome
Association with acne	Synovitis, hyperostosis, acne, pustulosis, osteomyelitis (SAPHO) syndrome
Overlap with vasculitis	Erythema elevatum diutinum
	Behçet's disease
	Pustular vasculitis of the hands
	Bowel-associated dermatosis–arthritis syndrome (BADAS)
	Pyostomatitis vegetans
Specific association with gastrointestinal diseases	Bowel-associated dermatosis–arthritis syndrome (BADAS)
	Pyostomatitis vegetans

Plaque type/dermal:

- *Pyoderma gangrenosum*: Chronic, ulcerative skin condition affecting the dermis
- *Sweet's syndrome*: Acute febrile neutrophilic dermatosis presenting with dermal plaques
- *Erythema elevatum diutinum*: Rare chronic condition presenting as papules and plaques on extensor surfaces

Superficial/epidermal:

- *Noninfectious pustulosis of the folds*: Pustules in skin folds, often associated with autoimmune diseases
- *Noninfectious pustulosis of the scalp/leg*: Localized pustular eruptions on the scalp or legs
- *Noninfectious subcorneal pustulosis*: Characterized by pustules just beneath the stratum corneum
- *Acute generalized exanthematous pustulosis (AGEP)*: Acute eruption of pustules following drug exposure
- *Pustular psoriasis (DIRA-DITRA)*: Rare genetic forms of pustular psoriasis
- *IgA pemphigus*: Autoimmune blistering disorder presenting with pustules and vesicles

Hypodermal/dermal/epidermal:

- *Pyoderma gangrenosum*: Can involve multiple skin layers from epidermis to hypodermis
- *Behçet's disease*: Multisystem inflammatory disorder with skin manifestations affecting all layers
- *Hidradenitis suppurativa*: Chronic inflammatory condition affecting apocrine gland-bearing areas, involving multiple skin layers

Association with acne and autoinflammatory syndromes:

- *SAPHO syndrome*: Involves synovitis, acne, pustulosis, hyperostosis, and osteomyelitis
- *PAPA syndrome*: Characterized by pyogenic arthritis, PG, and acne
- *PASH syndrome*: Includes PG, acne, and suppurative hidradenitis
- *PAPASH syndrome*: Combination of pyogenic arthritis, PG, acne, and suppurative hidradenitis

Overlapping forms:

- *Bowel bypass syndrome*: Skin eruptions following bowel bypass surgery
- *Bowel-associated dermatosis-arthritis syndrome (BADAS)*: Associated with gastrointestinal diseases and characterized by skin and joint involvement
- *Behçet's disease*: Features both skin and systemic involvement, affecting various organ systems
- *Acne due to epidermal growth factor receptor (EGFR) inhibitors*: Acneiform eruptions secondary to epidermal growth factor receptor inhibitors

COMMON FEATURES OF NEUTROPHILIC DERMATOSES

- Many cases of NDs, regardless of type, often have underlying systemic associations, such as hematologic or gastrointestinal diseases, infections, neoplastic processes, or medication reactions.
- Histologically, NDs are characterized by sterile perivascular or diffuse infiltrates primarily consisting of mature neutrophils.
- Although the reaction typically exhibits vasculopathic features, it may not reach the level of frank vasculitis in all cases.
- Extracutaneous infiltration is common and can affect various organs such as bones, lungs, joints, lymph nodes, liver, eyes, heart, and nerves.
- Systemic symptoms like fever, malaise, arthralgia, and myalgia may accompany the neutrophilic process.
- Coexistence or sequential occurrence of different types of NDs within the same individual is possible.
- Neutrophilic dermatoses are not contagious.
- Skin or blood cultures conducted to detect infectious agents typically yield negative results.
- Antibiotics are ineffective in treating these disorders.
- Immediate therapeutic response is often observed with systemic corticosteroids and other immunosuppressive medications.

PATHOPHYSIOLOGY

During a typical pregnancy, there exists a delicate equilibrium between cell-mediated immunity, dominated by T helper 1 cells (Th1), and humoral immunity, which is Th2-dominated. Initially, Th2 cytokines prevail, but as gestation progresses toward its conclusion, there is a gradual shift toward Th1 cytokines, especially toward the end of pregnancy when inflammation becomes desirable, possibly aiding in childbirth. Factors like parainflammatory conditions, tissue damage, alterations in the microbiome, and other immune system activators can further skew this balance toward Th1 dominance. By around the 30th week of gestation, there is a significant increase in the numbers of neutrophils and monocytes, which could contribute to a sustained inflammatory response, even in sterile injury sites.

The pathogenesis of NDs is intricate and not fully understood. Discrepancies in matrix metalloproteinases (MMPs) found in ND lesions compared to those in normally healing wounds, along with elevated expression of tumor necrosis factor-α (TNF-α), a Th1 cytokine, have been proposed as factors contributing to tissue damage. Elevated levels of interleukin-8 (IL-8), myeloperoxidase, and MMP-9 have also been detected in the wound beds of ND lesions. Moreover, ND lesions exhibit overexpression of IL-1β, IL-17 (the receptor of IL-1β), CXCL1, 2, and 3, and RANTES **(Table 2)**. Studies analyzing serum and lesions from ND patients suggest a predominance of Th1 and Th17 cytokine expression.

Another potential pathway in ND development involves granulocyte–macrophage colony-stimulating factor (GM-CSF), a cytokine essential for normal pregnancy. Low levels of GM-CSF during pregnancy have been linked to higher rates of recurrent spontaneous abortions. GM-CSF overexpression can trigger an abnormal inflammatory response by promoting the production of inflammatory mediators by macrophages and neutrophils, as well as stimulating the proliferation of Th-17 cytokines. There have been instances where subcutaneous injections of G-CSF were associated with ND development in patients with underlying malignancies.

TABLE 2: Cytokines and antigens having role in major neutrophilic dermatoses.

Neutrophilic dermatoses	Cytokines and antigens
Sweet's syndrome	G-CSF (cerebrospinal fluid), GM-CSF, IFN-γ, IL-1, IL-2, IL-3, IL-6, IL-8, IL-17, VEGF, TNF-α
Pyoderma gangrenosum	IL-1, IL-3, IL-6, IL-8, IL-17, TNF-α, ICAM-1, VCAM-1, aberrant integrins (CR4, CD11/CD18, a, B2), E-selectin, G-CSF, GM-CSF, IFN, VEGF
Behcet's disease	IL-1B, IL-6, IL-8, IL-12, IL-17, IL-23, HSP-60, VEGF, TNF-α, sIL-2r, MCP-1, IFN-γ, G-CSF, CD-29, E-selectin, P-selectin, thrombomodulin, endothelin-1
Subcorneal pustular dermatosis	Desmocollin1, IL-8, LTB4, C5a, C5a

(ICAM-1: intercellular adhesion molecule-1; IL: interleukin; IFN: interferon; TNF: tumor necrosis factor; VCAM-1: vascular cell adhesion molecule-1; VEGF: vascular endothelial growth factor)

The precise connection between inflammatory pathways in pregnancy and ND remains unclear, but a shift toward Th1 and Th17 expression may be a common factor. Notably, over half of ND cases during pregnancy occur in the third trimester or post-cesarean section, aligning with the shift toward proinflammatory Th1 cytokines toward the end of pregnancy, which further emphasizes the involvement of Th17 cytokines in the pathophysiology of ND. As pregnancy progresses, the number of young, overactive neutrophils—particularly band neutrophils—increases, especially in the second and third trimesters. Band neutrophils contain more myeloperoxidase, which causes them to be more active and bactericidal, possibly predisposing a pregnant woman to the overactive, neutrophil-dominant lesions found in ND.

Certain comorbidities may alter the normal response of the innate immune system, potentially increasing the likelihood of developing PG. Some gravid patients had inflammatory comorbidities such as relapsing polychondritis, antiphospholipid syndrome, Takayasu arteritis, systemic lupus erythematosus (SLE), and hidradenitis suppurativa.

- *Preeclampsia and inflammation*: Preeclampsia, characterized by sterile inflammation driven by a dysfunctional placenta, involves various factors such as lipid peroxides and damage-associated molecular patterns (DAMPs) affecting circulating granulocytes. Th17 cells and interleukin-17 (IL-17) also play significant roles in preeclampsia. While normal pregnancy shows an increase in serum IL-17, preeclampsia exhibits elevated IL-17 levels along with a decrease in T regulatory cells (Tregs). This imbalance may contribute to a chronic inflammatory response, similar to that seen in PG patients.
- *Abruptio placentae and inflammation*: Abruptio placentae, the premature detachment of the placenta, are closely associated with preeclampsia. It involves excess thrombin production from decidual cells expressing tissue factor. Thrombin can promote inflammation-associated preterm labor by enhancing the expression of MMPs and neutrophilic chemokines.

Several common features may play roles in both PG and the inflammatory comorbidities mentioned. These features include alterations in the innate immune system marked by overexpression of interleukin-8 (IL-8), increased neutrophil recruitment, and tumor necrosis factor-α (TNF-α) response. Additionally, increased expression of MMPs, thrombosis, and overexpression of Th17 cytokines are observed, indicating potential shared mechanisms in the pathogenesis of ND.

Adverse effects of NDs on pregnancy can vary depending on the specific dermatosis, the severity of symptoms, and individual patient factors. Here are some potential adverse effects **(Table 3)**:

- *Exacerbation of symptoms*: In some cases, pregnancy can exacerbate the symptoms of ND, leading to increased inflammation, pain, and discomfort for the mother. Flares of ND during pregnancy may be triggered by hormonal changes, altered immune responses, or other pregnancy-related factors.
- *Complications during delivery*: Certain NDs, such as PG, can pose challenges during delivery. Active lesions in the perineal or abdominal regions may complicate childbirth and increase the risk of complications such as delayed wound healing, infection, or excessive bleeding.

TABLE 3: Various types of neutrophilic dermatoses and their effects on pregnancy outcomes.

Neutrophilic dermatosis	Effect on pregnancy outcome
Sweet's syndrome	Variable impact; may worsen or improve
Pyoderma gangrenosum	Risk of exacerbation, especially postpartum
Behçet's disease	Potential for flares; may affect fertility
Acute generalized exanthematous pustulosis	Possible exacerbation during pregnancy
Subcorneal pustular dermatosis	Variable impact; may improve or worsen

- *Impact on maternal mental health*: The physical symptoms and emotional distress associated with ND during pregnancy can have a significant impact on maternal mental health. Coping with chronic skin conditions during pregnancy may increase stress, anxiety, and depression, affecting overall well-being and quality of life.
- *Risk of adverse pregnancy outcomes*: Although research on the specific effects of ND on pregnancy outcomes is limited, severe or uncontrolled inflammation associated with certain dermatoses may potentially increase the risk of adverse pregnancy outcomes such as preterm birth, low birth weight, or fetal growth restriction.
- *Challenges in treatment*: Managing ND during pregnancy can be challenging due to limitations on the use of certain medications, such as systemic corticosteroids and immunosuppressants, which may pose risks to the developing fetus. Finding safe and effective treatment options that provide symptom relief while minimizing fetal exposure to medications can be complex and may require close collaboration between dermatologists and obstetricians.
- *Impact on fetal health*: Although rare, there is a theoretical risk that severe or uncontrolled ND during pregnancy could impact fetal health. Factors such as maternal inflammation, medication use, and maternal stress may potentially affect fetal development and well-being, highlighting the importance of careful monitoring and management of ND during pregnancy.

DIAGNOSIS

Investigations for NDs during pregnancy aim to confirm the diagnosis, assess disease severity, and monitor treatment response while considering the safety of investigative procedures for both the mother and the fetus. Here are some key investigations commonly employed:

- *Skin biopsy*: A skin biopsy is often necessary to confirm the diagnosis of ND and rule out other dermatological conditions. Histopathological examination typically reveals a dense neutrophilic infiltrate in the dermis or epidermis, which is characteristic of ND.
- *Cultures*: Although NDs are primarily noninfectious, obtaining cultures (bacterial, fungal) from affected skin lesions may be warranted, especially if there is suspicion of secondary infection or atypical clinical presentation.

- *Blood tests*: Routine blood tests, including complete blood count (CBC) with differential, erythrocyte sedimentation rate (ESR), and C-reactive protein (CRP) levels, can help assess the systemic inflammatory response and monitor disease activity.
- *Serological testing*: Depending on clinical suspicion and associated symptoms, serological tests may be performed to evaluate for underlying autoimmune or systemic inflammatory conditions commonly associated with ND, such as autoimmune connective tissue diseases or inflammatory bowel disease.
- *Imaging studies*: In cases where extracutaneous involvement is suspected or to assess disease extent, imaging modalities such as ultrasound and magnetic resonance imaging (MRI) may be utilized.
- *Pregnancy-specific tests*: Special consideration is given to the safety of investigations during pregnancy. Pregnancy-specific tests, such as fetal ultrasound and fetal monitoring, may be performed to assess fetal well-being and ensure the safety of investigative procedures for both the mother and the fetus.
- *Monitoring*: Regular clinical assessments, including photographing skin lesions to document changes over time, are essential for monitoring disease progression and treatment response.

It is important to individualize the investigative approach based on the patient's clinical presentation, disease severity, and gestational age, while considering the safety of investigative procedures during pregnancy. Close collaboration between dermatologists, obstetricians, and other healthcare providers is essential to ensure optimal management of ND in pregnant patients.

TREATMENT

Treating patients with NDs during pregnancy and the postpartum period can be particularly challenging due to potential risks associated with medications for both the mother and fetus. Here is a summary of the treatment approaches and considerations:

- *Topical or intralesional corticosteroids*:
  - Safest approach whenever possible
  - May be used exclusively in some cases, although symptoms of ND can progress rapidly
- *Systemic corticosteroids*:
  - Common first-line therapy for disseminated ND
  - Prednisone, prednisolone, or methylprednisolone used in pregnancy with success
  - Considered first-line therapy in patients with ND during pregnancy and the postpartum period
- *Adjuvant therapy*:
  - Addition of adjuvant therapy in some cases
  - Topical intralesional corticosteroids or tacrolimus used in combination with systemic therapy
  - Ciclosporin commonly used as adjuvant therapy due to rapid onset of action
  - Known side effects of ciclosporin include hypertension and renal toxicity

- *Other systemic agents*:
    - Dapsone used in some cases to inhibit neutrophil chemotaxis
    - Side effects of dapsone include hemolytic anemia and methemoglobinemia
    - Azathioprine, with slower onset of action, used in cases with bone marrow suppression and gastrointestinal intolerance as main side effects
- *Intravenous immunoglobulin (IVIG)*:
    - Used successfully as adjuvant therapy in some cases
    - May act as an immunomodulator and could be considered when starting or continuing immunosuppressive therapy
- *Cyclophosphamide*:
    - Used in special cases, such as patients with SLE
    - Considered in situations where other therapies are ineffective or contraindicated
- *TNF-α inhibitors*: Infliximab, etanercept, and adalimumab or ustekinumab have been used to treat ND, especially PG in pregnant women or during the postpartum period, with successful outcomes reported. These medications are categorized as category B, with etanercept considered safe during lactation. Therefore, their use in pregnant patients with PG is considered a reasonable option for both the mother and the fetus.

Overall, the management of ND during pregnancy and the postpartum period requires a careful assessment of risks and benefits associated with various treatment options. Individualized therapy plans, close monitoring, and multi-disciplinary collaboration are essential to optimize outcomes for both mother and baby.

KEY POINTS

- Abnormalities in the immune system during pregnancy can alter the immunological response, potentially triggering neurodermatitis (NDs).
- The reason why some pregnant individuals are more susceptible to developing ND remains unclear.
- Understanding immune system imbalances, especially in the Th1/Th2 and Th17/Treg ratios, is essential for understanding inflammatory skin conditions like ND.
- ND typically responds well to topical and systemic corticosteroids. Successful use of other immunomodulatory medications, such as cyclosporine combined with corticosteroids, has been reported.
- Timely and appropriate therapy can lead to complete resolution of the disease, ensuring a healthy newborn.

SUGGESTED READINGS

1. Vigl K, Posch C, Richter L, Monshi B, Rappersberger K. Pyoderma gangrenosum during pregnancy—treatment options revisited. J Eur Acad Dermatol Venereol. 2016;30(11): 1981-4.
2. Villani A, Fabbrocini G, Napolitano M, Costa C, Megna M, Ferrillo M. Neutrophilic Dermatosis in Pregnancy: An Uncommon Course. Open Access Maced J Med Sci. 2018;6(12):2393-4.

3. Steele RB, Nugent WH, Braswell SF, Frisch S, Ferrell J, Ortega-Loayza AG. Pyoderma gangrenosum and pregnancy: an example of abnormal inflammation and challenging treatment [published correction appears in Br J Dermatol. 2016 Jul;175(1):227]. Br J Dermatol. 2016;174(1):77-87.
4. Cohen PR. Pregnancy-associated Sweet's syndrome: world literature review. Obstet Gynecol Surv. 1993;48(8):584-7.
5. Lo A, Thompson B, Sami N. Rare Autoinflammatory Neutrophilic Dermatoses in Pregnancy: Literature Review. Am J Clin Dermatol. 2024;25:227-42.
6. Wang W, Sung N, Gilman-Sachs A, Kwak-Kim J. T helper (Th) cell profiles in pregnancy and recurrent pregnancy losses: Th1/th2/th9/th17/th22/tfh cells. Front Immunol. 2020;11:2025.
7. Abu-Raya B, Michalski C, Sadarangani M, Lavoie PM. Maternal immunological adaptation during normal pregnancy. Front Immunol. 2020;11:575197.

CHAPTER 14

Vasculitis and Pregnancy

Vikram K Mahajan

INTRODUCTION

The vasculitides comprise a group of heterogeneous disorders characterized by inflammation, inflammatory cell infiltration, and necrosis of blood vessel walls and manifesting with a spectrum of clinical features ranging between cutaneous rash that may be mild and potentially life-threatening multisystem involvement. The systemic involvement and clinical outcome usually depend on the size of blood vessels (large, medium, and small) affected. The cutaneous and systemic involvement may be a primary event or occurs secondary to other well-established systemic disorders such as systemic lupus erythematosus (SLE), antiphospholipid syndrome (APS), rheumatoid arthritis, or infection(s) or a malignancy **(Table 1)**. The incidence of these disorders is 40–60 cases per million and majority affected are females often of childbearing age posing distinct challenges in reproductive health care **(Table 2)**. This necessitates a careful and appropriate assessment of pregnancy and all its related issues for an individual patient. Fortunately, vasculitis in pregnancy is uncommon and overall risk of poor pregnancy outcome does not seem to be as high as in SLE or APS, well known to complicate pregnancy in its all aspects. Nevertheless, the impact of vasculitis on pregnancy (from conception to the postpartum period), the management of pregnancy, and the impact of pregnancy on vasculitis as such vary among affected women. In patients with vasculitis, it is imperative to consider pregnancy as of high risk requiring meticulous planning and a multidisciplinary monitoring by proficient obstetricians and internists/rheumatologists maintaining high standards of care for good maternal and fetal outcomes. Since extensive review on individual types of vasculitis, clinical presentation, diagnosis, and management is beyond the scope of this chapter, interested readers can refer standard textbooks for details. Herein, only a brief overview of vasculitis is presented in the context of pregnancy.

- Vasculitis refers to a group of disorders characterized by inflammation of blood vessels, leading to vessel wall damage and ischemic tissue injury in pregnancy.
- It is more common in females especially of reproductive age group.
- It may be primary or secondary.

TABLE 1: Common causes of secondary vasculitis.

Collagen vascular disorders	Systemic lupus erythematosus, Sjögren's syndrome, rheumatoid arthritis
Inflammatory bowel disease	Ulcerative colitis, Crohn's disease, bowel bypass syndrome
Malignancies	Lymphomas (Hodgkin's disease, cutaneous T-cell lymphoma, adult T-cell leukemia, multiple myeloma, lymphosarcoma)
	Carcinoma of the lung, colon, prostate, breast, renal, head, and neck
Others	Primary biliary cirrhosis
Infections	Hepatitis B or hepatitis C, and human herpes virus, *Staphylococcus aureus*, *Streptococcus haemolyticus*, *Mycobacterium leprae*, *Candida albicans*, *Plasmodium*, and *Schistosoma*
Common drugs	Penicillin, sulfonamide, minocycline, PAS, phenytoin, thiazides, oral contraceptive, hydralazine, tamoxifen, thiouracil, penicillamine, allopurinol, and sulfasalazine
Miscellaneous	Vaccines and serum products, insecticides, milk protein, gluten, food additives, nutritional supplements, and drug (sympathomimetics) abuse

(PAS: para-aminosalicylic acid)

TABLE 2: Age and gender predilection of primary vasculitides.

Vasculitis		Age	Gender
Large-vessel arteritis	Takayasu's arteritis	<40 years (range 20–30 years)	F > M
	Giant cell arteritis	>50 years	F > M
Small and medium vessel vasculitis	Wegener's granulomatosis*	60–70 years	M > F
	Churg–Strauss syndrome*	60–70 years	M > F
	Microscopic polyangiitis*	60–70 years	
	Polyarteritis nodosa (PAN)	50–60 years	M > F
	Cutaneous PAN	Children	M > F
	Behçet's disease	20–30 years	M > F
	Nodular vasculitis	56 years (range 23–82 years)	F > M
	Henoch–Schönlein purpura (IgA vasculitis)	Children (4–7 years)	M > F
	Kawasaki disease	Children	M > F
	Urticarial vasculitis (UV)	Young adults	
	Normocomplementemic UV	30–40 years	F > M
	Hypocomplementemic UV		F > F

*These are antineutrophil cytoplasmic antibody (ANCA)-associated vasculitides.

OVERVIEW OF VASCULITIS

It is essential to recognize the size and location of the involved vessels within each disease for predicting organ involvement, the effect of the vasculitis on pregnancy, and for adequate monitoring. Chapel Hill Consensus Conference 2012 classifies vasculitides according to the size of the inflamed blood vessels. Large vessel vasculitis (LVV) comprises Takayasu's arteritis (TA) and giant cell arteritis (GCA) that affect the aorta and its major branches. Medium vessel vasculitides involving visceral arteries, veins, and initial branches include polyarteritis nodosa (PAN) and Kawasaki disease. The small vessel vasculitides affect arterioles, capillaries, venules, and veins and are subclassified into antineutrophil cytoplasmic antibody (ANCA)-associated vasculitis and immune complex vasculitides. ANCA-associated vasculitis includes granulomatosis with polyangiitis (GPA) or Wegener's granulomatosis, eosinophilic granulomatosis with polyangiitis (EGPA) or Churg–Strauss syndrome and microscopic polyangiitis (MPA). The immune complex vasculitides include IgA vasculitis, cryoglobulinemic vasculitis, and hypocomplementemic urticarial vasculitis. IgA vasculitis (Henoch–Schönlein purpura) affecting the small blood vessels manifests with palpable purpura **(Fig. 1)**, arthralgias, glomerulonephritis, and enteritis. Behçet's disease having variable vessel involvement is labeled as variable vessel vasculitis.

The classification for ANCA-associated vasculitis has been updated by ACR and EULAR recently in 2022 by assigning weightage to specific clinical and serological criteria for improved diagnostic sensitivity and specificity. Sinonasal

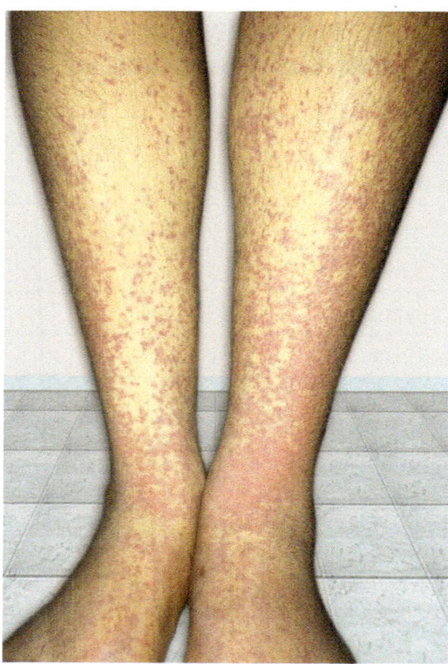

FIG. 1: Palpable and nonblanchable purpuric lesions over lower extremities and signifies small-vessel vasculitis. It can be a presenting sign in almost 50% of cases with Henoch–Schönlein purpura (IgA vasculitis). These lesions can evolve into nodular, vesicular, pustular, necrotic, or ulcerative lesions in severe form.

congestion and presence of cytoplasmic-ANCA (c-ANCA) and/or anti-proteinase 3 (PR3) antibodies are given highest value to diagnose Wegener's granulomatosis (GPA). Presence of perinuclear-ANCA (p-ANCA) and/or anti-myeloperoxidase (MPO) positivity followed by interstitial lung disease and pauci-immune glomerulonephritis are valued in that order to diagnose MPA. Eosinophilia, nasal polyps, and obstructive airway disease are essential diagnostic criteria for Churg–Strauss syndrome (EGPA) while ANCA positivity is a negative item for classifying it.

Takayasu's Arteritis

Takayasu's arteritis involves aorta and its major branches and the pulmonary arteries resulting in vessel fibrosis, stenosis, thrombosis, and aneurysm formation. Erythema nodosum-like cutaneous lesions are rare and hypertension, cardiac valve disease, retinopathy, and stroke remain its major complications. With an annual incidence of 2–3 cases per million, it affects women almost 10 times more often than men aged between 20 and 30 years at onset. Most patients are of Asian origin and various HLA class I and II molecules have been implicated in the susceptibility or development of TA. Inactive disease is compatible with favorable outcomes but active disease in pregnancy has worst maternal and fetal outcomes necessitating that the disease must be in remission prior to conception **(Box 1)**.

Polyarteritis Nodosa

Polyarteritis nodosa, a necrotizing vasculitis predominantly involving medium vessels, affects all major organ systems. With an annual incidence of 2 cases per million, it typically affects individuals of European decent aged between 50 and 60 years with a male to female ratio of 1.5:1. Arterial wall weakening and microaneurysm formation are hallmark features and digital gangrene is common. Arthralgia/arthritis is frequent. Livedo reticularis before and following nodules indicates larger vessel and systemic involvement. "Starburst" pattern of livedo reticularis that may ulcerate is a prominent cutaneous finding in cutaneous PAN. Orchitis/epididymo-orchitis may occur more classically when PAN is associated

BOX 1 Takayasu's arteritis.

- Inactive disease is compatible with favorable outcomes but active disease in pregnancy has worst maternal and fetal outcomes necessitating that the disease must be in remission prior to conception
- Maternal complications include hypertension (40%) and preeclampsia (35%) and less commonly congestive cardiac failure, progressive renal failure, intracranial hemorrhage, and death during the second stage of labor
- Maternal outcomes include spontaneous abortion (up to 30%), therapeutic abortions (15%), preterm deliveries (30%), and cesarean deliveries in 35–50%
- Intrauterine deaths (5%), low birth weight, and intrauterine growth retardation in 20% are common fetal outcomes

with hepatitis B infection. It appears that pregnancy does not have significant effect on PAN **(Box 2)**.

Antineutrophil Cytoplasmic Antibody-associated Vasculitis

Antineutrophil cytoplasmic antibody is an important diagnostic test in ANCA-associated systemic vasculitis and cANCA or pANCA is typically positive and helps in monitoring disease activity as well **(Box 3)**.

Wegener's granulomatosis and Churg–Strauss syndrome together with MPA are often classified as ANCA-associated systemic vasculitis as they affect the same sized vessels in the same internal organs, albeit upper airway involvement is characteristic of Wegener's granulomatosis.

Wegener's granulomatosis is predominantly a disease of small vessels manifesting with granulomatous vasculitis of the upper and lower respiratory tracts (pulmonary hemorrhage) and the kidneys (crescentic, necrotizing glomerulonephritis). Ulceronecrotic papules or nodules, perianal ulcers, persistent nasal polyps, oral and nasal ulcers, recurrent pansinusitis, septal perforation, and saddle nose deformity are strongly suggestive of Wegener's granulomatosis. Hyperplastic gingivitis with petechiae (strawberry gingival hyperplasia) and pyoderma gangrenosum-like ulcer lacking characteristic rolled-out borders are considered pathognomonic. The reported annual incidence is 5–12 per million

BOX 2 Polyarteritis nodosa.

- Polyarteritis nodosa predominantly involves medium vessels, affects all major systems
- It is a rare disease in patients of childbearing age. However, if occurs, it can affect all the major organs and it is recommended that the disease must be in complete remission prior to conception for better maternal/fetal outcomes
- Significant proteinuria, high serum creatinine, cardiomyopathy, and gastrointestinal or neurological involvement are major risk factors for poor prognosis requiring careful monitoring of these indicators throughout pregnancy
- Maternal deaths occur from renal failure or complication of hypertension associated with disease onset during pregnancy or active disease
- Maternal outcomes include—spontaneous abortion up to 16%, therapeutic abortions in 10%, preterm deliveries in 50–100%, and severe complications with disease onset during pregnancy
- Intrauterine fetal deaths are rare but low birth weight newborns are common fetal outcomes

BOX 3 Antineutrophil cytoplasmic antibody (ANCA).

There are two types of ANCA—pANCA (perinuclear staining pattern) and cANCA (cytoplasmic staining pattern) depending on immunofluorescent staining in ethanol-fixed neutrophils. cANCA pattern is most commonly produced by autoantibodies to antigen proteinase (PR)-3 and predominant pANCA antigen is myeloperoxidase (MPO). ANCA with PR3 positivity is occurs in 90–95% of Wegener's granulomatosis. Serial monitoring of cANCA is useful in predicting relapse and clinical course of Wegener's granulomatosis. Each cANCA with PR3 positivity and pANCA with MPO positivity occur in 45% of microscopic polyangiitis patients. pANCA also occurs with Churg–Strauss syndrome.

populations of both genders aged between 60 and 70 years but a notable number of young patients may also get it and pregnancy appears to affect it adversely and vice versa **(Box 4)**.

Churg-Strauss syndrome, a necrotizing vasculitis of medium and small arteries, manifests with late-onset asthma, nasal polyps, pulmonary infiltrates, and eosinophilia. Asthma is the major feature and always precedes other systemic manifestations while granulomatous myocarditis is characteristic. Renal involvement is comparatively less severe than Wegener's granulomatosis and MPA. Peripheral neuropathy and mononeuritis multiplex mainly involving lower limbs is frequent. It is often p-ANCA positive. Both men and women are affected equally in the fourth decade of life and annual incidence is 1-3 cases per million populations. Severe disease with heart, kidney, gut, or brain involvement is associated with a poor prognosis and necessitates treatment with immunosuppressive drugs. In general, pregnancy affects the disease adversely but when the disease is in remission, it does not affect pregnancy outcome significantly **(Box 5)**.

Microscopic polyangiitis is a necrotizing vasculitis predominantly affecting small vessels that mainly involves the kidneys and lungs. Arthralgia/arthritis is

BOX 4 Wegener's granulomatosis.

- Pregnancy has an adverse effect on Wegener's granulomatosis with possible increased risk of relapses
- Flare in 25–50% with exacerbation of asthma, lung infiltration, or neuropathy (90%)
- Cardiac involvement carries poor prognosis
- Poor maternal outcomes associated with preeclampsia (<5%), fetal loss (10–15%), and up to 50% in active disease. Therapeutic abortions (5–10%), preterm delivery (10–40%), and cesarean delivery (15–40%)
- Fetal outcomes are seen as low birth weight (10–30%) and intrauterine growth retardation (10–25%), but intrauterine fetal deaths are rare

BOX 5 Churg–Strauss syndrome.

- There is a risk of disease onset during pregnancy in 30%
- Risk of flares in 25–40% if disease in remission during conception and up to 100% if disease is active
- Flares (pulmonary involvement, skin lesions, and arthralgias) are mostly in first and second trimesters
- Eosinophilic myocarditis is a rare but serious complication of Churg–Strauss syndrome
- Abortions in 5–10% (up to 40–100% when disease is active)
- Therapeutic abortions in 10%
- Preeclampsia in 20%
- Preterm deliveries in 40%
- Cesarean delivery in 40–50%
- Maternal death rarely from intracranial bleed during vasculitis flare
- Low birth weight and intrauterine growth retardation in 10–25%
- Intrauterine fetal deaths—rare

frequent and pulmonary renal syndrome (crescentic, necrotizing glomerulonephritis, pulmonary hemorrhage, circulating ANCA) is comparatively more common than Wegener's granulomatosis and Churg-Strauss syndrome. ANCA (mostly p-ANCA with specificity for myeloperoxidase) is typically positive. It occurs with an annual incidence of 3-4 cases per million and both genders are affected equally with majority being in the fifth decade of life. The effect of MPA on pregnancy and vice versa remains underappreciated for want of more data. Few reports suggest that pregnancy has adverse effects on MPA and the latter affecting pregnancy outcomes adversely **(Box 6)**.

Behçet's Disease

Behçet's disease is usually more prevalent in men than women with few exceptions and male to female ratio varies from 1.5:1 to 5:1. The prevalence of Behçet's disease is highest across regions spanning the ancient Silk Road including eastern Mediterranean regions and China. It is one of the most common reported vasculitis in pregnancy with overall incidence of 1.4 per 100,000 with increasing trends. Behçet's disease improves during pregnancy in nearly 60% of cases while it worsens in 30% of patients affecting both maternal and fetal outcomes adversely **(Box 7)**.

BOX 6 Microscopic polyangiitis.

- Exacerbations are rare when the disease is in remission but occurs in <50% when the disease is active
- Associated with worse prognosis if diagnosed during pregnancy and postpartum.
- Preeclampsia occurs in up to 45%
- Therapeutic abortions occur in 5–10%, spontaneous abortions happen in 10%, and preterm deliveries occur in 30%
- Very rarely ends fatally for mothers
- Low birth weight neonates born in up to 65% reports
- Newborn developing pulmonary renal syndrome possible from placental transfer of anti-MPO antibodies

BOX 7 Behçet's disease.

- Spontaneous abortions are seen in 7–25% of cases
- Therapeutic abortions occur in <5% of cases
- Preterm deliveries happen in 12–25% of cases
- Increased number of cesarean deliveries is reported
- Increased thromboembolic events occur during postpartum
- Up to 30% neonates are born with low birth weight
- The rate of fetal deaths is <3%
- Transient neonatal Behçet's disease is reported in a few cases
- Congenital anomalies do not occur

Immunoglobulin A Vasculitis (Henoch–Schönlein Purpura)

The IgA vasculitis (Henoch-Schönlein purpura) mostly occurs in children aged between 4 and 7 years and remains very rare in adults. With an annual incidence of 0.1–1.8 per 100,000 individuals, it is common in males with a male to female ratio of 1.5:1. Palpable purpura mostly over dependent body parts and sparing mucosal surfaces is the hallmark cutaneous feature. Systemic features may occur and include arthralgia/arthritis, glomerulonephritis, gastrointestinal symptoms such as abdominal angina and/or obstruction, hematemesis, and melena. Its onset during pregnancy is seen in 50–75% patients and during postpartum period in 10% of the patients when it usually carries poor prognosis. Mild exacerbations are not uncommon in up to 38% patients **(Box 8)**. However, the reports of Henoch-Schönlein purpura during pregnancy remain contested.

Others

Giant cell vasculitis and Kawasaki diseases do not typically affect women of reproductive age. Giant cell vasculitis mainly occurs at the age of 50 years or above with the highest incidence in Northern Europe, particularly Scandinavian countries. It is unlikely to affect pregnancy. Kawasaki disease, a medium vessel disease of children younger than 5 years, affects visceral arteries, veins, and initial branches. High fever (38.8–40.0°C), lymphadenopathy, edema hands and feet, conjunctival congestion, red chapped lips and strawberry tongue, and ill-defined maculopapular rash subsiding with periungual and perineal desquamation are characteristic during acute phase and coronary aneurysms as late complication.

VASCULITIS IN PREGNANCY

Being uncommon, vasculitis in pregnancy is mostly underdocumented as the disease exacerbations may remain unrecognized in general. However, the impact of pregnancy and vasculitis on each other from preconception to delivery and postpartum period is likely to vary given that the prognosis for maternal and fetal outcomes depends largely on disease activity, extent and severity of end organ/ systemic involvement, and choice of pharmacotherapy during pregnancy. The overall effect of vasculitis on every aspect of pregnancy and pregnancy outcomes

BOX 8 Immunoglobulin A (IgA) vasculitis.

- Pregnancy outcomes are usually good
- There is increased risk of spontaneous absorptions, preterm delivery, and gestational hypertension
- Up to 50% cases end up with cesarean deliveries
- Eclampsia and severe renal complications (renal failure and necrotic ulcers) are rare
- The rate of low birth weight is 15–25%
- Fetal death due to rapidly progressive renal failure in a patient diagnosed during pregnancy
- No neonatal cases reported

(fertility to postpartum period and the neonate) and the vice versa is presented below.

VASCULITIS AND FERTILITY

Wegener's granulomatosis, PAN, or Behçet's disease rarely affects female reproductive organs and fertility. Vasculitis may cause transient dysregulation of the hypothalamic–pituitary–ovary axis. PAN can cause orchitis or epididymo-orchitis in men and possibly from Wegener's granulomatosis (because of testicular granulomatous inflammation and ischemia) and Behçet's disease. Testicular necrosis due to ischemia can occur even though testicular inflammation ameliorates with treatment without any clinical consequences. However, hypogonadism may manifest as increased follicle-stimulating hormone more than two times the upper reference limit and low serum testosterone level irrespective of type of previous treatment.

Although impact of vasculitis on fertility in young men and women is of significant concern, implications of the diagnosis for fertility are not immediately considered in view of potentially life-/organ-threatening complications of vasculitis. Nevertheless, it is imperative to identify and address these issues with patient at the earliest and before initiating pharmacotherapy and certainly at the time of planning for pregnancy. It is also important to assess current fertility status of the patient, implications of age, and to counsel for therapeutic options for fertility especially for negative effects of advanced age and immunosuppressive drugs on fertility/pregnancy.

VASCULITIS AND CONCEPTION

Renal impairment, cardiac insufficiency, and uncontrolled asthma in Churg–Strauss syndrome, poorly controlled blood pressure in PAN or TA with renal artery involvement, and pharmacotherapy that is not compatible with pregnancy remain major risk factors in addition to other common risk factors (alcohol consumption and low or excess maternal weight) for complicated pregnancy in these patients. The women with vasculitides are on average 5 years older than other healthy women, which can have an additional impact on pregnancy outcomes. Since the disease activity and prior organ damage are the major cause of maternal and obstetrical complications, it is ideal to plan pregnancy when the disease is in continuous remission or has minimal activity at least 6 months before conception and the woman is on pregnancy safe medications. In addition to clinical status, advancing maternal age with the time required to reach full versus partial disease remission must also be taken into consideration while counseling for conception.

Ideally, a multidisciplinary management of these high-risk pregnancies under a dedicated set-up of internists, rheumatologists, and obstetricians is highly desirable after a complete baseline assessment is performed for extent of disease especially for cardiac or renal impairment, hypertension, asthma tracheal or stenosis, which can affect the course of the pregnancy and/or its outcome.

VASCULITIS WITH IN PREGNANCY

Since most patients with Wegener's granulomatosis, Churg-Strauss syndrome, MPA, or PAN are about 50 years or above at the time of diagnosis and who for their severe disease often require intensive treatment with strong immunosuppressive regiments such as cyclophosphamide, data related to pregnancies in them is sparse. In comparison, pregnancies in patients with TA or Behçet's disease have been reported more frequently wherein, the average maternal age at disease onset is 20–30 years and treatment is primarily with pregnancy safe medications (corticosteroids and/or colchicines).

EFFECT OF PREGNANCY ON VASCULITIS

The pregnancy is not a recognized trigger for new-onset vasculitis or new flare up. When vasculitis is in remission with or without appropriate maintenance treatment before the pregnancy, the outcomes for the mother and newborn are usually favorable. But outcomes remain uncertain when the disease is still active at the time of conception and it becomes difficult to decide about treatment and/or pregnancy continuation.

With the exception of mild Behçet's disease, most vasculitides do not improve during pregnancy. However, vasculitis especially patients with PAN, ANCA-associated vasculitis, and IgA vasculitis have been diagnosed during pregnancy, postpartum, or postabortion. PAN and MPA diagnosed during pregnancy are associated with worst prognoses. A high rate (44%) of miscarriages is reported in women with pregnancies prior to the diagnosis of vasculitis. Outcomes in future pregnancies in a patient with vasculitis also remain uncertain.

Overall risk for new exacerbations seems low but variable depending on the type of vasculitis and higher with active or recently diagnosed disease. The risk for new exacerbations is <10–40% with Wegener's granulomatosis in remission at conception but increases up to 100% in patients with active disease; 25–50% in Churg-Strauss syndrome and less when in remission at conception; <50% in MPA and <5% in TA, but relapses are exceptional in PAN. Nonsevere Behçet's disease improves during pregnancy in up to 60% of patients but nearly 30% of patients can experience relapses which can be severe and complicated by cerebral venous thrombosis. The severity of exacerbation in Wegener's granulomatosis varies from recurrent or persistent rhinitis to pulmonary-renal syndrome, and minor asthma to severe cardiomyopathy in Churg-Strauss syndrome. Additionally, severe exacerbations especially in TA, PAN, and ANCA-associated vasculitis may end fatally prompting some workers to advocate avoidance of pregnancy especially in patients with severe renal impairment, cardiac insufficiency, uncontrolled asthma (Churg-Strauss syndrome), severe pulmonary hypertension, and uncontrolled hypertension with renal involvement. Moreover, monitoring can be challenging in view of pregnancy altering inflammatory biological parameters and utility of radioimaging studies remains limited because of contraindication.

EFFECT OF VASCULITIS ON PREGNANCY

Favorable outcomes are achieved in patients with systemic vasculitides when the disease is in remission and conception is well planned. Some of the potential pregnancy-related maternal complications are because of damage from earlier exacerbations. Hypertension is reported in up to 20% of these patients with systemic vasculitides. However, about 75% of patients with TA can develop severe complications of hypertension due to renal artery stenoses and/or aortic valve disease with cardiac insufficiency. Up to 5% of pregnancies end up with strokes, aortic dissection (spontaneous or in preexisting aneurysm), and rarely complications of pulmonary artery involvement. Patients with Wegener's granulomatosis and MPA can develop renal damage/insufficiency and hypertension. Asthma or cardiac damage can feature in Churg–Strauss syndrome and subglottic and/or bronchial stenosis happen in Wegener's granulomatosis. Gestational diabetes when present in these patients is usually because of corticosteroids therapy.

The risk of preeclampsia is up to 45% in TA, and 15–20% in Wegener's granulomatosis. When combined with vasculitis damage including hypertension, therapeutic abortions may be needed in up to 15% patients with TA, 5–10% in PAN, Wegener's granulomatosis, Churg–Strauss syndrome, and MPA. Many studies report high rates of preterm birth; up to 40% in vasculitis not in remission, 15–20% in TA, <10–30% in Wegener's granulomatosis, 15–40% in Churg–Strauss syndrome, and 5% in Behçet's disease. Intrauterine growth retardation and low-birth weight happen in up to 40–50% Wegener's granulomatosis and Churg–Strauss syndrome. Premature rupture of membranes occurs in up to 30% in Wegener's granulomatosis and Churg–Strauss syndrome and MPA. Preeclampsia is not uncommon in such cases with pregnancy loss in up to 25–35% in TA, Wegener's granulomatosis, and Churg–Strauss syndrome. High rate of cesarean deliveries has been reported in all vasculitis and is preferred procedure in TA because of hypertension, although spinal blocks may lead to lower limb artery stenosis and ischemic complications. Similarly, due to major artery stenosis and/or use of hypotensive and anesthetic drugs, the risk of hemodynamic instability remains due to cerebral or cardiac hypoperfusion during labor necessitating epidural block rather than general anesthesia.

VASCULITIS AND PREGNANCY OUTCOMES

Although some genetic predisposition and associations have been observed, vasculitis is neither heritable nor transmissible to the newborn. However, transient vasculitic manifestations may occur in newborns of these mothers. However, risks of pregnancy for the mother with vasculitis and the newborn(s) differ by type of vasculitis and single pregnancy outcome is not predictive of subsequent ones. Pregnancy, postpartum, or postabortion associated cases of vasculitis including TA, PAN, Wegener's granulomatosis, MPA, and Churg–Strauss syndrome tend to have worse prognosis in general than those with an earlier diagnosis of vasculitis, especially PAN and MPA are more fatal. Treatment of

Wegener's granulomatosis with cyclophosphamide is avoided during conception and the first trimester as it often leads to miscarriage and/or therapeutic abortion. However, remission was achieved in 50% women, delivering healthy but often premature newborns in cases treated with corticosteroids combined with intravenous cyclophosphamide during the second and/or third trimesters. Some of these cases had also received intravenous immunoglobulins and plasma exchange.

VASCULITIS AND POSTPARTUM PERIOD

The association between vasculitis and postpartum period remains tenuous for want of robust evidence given that the number of cases reported with new-onset vasculitis including TA, Wegener's granulomatosis, MPA, Churg-Strauss syndrome, and PAN during the postpartum period remains limited. However, it will be prudent to monitor patients with vasculitis for 6–12 weeks after delivery and any treatment prescribed during pregnancy should not be discontinued abruptly as flares have been reported in 20–40% of patents, more frequently in Behçet's disease. Additionally, patients with worsening of vasculitis during pregnancy and partially controlled with pregnancy compatible medications (corticosteroids alone or in combination with other immunomodulators, colchicine) may be treated aggressively after delivery. Outcome is different in patients developing postpartum reversible cerebral vasoconstriction syndrome or postpartum cerebral angiopathy mimicking cerebral vasculitis characterized clinically by headache and focal neurologic deficits, and angiographically by transient, fully reversible cerebral vasoconstriction requiring a different therapeutic approach.

PHARMACOTHERAPY RELEVANT TO PREGNANCY AND LACTATION

In general, systemic glucocorticoids remain cornerstone for the treatment of vasculitis and are used as first-line treatment for mild disease; whereas, cyclophosphamide, azathioprine, and mycophenolate mofetil are second-line treatments needed for more severe disease **(Table 3)**. Tumor necrosis factor (TNF) inhibitors or anti-B cells (rituximab) are recent addition to therapeutic armamentarium.

Only corticosteroids, intravenous immunoglobulin (IVIg), colchicine, hydroxychloroquine, cyclosporine, tacrolimus, and azathioprine are considered pregnancy compatible and can be used safely before or for limited disease exacerbations during pregnancy and for continuous remission of vasculitis. However, they must be taken continuously to limit the risk of disease exacerbations associated with their abrupt withdrawal. Although transplacental absorption of oral prednisone is low, there is an increased risk of preterm deliveries and intrauterine growth retardation; whereas, prolonged use may be associated with maternal hypertension and gestational diabetes. The reported

TABLE 3: Therapies for the treatment of vasculitis.

Drugs and dose		Remarks
Corticosteroids	Prednisolone: • 1 mg/kg/day for ANCA-associated vasculitis; and to treat renal and central nervous system manifestations • Equivalent doses of other corticosteroids	• First-line treatment in Takayasu's arteritis, ANCA-associated vasculitides, polyarteritis nodosa, and microscopic polyangiitis • Risk of intrauterine growth retardation with prolonged therapy • Dexamethasone and betamethasone cross the placenta and suitable for fetal indications only • Methylprednisolone 1 g/day for 3 days intravenous pulse for life-threatening organ involvement
Cytotoxic drugs	Azathioprine [2–3 mg/kg/day (50–200 mg/day)]	• Pregnancy category X drug • No evidence of teratogenicity but sporadic anomalies reported • No effect on ovarian function or spermatogenesis • Intrauterine growth retardation reported in 40% cases • Best used as steroid-sparing drug
	Methotrexate [10–15 mg/week (maximum 25 mg/week)]	• Pregnancy category X drug • No effect on ovarian function, causes reversible oligospermia in men • Highly teratogenic (embryolethal, abortifacient) during the first trimester, should be avoided throughout pregnancy where possible • Low-birth weight neonate • Add folic acid or folinic acid to minimize toxicity
	Cyclophosphamide (50–100 mg/day or 500–2,000 mg intravenous every 2 weekly)	• Pregnancy category X drug • Risk of ovarian failure in women and irreversible azoospermia in men • A known teratogenic (congenital malformations in 22%, intrauterine growth retardation and transient bone marrow suppression) with highest rates of malformation during the first trimester and remains absolutely contraindicated • Associated with higher efficacy and adverse effects. But has been used for treatment of severe Wegener's granulomatosis/life-threatening maternal disease in late pregnancy without short-term complication

Continued

Continued

Drugs and dose		**Remarks**
	Mycophenolate mofetil (500–3,000 mg/day)	• Pregnancy category D drug • Toxicity has been demonstrated in animal studies • Few reports suggest fetal toxicity in humans; preferably should be avoided until more information
Anti-inflammatory agents	Hydroxychloroquine (HCQs) (200–400 mg/day)	• Pregnancy category C drug • Eye examination recommended at baseline and every 6-month interval
	Colchicine (0.5 mg × 2–3 times/day)	• Pregnancy compatible • Used effectively and safely in Behçet's disease
	Thalidomide	• Pregnancy category X drug • Absolutely contraindicated in women of childbearing age
Biologics	Rituximab (650 mg or 375 mg/m^2 intravenous, weekly for 4 weeks)	• A third-line agent in the treatment of Wegener's granulomatosis • The risk of toxicity in pregnancy is not quantified • There is a risk of B-cell depletion in the fetus
Others	Intravenous immunoglobulin (2 g/kg body weight in single dose)	Considered safe
	Plasma exchange	
Emerging/evolving treatment modalities		*Biologics*: Anakinra, abatacept, belimumab, tocilizumab, secukinumab, ustekinumab *Small molecules*: Tofacitinib, baricitinib, upadacitinib, avacopan
(ANCA: antineutrophil cytoplasmic antibody)		

association between glucocorticoids intake and fetal malformations, especially orofacial clefts, remains contested in recent studies.

Cyclophosphamide, methotrexate, and mycophenolate remain contraindicated especially in first trimester of pregnancy for their teratogenicity. However, severe life-threatening disease exacerbations may need treatment with cyclophosphamide necessitating therapeutic abortion or premature delivery at best. Leflunomide is detrimental to the fetus and must be stopped 24 months prior to conception or a cholestyramine washout should be given.

Severe ANCA-associated vasculitides, severe cases with pulmonary–renal syndrome or anti-glomerular basement membrane antibody disease, and hepatitis B-associated PAN have been treated with plasma exchange despite inadequate evidence for survival and long-term organ recovery in controlled trials. In general, its therapeutic potential remains underevaluated. IVIg has been used safely to treat relapses in Churg–Strauss syndrome.

The reported 30% increased risk for congenital anomalies and 68% increased risk of low-birth weight babies or serious infection in neonates during 1st year of life from exposure to biologics in vasculitis were not found significant in a recent meta-analysis including studies for Behçet's disease and TNF-inhibitors or rituximab. Unlike other TNF inhibitors, certolizumab has limited placental transfer and fetal exposure. However, live vaccines for infants born to mothers exposed to TNF-inhibitors during the first 6 months of life need to be avoided. Although rituximab can be continued safely during pregnancy, it crosses the placenta and there is a risk of infant being born with B-cell depletion persisting for months.

Prophylactic use of aspirin in a dose of ≥100 mg when initiated before 16 weeks of gestation and continued until delivery has been associated with a 62% reduction in preterm preeclampsia in women at high risk and with chronic hypertension in addition to reduction in intrauterine growth retardation. Thus, prescription of aspirin has been advocated by some experts because of increased risk of preeclampsia in patients with vasculitides especially TA and preexisting hypertension or chronic renal disease despite there are not many studies assessing the potential reduction of preeclampsia in these patients.

Data on potential use and safety of some newer therapeutic modalities including apremilast, biologics (mepolizumab, abatacept, belimumab, and tocilizumab), and small molecules (tofacitinib and avacopan) during pregnancy and/or lactation remains limited. However, according to ACR reproductive guidelines, all biologics are expected to have minimal secretion in breast milk owing to large molecular size and can be conditionally recommended during breastfeeding.

ADJUVANT TREATMENT

Pregnant patients with vasculitis need additional general care and regular follow-up. Patients under treatment with corticosteroids and other immunosuppressive(s) or rituximab and having low CD4+ cell counts will need cotrimoxazole prophylaxis for pulmonary pneumocystis and folate supplementation after first trimester.

Monitoring and ensuring satisfactory blood pressure control during pregnancy with nifedipine, hydralazine, or labetalol is recommended particularly in cases with TA and ANCA-associated vasculitis while patients with preeclampsia may need treatment with methyldopa. Angiotensin-converting enzyme inhibitors and angiotensin II receptor blockers can cause renal toxicity to the fetus and remain contraindicated. Antibiotic prophylaxis against endocarditis at the time of delivery is recommended in TA in the presence of aortic regurgitation.

CONCLUSION

Pregnancy in women with systemic vasculitides is relatively uncommon but must be considered of high risk. Apparently, pregnancy has an adverse effect on vasculitis and vice versa is also true. Pregnancy outcome is generally poor where vasculitis is uncontrolled at the time of conception. However, with increasing awareness and understanding of the disease, improved maternal and fetal outcomes have been reported with planned pregnancies and when the disease is in sustained remission. Patients should be counseled for timing of conception and significance of close monitoring for the disease status as life-threatening complications may happen especially when involvement of cardiac or renal systems occurs. However, more data are needed to improve pregnancy outcomes and identify and evaluate best predictors of disease exacerbations and best therapeutic options. The role of aspirin in the prevention of preeclampsia in these patients needs to be further evaluated. Nevertheless, need-based appropriate therapy conducive to conception and pregnancy must be initiated early and such patients managed by a multidisciplinary team of experts comprising obstetricians, rheumatologists/internists, and pediatricians having experience in managing vasculitis and high-risk pregnancies.

KEY POINTS

Takayasu's arteritis:

- Assessment and monitoring of disease severity is a must prior to conception and when needed MRI scanning should be performed before conception.
- The patient must be counseled about the unfavorable pregnancy outcome especially in extensive disease with involvement of abdominal aorta.
- Regular monitoring of blood pressure, cardiac and renal failure is imperative throughout pregnancy. There is increased risk of intracranial hemorrhage during labor necessitating strict vigil for blood pressure monitoring during this time; may need central arterial monitoring.
- Corticosteroids are the first-line treatment option.

Wegener's granulomatosis:

- The women with Wegener's granulomatosis must be counseled before pregnancy as pregnancy has an adverse effect on Wegener's granulomatosis with possible increased risk of relapses.

Continued

Continued

- Relapses during pregnancy require aggressive treatment to avoid maternal and/or fetal death. It is a serious condition and may need pharmacotherapy with pregnancy-incompatible drugs.
- The disease must be in remission prior to conception and she should not be on treatment with therapy with potentially teratogenic drugs. When conception is desired, treatment with prednisolone with or without azathioprine will be safe choice.
- Monitoring early in the pregnancy and during antenatal period by a multidisciplinary team comprising rheumatologist/internist, obstetrician, and pediatrician is highly desirable and recommended.
- There is an increased risk for spontaneous abortion, preterm birth, therapeutic abortion, cesarean delivery, and maternal death.
- Regular testing for complete blood counts, ANCA, erythrocyte sedimentation rate (ESR), C-reactive protein (CRP), and monitoring of renal functions (blood urea, electrolytes, proteinuria, and blood pressure) is highly important.
- Any relapses need effective and aggressive treatment with pregnancy drugs.

Churg–Strauss syndrome:

- The disease must be in complete remission prior to conception.
- Eosinophilic myocarditis is a rare but serious complication of Churg–Strauss syndrome and assessment of left ventricular function by echocardiography is imperative prior to pregnancy.
- Monitoring of pulmonary functions is of paramount significance all through pregnancy and postpartum period.
- Relapses are not uncommon and need to be affectively controlled with corticosteroid therapy with or without pregnancy safe second-line agents.

Microscopic polyangiitis:

- Microscopic polyangiitis predominantly affects liver and lungs necessitating regular monitory for liver and lung functions.
- Therapeutic options and drugs do not differ much from those used for Wegener's granulomatosis.
- Plasma exchange, methylprednisolone, and cyclophosphamide have been used with variable efficacy.

Polyarteritis nodosa:

- Polyarteritis nodosa is a rare disease in patients of childbearing age. However, if occurs, it can affect all the major organs and it is recommended that the disease must be in complete remission prior to conception for better maternal/fetal outcomes.
- Significant proteinuria, high serum creatinine, cardiomyopathy, and gastrointestinal or neurological involvement are major risk factors for poor prognosis requiring careful monitoring of these indicators throughout pregnancy.
- Maternal deaths from renal failure or complication of hypertension associated with disease onset during pregnancy or active disease.
- Maternal outcomes include spontaneous abortion up to 16%, therapeutic abortions in 10%, preterm deliveries in 50–100%, and severe complications with disease onset during pregnancy.
- Intrauterine fetal deaths are rare but low-birth weight newborns are common fetal outcomes.

SUGGESTED READINGS

1. Pagnoux C, Mahendira D, Laskin CA. Fertility and pregnancy in vasculitis. Best Pract Res Clin Rheumatol. 2013;27:79-94.
2. Sims C, Clowse MEB. A comprehensive guide for managing the reproductive health of patients with vasculitis. Nat Rev Rheumatol. 2022;18:711-23.
3. Andreoli L, Bertsias GK, Agmon-Levin N, Brown S, Cervera R, Costedoat-Chalumeau N, et al. EULAR recommendations for women's health and the management of family planning, assisted reproduction, pregnancy and menopause in patients with systemic lupus erythematosus and/or antiphospholipid syndrome. Ann Rheum Dis. 2017;76:476-85.
4. Foster R, D'Cruz DP. Vasculitis in pregnancy. Expert Rev Obstet Gynecol. 2007;2:681-8.
5. Lee S, Czuzoj-Shulman N, Abenhaim HA. Behcet's disease and pregnancy: obstetrical and neonatal outcomes in a population-based cohort of 12 million births. J Perinat Med. 2019;47:381-7.
6. Clowse ME, Richeson RL, Pieper C, Merkel PA, Vasculitis Clinical Research Consortium. Pregnancy outcomes among patients with vasculitis. Arthritis Care Res (Hoboken). 2013;65:1370-4.
7. Machen L, Clowse ME. Vasculitis and pregnancy. Rheum Dis Clin N Am. 2017;43:239-47.
8. Fredi M, Lazzaroni MG, Tani C, Ramoni V, Gerosa M, Inverardi F, et al. Systemic vasculitis and pregnancy: a multicenter study on maternal and neonatal outcome of 65 prospectively followed pregnancies. Autoimmun Rev. 2015;14:686-91.
9. Chen JS, Roberts CL, Simpson JM, March LM. Pregnancy outcomes in women with rare autoimmune diseases. Arthritis Rheumatol. 2015;67:3314-23.
10. Sangle SR, Vounotrypidis P, Briley A, Nel L, Lutalo PM, Sanchez-Fernandez S, et al. Pregnancy outcome in patients with systemic vasculitis: a single-centre matched case-control study. Rheumatology (Oxford). 2015;54:1582-6.
11. Tsao NW, Rebic N, Lynd LD, De Vera MA. Maternal and neonatal outcomes associated with biologic exposure before and during pregnancy in women with inflammatory systemic diseases: a systematic review and meta-analysis of observational studies. Rheumatology (Oxford). 2020;59:1808-17.
12. Pefanis A, Williams DS, Skrzypek H, Fung A, Paizis K. A case of ANCA-associated vasculitis presenting de novo in pregnancy successfully treated with rituximab. Obstet Med. 2020;13:41-4.
13. Roberge S, Bujold E, Nicolaides KH. Aspirin for the prevention of preterm and term preeclampsia: systematic review and meta-analysis. Am J Obstet Gynecol. 2018;218:287-93.e1.

CHAPTER 15

Metabolic Disorders—Porphyria Cutanea Tarda, Acrodermatitis Enteropathica, etc.

Payal Chauhan, Pratika Goyal

INTRODUCTION

Pregnancy involves a variety of physiological and pathological processes driven by hormonal, vascular, metabolic, and immunological changes, many of which manifest in the skin. The cutaneous changes observed during pregnancy can generally be categorized into three groups: Normal physiological changes due to hormonal fluctuations, alterations in preexisting skin conditions that may either improve or worsen, and the development of specific dermatoses unique to pregnancy or the postpartum period.

Metabolic disorders refer to a group of inherited or acquired diseases caused by disrupted biochemical processes of the body. Inherited metabolic disorders are relatively rare and are caused by genetic factors that affect metabolic pathways, whereas acquired disorders are more common and are influenced by external factors such as environment, sedentary lifestyle, dietary habits, and other stimulants.

The various metabolic disorders associated with pregnancy and postpartum include:

- Acrodermatitis enteropathica (AE)
- Porphyria cutanea tarda (PCT)
- Glucose intolerance and gestational diabetes mellitus (GDM)
- Gestational hypertriglyceridemia and xanthomatosis
- Thyroid disorders
- The various other inherited disorders of metabolism which although can have adverse effects on both the mother and fetus include the following:
    - *Carbohydrate disorders*: Glycogen storage diseases types I and III
    - *Disorders of amino acid metabolism*: Cystinuria and homocystinuria
    - *Organic acid disorders*: Maple syrup urine disease
    - Fatty acid oxidation defects with deficiency of carnitine palmitoyltransferase type I, long-chain 3-hydroxyacyl-CoA dehydrogenase, medium-chain acyl-CoA dehydrogenase, short-chain acyl-CoA dehydrogenase

- *Lysosomal disorders*: Gaucher's disease and Niemann–Pick disease
- *Urea cycle defects*: Argininemia, argininosuccinic aciduria, carbamoyl phosphate synthetase deficiency, citrullinemia, lysinuric protein intolerance, and ornithine transcarbamylase deficiency
- *Miscellaneous*: Congenital adrenal hyperplasia, mitochondrial deoxyribonucleic acid (DNA) disorders, and Wilson's disease

These listed disorders are beyond the scope of this chapter since they do not present primarily with cutaneous changes. The first two disorders have metabolic changes associated with predominant cutaneous manifestations and both are known to worsen during pregnancy.

ACRODERMATITIS ENTEROPATHICA

Acrodermatitis enteropathica is an inherited zinc deficiency disorder first described by Brandt in 1936. AE is classified into three types. Type I, or classical AE, is an autosomal recessive disorder caused by a mutation in the *SLC39A4* gene on chromosome 8q24.3. This mutation results in a total or partial deficiency of the zinc-binding protein ZIP4, leading to zinc deficiency due to impaired intestinal absorption of zinc. It is clinically characterized by diarrhea, alopecia, and dermatitis (predominantly affecting the acral and periorificial areas) with the latter presenting as erythematous erosions with or without blister formation.

Type II AE typically appears within the first 6 months of life in infants who are exclusively breastfed. It is caused by a mutation in the *SLC30A2* gene on chromosome 1p36.11, leading to a deficiency of the zinc-binding protein in breast milk. Type III, or acquired AE, is observed in preterm infants receiving parenteral nutrition, as well as in adults with malabsorption syndromes, liver or kidney disease, or specific dietary habits, such as a vegetarian diet high in cereals that contain phytates, which can interfere with zinc absorption.

Acrodermatitis enteropathica is most commonly seen in children, with the severity of the disorder typically decreasing as they age, and complete remission often occurring during puberty. In adults, the symptoms may be nonspecific, making diagnosis challenging due to a low index of suspicion and subtle clinical features.

- AE is an inherited zinc deficiency disorder.
- Classical AE primarily affects children, with the severity typically decreasing with age, often leading to complete remission during puberty.
- In adults, AE symptoms may be nonspecific, making diagnosis difficult due to a low index of suspicion and subtle clinical features.

During pregnancy, AE typically presents in the late first or early second trimester and progressively worsens until delivery. Zinc levels may drop to nearly 35% of nonpregnant levels, but a rapid, spontaneous recovery usually occurs during the postpartum period. Acute zinc deficiency can result in symptoms such as diarrhea, dermatitis, and alopecia, and may also cause anorexia, impaired wound healing, altered immune function, and behavioral changes such as lethargy and depression. AE may worsen during pregnancy, which is a characteristic feature, although it generally improves after childbirth. However, postpartum depression has been associated with low zinc levels. Additionally, about 20% of total zinc is utilized by intestinal bacterial flora, so zinc deficiency can alter this flora, leading to diarrhea.

The worsening during pregnancy can be attributable to:
- *Nutritional deficit*: It is estimated that about 82% of the pregnant women worldwide have decreased intake of zinc.
- Hemodilution
- Requirement of zinc by fetus
- Hormonal influence of estrogen which increases copper but decreases zinc levels (estrogen receptor has a zinc finger binding protein).
- Decreased zinc binding protein
- Iron, folic acid, and calcium given during pregnancy may decrease intestinal zinc absorption.
- High cereal consumption which is rich in phytates may decrease zinc absorption.

The differential diagnosis includes:
- Impetigo herpetiformis
- Pemphigoid gestationis

Acrodermatitis enteropathica should be considered in cases of nonresponsive bullous dermatoses of pregnancy. Measurement of serum zinc levels is therefore important to rule in the diagnosis of AE.

Maternal Complications

Deficiency of zinc may increase proinflammatory activity, cause insulin resistance, pregnancy-induced hypertension, premature rupture of membrane, abruptio placentae, prolonged labor, and infections.

Impact on Fetus

Even in pregnant ladies who are not zinc deficient, any stress/infection may lead to sequestration of zinc, hence, it is not available for the growing fetus. Such an event occurring during organogenesis can lead to teratogenicity.

It can cause preterm delivery, low birth weight, and congenital abnormality. These malformations most commonly include abnormalities of the skeleton and central nervous system. Adverse fetal outcomes have been reported in untreated cases of maternal AE in the form of anencephaly, achondroplastic dwarfism, and neonatal death. Appropriate diagnosis and treatment are therefore important.

Management

Maintaining normal serum zinc levels through zinc supplementation is effective in both maternal AE and preventing adverse fetal outcomes. Usually, the treatment of AE requires indefinite therapy with daily administration of 3 mg/kg of elemental zinc in affected children. The preferred formulations include oral zinc gluconate/zinc sulfate or parenteral zinc chloride. Supportive therapy in the form of compresses and emollients helps in re-epithelialization. 3–6 monthly monitoring of serum zinc and copper levels, complete blood counts, erythrocyte indices, occult blood in the stool, and alkaline phosphatase levels are important. Clinical improvement usually occurs within a few days to weeks of initiating the treatment. However, increase in therapy may be required for the treatment of AE during pregnancy or states of stress. However, with appropriate oral zinc administration, the lesions begin to heal and may resolve completely post pregnancy. During pregnancy 300 mg/day (68 mg of elemental zinc) of supplementation with zinc sulfate may be required to prevent maternal complications and fetal risk.

- AE often worsens during pregnancy, especially in the late first or early second trimester, due to increased zinc demands and hormonal changes.
- Zinc deficiency in pregnancy can lead to serious complications such as pregnancy-induced hypertension, premature rupture of membranes, prolonged labor, and increased risk of infections.
- Zinc deficiency can result in preterm delivery, low birth weight, and congenital abnormalities, particularly affecting the skeleton and central nervous system.
- Accurate diagnosis through serum zinc level measurement is crucial to prevent adverse outcomes.
- During pregnancy, a daily supplementation of 300 mg of zinc sulfate (68 mg of elemental zinc) may be required to prevent complications for both mother and fetus.
- Monitoring zinc levels postpartum is still important to manage any lingering deficiency.

PORPHYRIA CUTANEA TARDA

Porphyria cutanea tarda is a metabolic disorder characterized by the deficiency of the enzyme uroporphyrinogen decarboxylase (UROD), which is involved in the heme biosynthesis pathway. There are two major types of PCT, i.e., acquired (type I or sporadic) and autosomal dominant (type II or familial). The acquired form is more common and typically affects middle-aged individuals, with UROD deficiency limited to liver cells, while the inherited form affects all tissues. The disease primarily manifests with skin-related symptoms, particularly in areas exposed to sunlight, such as blistering, hyperpigmentation, and increased skin fragility.

Porphyria cutanea tarda was first described by Waldenström in 1937 and is the most common type of porphyria, with an estimated prevalence of 1 in 10,000–25,000 individuals in the general population. It is more frequently observed in middle-aged males.

Pregnancy itself does not increase the likelihood of developing PCT, but the hormonal changes associated with pregnancy, particularly elevated estrogen levels, can exacerbate the symptoms in women who already have the underlying genetic or acquired susceptibility to PCT.

- PCT is a metabolic disorder caused by a deficiency of the enzyme UROD.
- Elevated estrogen levels during pregnancy can worsen symptoms in women with existing genetic or acquired susceptibility to the disorder.

Aggravating Factors

Patients taking oral contraceptives containing estrogen, as well as those with hepatitis C, hepatitis B, human immunodeficiency virus (HIV), iron overload or supplementation, and alcohol intake, have been implicated in the development of both types of PCT. Exogenous estrogen is more likely to trigger PCT than endogenous estrogen from pregnancy, as it increases levels of renin substrate, thyroxine-binding globulin (TBG), and cortisol-binding globulin through hepatic metabolism. The extent to which pregnancy-related estrogen influences PCT is debated, but the first trimester and postpartum period are known to exacerbate the condition. Hemodilution during the second trimester, leading to a decrease in serum iron, may contribute to an improvement in PCT symptoms.

Complications of Porphyria Cutanea Tarda in Pregnancy

Pregnant females with PCT may experience chemical and biochemical deterioration. The various effects include:

- Liver dysfunction and chronic liver disease with benign elevated levels of aspartate aminotransferase (AST) and alanine aminotransferase (ALT) that spontaneously resolve or improve during the postpartum period.
- Increased risk of abnormal glucose tolerance and overt diabetes. This may be seen in 60% patients.
- Antinuclear antibody, lupus anticoagulant, and anticardiolipin antibodies may be positive.
- Increased incidence of preeclampsia.

Monitoring

- It is important to appropriately monitor the patient, newborn, and staff for hepatitis B and C due to their high incidence associated with PCT.
- Screening of blood glucose levels.
- Testing for lupus anticoagulant and anticardiolipin antibodies.
- Blood pressure monitoring.
- Screening for HIV in pregnant patients of PCT presenting with risk factors for HIV.

Management

Management includes the avoidance of risk factors such as alcohol intake, iron supplementation in absence of iron deficiency anemia, and sun exposure.

Drugs such as estrogen, diethylstilbestrol, valproic acid, barbiturates, sulfonamides and hydantoins which may precipitate PCT must be avoided.

The mainstay of treatment is:

- Sun protection
- Low dose aspirin can be prescribed as preeclampsia is common complication of PCT in pregnancy.
- *Phlebotomy*: It involves biweekly venesection of about 500 mL of blood with clinical improvement evident in 2–3 months. However, in patients

with no improvement by second trimester/multiple recurrences, repeated phlebotomies with careful monitoring of hematocrit levels have been successful. While no adverse effects have been seen, venesection in pregnancy should be avoided.

- Low-dose chloroquine in refractory cases/acute exacerbations after considering the risk-benefit ratio since it is known to be cause birth defects and with appropriate ophthalmological clearance to rule out maculopathy.

Porphyria cutanea tarda aggravates during the first trimester and improves with advancing gestation. However, the fetal prognosis is excellent. There is no known adverse effect of PCT in mother reported in fetus.

- Pregnancy itself does not increase the risk of developing PCT, but elevated estrogen levels, particularly in the first trimester and postpartum, can worsen symptoms in women with preexisting PCT.
- PCT in pregnancy can lead to liver dysfunction, abnormal glucose tolerance, and an increased risk of preeclampsia.
- Management includes avoiding triggers such as alcohol, iron, and certain medications, monitoring blood glucose and blood pressure, and considering low-dose aspirin.
- Despite the aggravation of PCT symptoms, fetal prognosis generally remains excellent.

GLUCOSE INTOLERANCE AND GESTATIONAL DIABETES MELLITUS

Glucose intolerance is mainly divided into three broad categories, i.e., types 1, 2, and GDM. While GDM refers to diabetes mellitus (DM) that is diagnosed for the first-time during pregnancy (gestation) with a known prevalence of 1–14%, but also 10–12% of gestational cases may also be of type 1 or type 2 DM. The pathogenesis of GDM combines inadequate insulin secretion and responsiveness (insulin resistance) similar to type 2 DM. The various risk factors include ethnicity, obesity, childbearing at a late age, previous history of GDM, family history of type 2 DM, and polycystic ovarian syndrome (PCOS).

Cutaneous Manifestations

Gestational diabetes mellitus may present with or without cutaneous manifestations of DM. Skin changes with type 2 DM such as skin tags and acanthosis nigricans (AN) may have a predictive role for early diagnosis for GDM. The possibility of association of skin tags with DM was first explored in 1951. However, the studies of correlation between the number of skin tags and DM have also not yielded any specific results. Although AN is a known marker for insulin resistance and DM, with relatively less clear association with GDM, it has also been found that the probability of pregnant women with AN having GDM is 5.5 times more as compared to pregnant women without AN.

The density of Demodex folliculorum mite has also been shown to be increased in GDM patients, possibly due to poor glucose regulation in these patients as compared to the patients with regulated glucose levels.

Management

Gestational diabetes mellitus is associated with profound maternal and fetal morbidity, and therefore, early diagnosis and treatment is important to prevent the complications. Identification of individual risk factors is important for appropriate interventional strategies. Although, it is a very commonly encountered problem during pregnancy, there is lack of a worldwide consensus about threshold hyperglycemic levels that merit the diagnosis and treatment of GDM. It is fully treatable but requires careful supervision throughout pregnancy.

- Gestational diabetes is raised blood sugar which develops in pregnancy.
- Various cutaneous manifestations such as AN and acrochordon may be seen due to insulin resistance.
- Other such as increased risk of pyogenic infection, pruritus, and xerosis diabetic dermopathy may be seen.
- Risk factors for gestational diabetes include obesity or overweight, advanced maternal age (particularly over 35 years), family history of diabetes, previous history of gestational diabetes, or delivering a large baby.

GESTATIONAL HYPERTRIGLYCERIDEMIA AND XANTHOMATOSIS

Xanthomas are the well-circumscribed local accumulations of foam cells in the dermal tissue or the tendons, histologically characterized by the presence of histiocytes, fibroblasts, macrophages, and Touton cells full of lipids, clinically expressed as yellowish papules and plaques, nodules, and tumors.

The most common type of xanthomatosis associated with pregnancy is eruptive xanthomatosis, as reported in literature. The primary triggers include mutations in familial *lipoprotein lipase (LPL)* gene and familial dysbetalipoproteinemia.

Etiopathogenesis

Early pregnancy and increased insulin sensitivity promotes lipid synthesis and fat storage. In the third trimester, shifts to a catabolic state due to rising levels of hormones such as human placental lactogen (HPL), cortisol, and estrogen, which enhances maternal glucose production for the fetus. As pregnancy progresses, increasing insulin resistance reduces glucose uptake in muscles, leading to fatty acid oxidation and increased lipolysis, releasing free fatty acids (FFAs) and glycerol. The liver re-esterifies excess FFA into triglycerides (TGs) and releases them as very-low-density lipoprotein (VLDL), raising maternal lipid levels to meet fetal and maternal demands. Lipid levels, particularly TGs, significantly rise during pregnancy, with the peak occurring before delivery. HPL reduces LPL activity and increases lipolysis in adipose tissue. While the TG levels increase two- to threefold by the third trimester, they almost never exceed 300 mg/dL xanthomas in pregnancy.

Familial combined hyperlipidemia typically results in only mild TG elevation. However, additional risk factors, such as elevated estrogen levels during pregnancy, can lead to significant hyperlipidemia. Complications such as pancreatitis and acute respiratory distress syndrome can occur if TG levels exceed 2,000 mg/dL, eruptive xanthomas which may appear generally resolve within weeks after correcting hypertriglyceridemia. Obesity, uncontrolled DM, hypothyroidism, nephrotic syndrome, and alcohol abuse further aggravate the problem.

Management

There is also a risk of developing materno-fetal systemic complications such as fulminant pancreatitis, acute respiratory distress syndrome, preeclampsia, and preterm labor. It is therefore important to monitor the TG levels in pregnancy.

It is important to elicit appropriate history of dyslipidemia in expectant mothers and aggressive multidisciplinary management should be undertaken to prevent complications for both the mother and baby. The decrease in TG levels is associated with resolution of xanthomas.

- Early pregnancy is an anabolic state, while third trimester catabolism is seen.
- Insulin resistance and decreased utilization of glucose leads to increase breakdown of lipids to be used as a source of energy.
- There is moderate hypertriglyceridemia during normal pregnancy.
- In patients of familial combined lipidemia, there is mild increase of TGs.
- Pregnancy in these patients may lead to severe hypertriglyceridemia which may increase maternal mortality and compromise the fetus.
- Eruptive xanthomas may be seen.

THYROID DISORDERS

The thyroid gland undergoes changes during pregnancy to meet the increased metabolic demands of the maternal body and this reflects in the alteration of thyroid function tests. Thyroid disorders can present as either hypo-or-hyperthyroidism. There occurs an increase in thyroid hormones (T3 and T4) and reduced thyroid-stimulating hormone (TSH) secretion from second trimester until delivery. This along with increased renal iodine clearance results in increased iodine requirement of both the mother and fetus.

Clinical Features

The cutaneous features of thyroid disorder in pregnancy are similar to those of nonpregnant females.

Cutaneous Manifestations in Hyperthyroidism

The skin in hyperthyroidism is warm, moist, soft, and velvety smooth resembling the texture of an infant skin. This also manifests as facial flushing, palmar erythema, and heat intolerance. It occurs because of increased cutaneous blood flow and peripheral vasodilation. There is increased eccrine sweating progressively near the end of pregnancy because of increase in both thyroid gland and vasomotor activity due to which there is increased incidence of hyperhidrosis, miliaria, and dyshidrotic eczema which manifest as physiological adaptations of pregnancy. The appendageal changes include Plummer nails and diffuse nonscarring alopecia. Rarely, the occurrence of generalized hypermelanosis suggests the presence of hyperthyroidism. Other features include pretibial myxedema, palpitations, anxiety, weight loss, insomnia, tremors, tachycardia, lid lag, and hyperreflexia.

Cutaneous Manifestations in Hypothyroidism

In hypothyroidism, the skin is cold, dry, pale, thickened, and hyperkeratotic, especially along the extensor surfaces. The face may be puffy with large tongue and coarse features presenting as myxedematous facies. The involvement of appendages results in diffuse loss of scalp hair, loss of lateral third of eyebrows, onycholysis, and atrophy of nails. Other features include puffiness of faces, periorbital edema, delayed relaxation of deep tendon reflexes and bradycardia, fatigue, weight gain, and constipation.

Thyroid disorder may occur in association with other cutaneous disorders particularly vitiligo, alopecia areata, and urticaria.

Management

Iodine deficiency can result in poor fetal outcomes in form of poor neurological and cognitive development. Therefore, a complete and thorough assessment of clinical features and laboratory parameters is mandatory for appropriate management and preventing fetal complications.

The treatment of hyperthyroidism in pregnancy requires to maintain mild maternal hyperthyroidism while avoiding fetal hypothyroidism. Therefore, maternal free T4/total T4 should be maintained at the upper limit of normal reference range through the use of antithyroid drugs in their lowest effective doses. The treatment is based on etiology as well as the severity of hyperthyroidism and it includes the following:

- Graves' disease is the most common cause of thyrotoxicosis during pregnancy. The treatment includes the use of antithyroid drugs, beta-blockers, and surgical management. However, the use of radioactive iodine ablation is contraindicated.
- Subclinical and gestational thyrotoxicosis does not require treatment during pregnancy. Observation with periodic monitoring of thyroid function tests every 4–6 weeks is recommended.

Overt hypothyroidism requires thyroid hormone replacement to keep TSH levels in trimester specific range (reference range for TSH is 0.1–4.0 mU/L during the first trimester with a gradual return to the nonpregnant range during second and third trimesters. When the trimester specific range is not available, an upper reference range > 4.0 mU/L should be used. However, there is insufficient evidence about the treatment of subclinical hypothyroidism in pregnancy. The recommendations of the American Thyroid Association (ATA) guidelines require the treatment of subclinical hypothyroidism in females with positive thyroid peroxidase (TPO) antibodies and TSH > 2.5 mU/L.

- Pregnancy stimulates the thyroid gland to produce more thyroid hormones due to elevated human chorionic gonadotropin (hCG) levels.
- TSH levels decrease in the first trimester due to hCG stimulation, then rise but remain slightly lower than nonpregnant levels in the second and third trimesters.
- Graves' disease, an autoimmune disorder where antibodies stimulate the thyroid gland, is the most common cause of thyrotoxicosis during pregnancy, while subacute thyroiditis, an inflammation of the thyroid gland, can also cause transient thyrotoxicosis.

CONCLUSION

- Metabolic disorders are associated with adverse materno-fetal outcomes.
- Both AE and PCT show a flare during pregnancy. PCT is also known to be associated with GDM and preeclampsia. While no known adverse effect of maternal PCT is known to occur in the fetus, AE is associated with adverse fetal outcome.
- GDM may present with or without cutaneous manifestations. Therefore, it is important to elicit appropriate history to rule out any precipitating risk factors.
- The aggressive management of dyslipidemia is important through a multidisciplinary approach to avoid the systemic complications in both mother and child.
- Since iodine deficiency affects neurological and cognitive development, appropriate evaluation of laboratory parameters is essential for appropriate management.

KEY POINTS

- It is important to elicit a detailed past history from any patient presenting with cutaneous signs/symptoms during pregnancy.
- Appropriate monitoring and early management are important to ensure an uneventful childbirth and to avoid any complications during pregnancy, labor, and postpartum period.

SUGGESTED READINGS

1. Pérez-Maldonado A, Kurban AK. Metabolic diseases and pregnancy. Clin Dermatol. 2006;24(2):88-90.
2. Preece MA, Green A. Pregnancy and inherited metabolic disorders: maternal and fetal complications. Ann Clin Biochem. 2002;39(5):444-55.
3. Ford D. Intestinal and placental zinc transport pathways. Proc Nutr Soc. 2004;63(1):21-9.
4. Bronson DM, Barsky R, Barsky S. Acrodermatitis enteropathica. J Am Acad Dermatol. 1983;9(1):140-4.
5. Verburg DJ, Burd LI, Hoxtell EO, Merrill LK. Acrodermatitis enteropathica and pregnancy. Obstet Gynecol. 1974;44(2):233-7.
6. Brenton DP, Jackson MJ, Young A. Two pregnancies in a patient with acrodermatitis enteropathica treated with zinc sulphate. Lancet. 1981;2(8245):500-2.

7. Aziz Ibrahim A, Esen UI. Porphyria cutanea tarda in pregnancy: a case report. J Obstet Gynaecol. 2004;24(5):574-5.
8. Urbanek RW, Cohen DJ. Porphyria cutanea tarda: pregnancy versus estrogen effect. J Am Acad Dermatol. 1994;31(2 Pt 2):390-2.
9. Loret de Mola JR, Muise KL, Duchon MA. Porphyria cutanea tarda and pregnancy. Obstet Gynecol Surv. 1996;51(8):493-7.
10. Yılmaz E, Kelekci KH, Kelekci S. Skin Tag and Acanthosis Nigricans: Do they have a Predictive Value for Gestational Diabetes Mellitus? Exp Clin Endocrinol Diabetes. 2011;119:419-22.
11. Mathur SK, Bhargava P. Insulin resistance and skin tags. Dermatology. 1997;195(2):184.
12. Keskin Kurt R, Aycan Kaya O, Karateke A, Silfeler DB, Soylu Karapınar O, Akkoca AN, et al. Increased Density of Demodex folliculorum Mites in Pregnancies with Gestational Diabetes. Med Princ Pract. 2014;23(4):369-72.
13. Bashir M, Navti OB, Ahmed B, Konje JC. Hyperlipidaemia and severe hypertriglyceridaemia in pregnancy. Obstet Gynaecol. 2023;25:196-209.
14. Jaber PW, Wilson BB, Johns DW, Cooper PH, Ferguson JE. Eruptive xanthomas during pregnancy. J Am Acad Dermatol. 1992;27(2 Pt 2):300-2.
15. Singh S, Sandhu S. Thyroid Disease and Pregnancy. Treasure Island (FL): StatPearls Publishing; 2024.
16. Puri N. A Study on Cutaneous Manifestations of Thyroid Disease. Indian J Dermatol. 2012;57(3):247-8.
17. Elling SV, Powell FC. Physiological changes in the skin during pregnancy. Clin Dermatol. 1997;15(1):35-43.

CHAPTER 16

Nipple Dermatitis

Nidhi Jindal, Aakansha Sharma, Mudita Gupta

INTRODUCTION

Nipple eczema (NE) and nipple dermatitis (ND) are interchangeably used terms. Eczema is derived from a Greek word "*ekzein*" which means to boil over or break out; it lacks accuracy and histopathologically correlates with "*spongiotic dermatitis*". It has vacillating clinical presentation that varies from pruritic erythematous papules, papulovesicles, vesiculobullous lesions, or oozing to crusted patches and plaques. NE is localized inflammation of nipple and/or areola which manifest as erythema, scaling, soreness, or cracking of the involved area. It may present as itching, burning, and less often pain. It can be unilateral or bilateral. Adolescent girls and lactating females are commonly affected. Males and infants are rarely affected.

- NE has variable clinical presentation.
- NE is usually bilateral.
- NE represents a minor criterion for atopic dermatitis (AD).
- NE usually spares the nipple and immediately surrounding skin, affects mostly the areola.

PHYSIOLOGICAL CHANGES OF NIPPLE AND AREOLA IN PREGNANCY

Nipple areolar complex is important and unique with respect to disease involvement. Few diseases such as eczema and Paget's disease preferably involve the nipple region; on the contrary it is spared by certain diseases such as morphea, cutaneous systemic sclerosis, and graft-versus-host disease. Inflammatory diseases involving the nipple areolar complex can lead to untimely seizing of lactation and can severely deteriorate quality of life of the individual.

Pregnancy brings anatomic and physiologic change in breast to prepare it for lactation. Breast enlargement, tenderness, nipple and areolar hyperpigmentation, pinkish areola, prominent veins, striae, and Montgomery's tubercle are the predominant changes. Montgomery's tubercles are hypertrophied areolar sebaceous glands called after obstetrician William Fetherstone Montgomery, 30–50% women experience it in first trimester.

All physiological breast changes in pregnancy results from increased adrenal, ovarian, placental, and pituitary hormones leading to sodium and water retention, melanocyte excitement, and overactivity of sebaceous gland.

- Few dermatosis specifically involve nipple region, while others show sparing.
- Physiological changes in breast to adjust for lactation are seen in pregnancy. These physiological changes are under hormonal control.
- Montgomery tubercles result from lactiferous ducts associated hypertrophied sebaceous glands on the areola. They tend to shrink back in postpartum.

PATHOPHYSIOLOGY/ETIOPATHOGENESIS

Dermatitis is characterized by swelling and irritation of the skin which can be secondary to multiple causes.

Atopic Dermatitis

Nipple dermatitis is a common manifestation (seen in 6–23%) of AD. Hanifin and Rajka mentioned NE as one of the minor criteria for AD. Involvement of bilateral nipples and adjacent breast among postpubertal girls and young adults is characteristically witnessed in AD. As there is shift from T helper type 1 (Th1) to T helper type 2 (Th2) in pregnancy so NE associated with AD increases.

Allergic Contact Dermatitis

Allergic contact dermatitis (ACD) is a type IV delayed hypersensitive response to various antigens nickel, poison ivy, etc., by an individual's immune system. Skin lesions usually appear 24–48 hours after the exposure, which can manifest as erythema, edema, intensely pruritic weeping plaques, or papulovesicular lesions. Dyes, clothing component, remnant of detergent, fragrances, chlorine, and fabric softeners in brasseries can cause ACD.

Irritant Contact Dermatitis

Irritant contact dermatitis (ICD) is a nonimmunological inflammatory reaction to various irritant agents such as friction, water, soaps, or washing detergents and depends on various factors such as skin sensitivity, duration of exposure, nature of irritant, and duration of exposure. The diagnosis of ICD is requiring comprehensive history and physical examination is often clinical. Cutaneous manifestation can vary from mild erythema and edema to eczematous reactions, vesicles or bullae, and occasionally epidermal necrosis with ulceration.

Frictional Contact Dermatitis

Fissure of the nipple/jogger's nipple or runner's nipple is the form of contact dermatitis secondary to repeated and continuous friction or rubbing of the T-shirt or upper body clothing against nipples after prolonged running, brisk walking, or exercise.

Psoriasis

Psoriasis is an immune-mediated chronic and inflammatory disease that affects approximately 2–3% of the world's population. Psoriasis of the nipple-areola complex has been rarely reported in the literature. Nipple psoriasis can develop after breastfeeding as koebnerization phenomenon, these nipple lesions are infamous for impersonating as dermatitic conditions. Psoriatic plaques are generally more demarcated and should always be suspected in conditions not responding to long-term treatment.

Lichen Simplex Chronicus

Lichen simplex chronicus (LSC) is an idiopathic chronic neurodermatitis that presents as extremely itchy condition in which dry, scaly, and thickened plaques develop in response to repetitive rubbing. LSC can occasionally be seen in the nipple due to persistent scratching or rubbing (e.g., running). It typically presents as a lichenified or excoriated erythematous or hyperpigmented plaque that is relatively well demarcated.

Nipple dermatitis in breastfeeding mother may become superinfected with yeast. A treatment nonrespondent NE should arouse suspicion for a rare skin cancer called Paget's disease.

Paget's Disease of Breast

Paget's disease of breast (PDB) is a rare cutaneous disease of the nipple-areola complex that contributes to 1.0–4.3% of all breast cancers. Though more common in postmenopausal women but may occasionally present in young. Nearly all PDBs are associated with underlying intraductal breast cancer, either invasive or in situ. Patients may present with itchy, red, or painful sensations before or after the lesions appear. Lesions of PDB slowly involve into unilateral, well delineated, erythematous, and scaly plaque on the nipple typically extending to areola but rarely to the skin. Later stages of the disease can also show ulceration, destruction of the nipple-areola complex, nipple retraction, and serous or bloody discharge.

- Pregnancy has a variable effect on AD, though tend to increase mostly.
- Contact dermatitis is exacerbated during third trimester of pregnancy. It is usually not advised to perform patch test in pregnant women.
- Most of the diseases can be distinguished on the basis of history and clinical examination.
- Skin biopsy is required to rule out the diagnosis of PDB.
- Clinico-histopathological correlation supports accurate diagnosis.

PATHOGENESIS OF NIPPLE DERMATITIS IN LACTATION

Nipple dermatitis during lactation is a common issue that causes discomfort and can hinder breastfeeding, particularly in the first 1–8 weeks postpartum due to pain and skin problems. The pathogenesis of ND in lactation is multifactorial, involving a combination of physical, immunological, and microbial factors.

Mechanical Trauma and Friction

During breastfeeding, the nipples are subjected to repeated mechanical stress from the infant's sucking, which can cause irritation and trauma. Improper latch, incorrect positioning, or vigorous sucking can exacerbate this stress, leading to microtears in the skin of the nipple and areola. Continuous mechanical trauma weakens the skin barrier, making it more susceptible to inflammation and secondary infection. Cracks and fissures may develop, which can lead to further irritation and dermatitis.

Moisture and Occlusion

Breastfeeding frequently exposes the nipples to moisture from breast milk, saliva, and sweat. Prolonged moisture exposure can macerate the skin, compromising its integrity and making it more vulnerable to dermatitis. The use of breast pads to absorb leaking milk can create a moist environment that promotes skin breakdown. In addition, friction from the pads can further irritate the skin.

Immune System Changes

Mechanical and moisture-induced damage to nipple skin can trigger a localized inflammatory response, characterized by the activation of immune cells and the release of inflammatory mediators such as cytokines, resulting in redness, swelling, and itching. Additionally, hormonal changes during pregnancy and lactation, especially elevated levels of estrogen and prolactin, increase skin sensitivity and reactivity, further raising the risk of developing dermatitis.

Microbial Factors

The compromised skin barrier in ND creates an entry point for microbial invasion. The skin can become colonized by bacteria (e.g., *Staphylococcus aureus*) and yeast (e.g., *Candida albicans*), which can lead to secondary infections and exacerbate inflammation. Thrush can cause additional pain and inflammation, making it more difficult for mothers to continue breastfeeding comfortably.

Allergic and Irritant Contact Dermatitis

In addition to antigens causing ACD as described earlier, certain other products are also implicated during lactation. The use of topical products, such as nipple creams, ointments, or lotions, may cause allergic reactions or ICD. The skin of the nipple and areola is particularly sensitive, and exposure to certain ingredients (e.g., fragrances, preservatives, or lanolin) can lead to dermatitis. Peppermint oil may present safety hazards for young nursing infants such as seizures and respiratory distress. It can temporarily provide a "cooling" effect, but has a drying effect on skin that leads to further weakening of the skin barrier. Breast creams contain lanolin (a purified anhydrous waxy substance obtained from the wool of sheep) preservatives, fragrances, *Aloe vera*, etc., and can cause ACD.

CLINICAL PRESENTATION

Dermatitis can present in acute, subacute, or chronic stage depending on the chronicity of the disease. Though it can present in pregnancy but is more common in lactation.

Redness and Inflammation

The nipples and areolae typically appear erythematous and inflamed. This redness is a hallmark of the inflammatory response and may extend beyond the nipple area, affecting the surrounding skin. Unlike dermatitis, mammary candidiasis does not spare the area of the areola immediately adjacent to the nipple. Indeed, fine hairline cracks at the base of the nipple may also develop in severe cases.

Itching and Burning Sensation

A common symptom of ND is an intense itching or burning sensation, which can lead to scratching and further irritation of the affected area.

Pain and Tenderness

Pain is a significant feature of ND, particularly during breastfeeding. The pain may be sharp, shooting, or throbbing and can occur during or between feedings. The presence of cracks or fissures can exacerbate pain, making breastfeeding uncomfortable or even intolerable.

Dryness and Scaling

The affected skin may become dry and scaly in subacute stage. Scaling is a result of the disrupted skin barrier, leading to increased water loss from the epidermis and resulting in dry and flaky skin.

Cracking and Fissures

In more severe cases, the skin may crack or develop fissures, which can be painful and bleed. These cracks provide an entry point for pathogens and increase the risk of secondary infection.

Exudation and Crusting

The inflamed skin may ooze serous fluid, leading to crust formation. This exudation is a sign of severe inflammation and skin breakdown. Crusts may be seen around the nipple area, particularly where the skin has been damaged.

Edema

Swelling of the nipple and areola may occur due to the underlying inflammation. The skin may feel thickened and appear puffy.

Blisters or Vesicles

In some cases, small blisters or vesicles may form on the surface of the skin. These can rupture, leading to further irritation and discomfort.

Secondary Infection Signs

If a secondary bacterial or fungal infection occurs, additional symptoms may develop. For example, in bacterial infection, the skin may become more red and swollen, with the presence of pus or yellowish crusts. In the case of a fungal infection, such as thrush, the nipples may appear shiny and have a white and curd-like discharge.

Nipple Discoloration

Changes in pigmentation may occur, with nipples becoming darker or lighter than usual. This can result from chronic inflammation or postinflammatory hyperpigmentation.

DIFFERENTIAL DIAGNOSIS

Differential diagnosis of eczematous and noneczematous nipple dermatitis is depicted in **Flowchart 1**.

INVESTIGATIONS AND DIAGNOSIS

Detailed history and clinical inspection are sufficient to diagnose ND.

Dermatoscopy

Dermatoscopy can be done, which might add to the clinical diagnosis. Dermatoscopy reveals characteristic serocrusts, patchily arranged dotted vessels, and dull red background. The color varies with the stage of the disease. In acute exudative lesions, yellow-brown to dark-brown colored serocrusts predominate (yellow clod sign).

Dermatoscopy in subacute stage reveals red color faint background with a variegated appearance corresponding to spongiosis. This pattern is interspersed

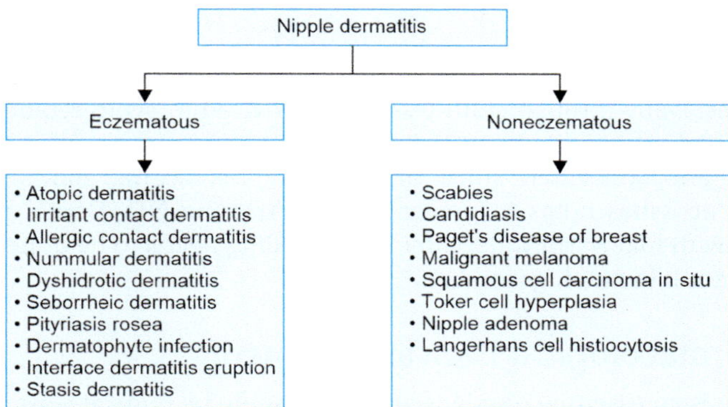

FLOWCHART 1: Differential diagnosis of eczematous and noneczematous nipple dermatitis.

with brown pigmented structures suggesting evolving pigmentary incontinence. Patchily distributed dotted vessels and other vascular patterns such as red globules, linear, curvilinear, arborizing, and looped vessels are routinely seen with fabric fibers.

Histopathology

Skin biopsy with histopathological examination may be required in nonrespondent cases of long duration to rule out malignancies like PDB.

Histopathology examination in acute stages show spongiosis with or without vesiculation, lymphocytic exocytosis, superficial perivascular infiltrate with lymphocytes, macrophages, and rare eosinophils. Whereas subacute/chronic phase show irregular acanthosis, hyperkeratosis, increased eosinophils within the perivascular infiltrate, and Langerhans cell in the epidermis and dermis. PDB show enlarged and pale, solitary or nested keratinocytes scattered through the upper layers of the epidermis.

- Diagnosis
- History and clinical examination
- Dermatoscopy
- 10% KOH to rule out fungal infection
- Skin biopsy in cases of suspicion for malignancy

TREATMENT

Pregnancy is a state of hormonal change that exacerbates eczema; hence a preconception counseling discussing the ways to prevent eczema is essential. Treatment depends primarily upon the underlying causative factor. Avoidance of irritants and allergens and frequent use of emollients, topical anti-inflammatory, and anti-infectious treatment, if required, form the essential part of treatment.

General Measures

Primary care includes avoidance of implicated allergen, use of padded bras, and tight clothes. Daily through cloth washing is advised to avoid retention of surf, detergent, and other irritants in the clothes. Dressing up oneself in noncotton, absorbent, and well-fitted shirts and sports bras during sports and other exhaustive activities helps in preventing and treating ND. Gentle cleaning of the nipple with lukewarm water after breastfeeding needs to be done to prevent nipple irritation in nursing women.

Nonpharmacological Topical Treatment

Emolliation is an essential nipple (skin) care, should be done at least once a day. *Emollient,* pH neutral wash products should be preferred over harsh detergents.

Nonfragrant, paraben-free, nonallergenic, and high lipid content emollients are preferred. Emollients plus are topicals containing additional active, but nonmedicated substances, which is supposed to have an anti-inflammatory or moisturizing effect.

Warm water compresses are easily available inexpensive treatment for nipple soreness. *Black tea compresses* can also be effective, since the tannins found in tea extracts are natural astringents and have anti-inflammatory effects. Nipple shields are nipple-shaped devices with holes at the apex allowing the infant to receive breast milk when sucking and are made from silicone, plastic, or rubber can be used in breastfeeding mothers.

Anti-inflammatory Treatment

Topical corticosteroids are the mainstay of the treatment. Ointments are preferred over creams, since they have less water and are preservative free, they are better tolerated and their occlusive effect improves steroid absorption too. Mostly class II or class III agents are used. Class IV topical steroids are generally avoided in nipple area.

Topical calcineurin inhibitors are also useful in the treatment of NE. They can be used as steroid sparing agents once the acute phase is over.

The role of newer topical products, such as *PDE4 inhibitors* and *JAK inhibitors,* in the treatment of NE during pregnancy/lactation remains to be determined. Phototherapy and systemic anti-inflammatory treatment for an underlying atopic eczema will also improve NE.

Anti-infectious Treatment

Candida superinfection is seen in lactating mothers, if suspecting antifungal treatment can be started. Antibiotics should be considered in case of superficial bacterial infection.

Eczema Treatment in Pregnancy

General measures:

- Emollients
- Topical steroids
- Ultraviolet B (UVB)
- Anti-infectious treatment
- Topical calcineurin inhibitors
- Oral steroids (in third trimester)

CONCLUSION

Literature on ND in pregnancy is scarce. All three types of eczema such as atopic eczema, ACD, and ICD are among major reasons for ND. It is essential to exclude Paget's disease, for which a biopsy is required, as it is still the gold standard to confirm diagnosis. Hygiene maintenance and general measures play key role in remission and preventing relapse of eczema. Topical steroids and calcineurin inhibitor can effectively control the dermatitis. Oral treatment can be considered in severe or nonrespondent cases.

SUGGESTED READINGS

1. Song HS, Jung SE, Kim YC, Lee ES. Nipple eczema, an indicative manifestation of atopic dermatitis? A clinical, histological, and immunohistochemical study. Am J Dermatopathol. 2015;37(4):284-8.
2. Leung AKC, Hon KLE. Atopic Dermatitis: a Review for the Primary Care Physician. New York, NY: Nova Science Publishers; 2012.
3. Hanifin JM, Rajka G. Diagnostic features of atopic dermatitis. Acta Derm Venereol Suppl (Stockh). 1980;60(92):44-7.
4. Waldman RA, Finch J, Grant-Kels JM, Whitaker-Worth D. Skin diseases of the breast and nipple: inflammatory and infectious diseases. J Am Acad Dermatol. 2019;80:1483-94.
5. Waldman RA, Finch J, Grant-Kels JM, Stevenson C, Whitaker-Worth D. Skin diseases of the breast and nipple: benign and malignant tumors. J Am Acad Dermatol. 2019;80:1467-81.
6. Zengin HB, Tan PH, Liu R, Smoller BR. 'Eczematous' dermatitis of the nipple: clinical and histopathological differential diagnosis of Paget disease. Pathology. 2024;56(3):300-12.
7. Weatherhead S, Robson SC, Reynolds NJ. Eczema in pregnancy. BMJ. 2007;335(7611):152-4.
8. Reynaert V, Gutermuth J, Wollenberg A. Nipple eczema: A systematic review and practical recommendations. J Eur Acad Dermatol Venereol. 2023;37(6):1149-59.

CHAPTER 17

Lifestyle Factors and Skin Health during Pregnancy; Skincare Routine during Pregnancy

Hima Gopinath, Sunita Gupta

INTRODUCTION

Pregnancy is a critical period in a woman's life. A healthy pregnancy requires harmony of mind, body, and thought. The increasing research on lifestyle and well-being parallels the rise in unhealthy lifestyles and chronic diseases in women. Minor changes in the woman's health or environment during pregnancy can have long-lasting implications on both the mother and her progeny. Many chronic adult diseases have fetal origins. Pregnant women may face the challenges of physiological changes in appearance, new dermatoses, or flare-ups of preexisting dermatoses. Many autoimmune and inflammatory skin disorders may be associated with adverse pregnancy outcomes. Pharmacological options may be limited during this phase.

Patients may neglect health even during pregnancy. For example, in the pregnancies registered in the Swedish hidradenitis suppurativa pregnancy register, 31% were overweight and 27% were obese. Smoking and drinking were reported both before and during pregnancy. Thus, a holistic approach during pregnancy focused on primary prevention and incorporating nonpharmacological interventions to mitigate any disease's systemic and psychological impact is crucial. This chapter will review lifestyle interventions such as nutrition, exercise, sleep, and stress management that can influence pregnancy outcomes.

DIET IN PREGNANCY

Maternal nutrition influences fertility, pregnancy outcomes, fetal development, and long-term health of the child. Preconceptional nutritional status, undernutrition, obesity, diabetes, and deficiency of key nutrients influence health outcomes through epigenetic mechanisms. Deoxyribonucleic acid (DNA) methylation is the most well-studied epigenetic change in pregnancy. Paternal diet also affects the fetus through epigenetic changes in the sperm. Epigenetic changes can affect several generations, mainly through the paternal side.

Diet plays a crucial role in modulating the skin through the skin-gut axis. It can influence blood sugars and lipids, oxidative stress, systemic inflammation, and skin flora. The Western diet, rich in red meat, dairy, and eggs, and a high-glycemic diet, is known to increase mTORC1 signaling, which is implicated in several chronic diseases. Dairy products increase insulin and insulin-like growth factor levels and contain exogenous androgens. High-glycemic food increases insulin and insulin-like growth factors. The Western diet is implicated in flares of acne. This understanding of the skin-gut axis highlights the importance of a balanced diet. However, the current body of knowledge on diet and acne in pregnancy is insufficient.

- Proper nutrition of mother is important for fertility, pregnancy outcome, fetal development, and future development of child.
- Paternal diet also may affect sperms through epigenetic changes in sperms.

Nutritional aspects that need to be addressed in pregnant women include the following:

- Nutritional status and body weight should be optimized prepregnancy.
- There is no need to eat for "two" people.
- There is no single best dietary pattern.
- A predominantly plant-based Mediterranean diet with low glycemic index (GI) foods, such as nuts, seeds, and legumes, is associated with a lower risk of diabetes. The diet should have adequate protein and fiber and be rich in iron and calcium. Dietary advice has to be customized according to culture and national guidelines.
- High-fat, high-sugar, sweetened beverages, and highly processed modern diets should be avoided.
- Focus on "ancestral eating" with nutrient-dense food. Food should be fresh, local, and seasonal.
- It may be ultraprocessed if the food label has more than five ingredients. Ultraprocessed food high in trans fats, sugar, and salt activates the brain's reward systems, leading to physiological dependence.
- Less than 10% of the total energy should be from free sugars.
- Fresh fruit can be consumed as dessert.
- Sugary beverages are high in calories, low in nutrients, and worse than sugary foods because of a quick rise in blood sugars.
- Low GI foods cause lower postprandial glucose spikes. For example, parboiled rice, basmati rice, brown rice, and rice with curd have a lower GI when compared to refined white rice. High-quality complex carbohydrates should be increased. Food with fructose (fruits) and galactose (milk) have lower glucose and GI. Fiber (e.g., from beans and seeds) lowers GI. Viscous soluble fiber (e.g., beans and rolled oats) also slows glucose absorption. The higher amylose; amylopectin ratio in basmati rice and legumes, organic acids in oranges and legumes, and acetic acid reduce glucose absorption. Starchy food should not be overcooked. For example, pasta should be cooked "al dente".
- Dysbiosis can lead to adverse pregnancy outcomes. Prebiotics, probiotics, and synbiotics may be beneficial, but more research is needed.

- Prebiotics such as fiber and probiotics like fermented foods are beneficial for the gut.
- Saturated fat should be limited and replaced with monounsaturated and polyunsaturated fats.
- Low-mercury fish may be consumed two to three times per week.
- Caffeine intake below 300 mg may be safe. However, daily consumption has to be limited. Caffeine is found in tea, coffee, cola, chocolates, cocoa, and energy drinks.
- Avoid food that causes gastrointestinal discomfort.
- Avoid taking supplements without consultation.
- Salt consumption should not exceed 5 g per day
- Myo-inositol is found in fresh fruits (e.g., citrus) and vegetables (e.g., beans and peas). It may be beneficial in preventing gestational diabetes mellitus (GDM), but more large controlled trials are needed.
- Earlier, iron was the only nutrient in focus. Now, iodine, vitamin D, and the one-carbon nutrients (folate, vitamin B12, vitamin B6, and choline) are increasingly being explored. Lower intake has been associated with neural tube defects, preeclampsia, and abortions. Several environmental factors, including diet, age, obesity, and smoking, can affect one carbon metabolism for 6 months around conception, influencing fertility, and pregnancy outcomes. Choline and vitamin B12 intake may be low in pregnancy. Vitamin B6 is present in fruits, grains, and legumes. Choline is rich in animal food but is also found in legumes and vegetables. Vegan and vegetarian patients may need supplementation or fortification to meet vitamin B12 requirements.
- A high dietary fiber and plant-based diet may be beneficial in preventing excessive weight gain. A diet high in calories, sucrose, and polyunsaturated fatty acid intake has been linked to preeclampsia. High potassium, fiber, and calcium supplementation in patients whose calcium intake is low may be beneficial in preventing preeclampsia.

A healthy diet in pregnancy should have foods with:
- A low GI and high fiber
- Minerals (iron, calcium, and one carbon nutrients)
- Proteins
- <10% energy from free sugars
- Pre/probiotics
- Myo-inositol
- High amylose:amylopectin ratio
- Mono saturated fatty acid
- Less salt/caffeine
- Smoking and alcohol should be avoided

DIET IN PREGNANCY AND SKIN

Minerals and vitamins play a crucial role in promoting skin health for both the mother and the fetus during pregnancy. Vitamins C and E are essential for collagen production and act as antioxidants, potentially preventing various autoimmune and inflammatory diseases. Nuts and seeds are packed with essential nutrients, including vitamin E, magnesium, and fiber, all known for their anti-inflammatory properties

Omega-3 fatty acids help reduce inflammation and maintain the integrity of the skin barrier. Additionally, omega-3 fatty acids found in fish and seafood also exhibit anti-inflammatory effects and may help lower the risk of allergic diseases like atopic dermatitis. Green leafy vegetables, flaxseed, linseed, and chia seeds are a rich source of alpha-linolenic acid (ALA), a type of omega-3 fatty acid. Walnuts, rapeseed oil, and soybeans have about 10% ALA. Omega-3 fatty acids and its metabolites reduce proinflammatory activity and are beneficial in atopic dermatitis, contact dermatitis, psoriasis, and for photoprotection.

As observed by Adineh et al., intake of nuts, vegetables, fruits, and protein in diet during pregnancy decreases risk of childhood allergies. Yogurt, a rich source of pre- and probiotics, is also reported to decrease incidence of allergic disease in the child.

Zinc serves as an immune modulator and can be beneficial in managing conditions such as acne and warts. Iron is vital for ensuring a proper oxygen supply to both mother and fetus, while folic acid is necessary to prevent neural tube defects. A balanced diet rich in these nutrients supports healthier skin and overall well-being during pregnancy. The mother's diet during pregnancy can influence the nutrient composition of breast milk, which in turn can impact the development of the immune system in the child.

Smoking has a negative impact on collagen production, and impairs wound healing and immune function both in the mother and the fetus.

- Intake of proper diet during pregnancy influences skin health and prevents many dermatological diseases in both the mother and the fetus.
- Vitamins and minerals may help in collagen synthesis in the developing fetus.
- Vitamins and minerals also have an anti-inflammatory effect.
- Consumption of diets rich in omega-3 fatty acids help in reducing inflammation, prevent allergic disease in the child, and maintain integrity of skin.
- Increase in weight during pregnancy may precipitate diseases like psoriasis.

A referral to a nutritionist may be needed to understand risk factors and provide individualized medical nutrition therapy. Comprehensive nutritional advice should not be given in one sitting as it may confuse the patient.

Adherence to dietary interventions is often poor. Cognitive behavior therapy and social cognitive theory principles can improve adherence. Social cognitive therapy is based on the principle that people learn by observing others. Group education strategies and sharing stories of success help manage diabetes. Motivational interviewing is a patient-centric approach based on the patient's motivations, feelings, goals, attitudes, and barriers. It is a collaborative approach with reflective listening to understand patient perspectives and supports patient autonomy and control. The counseling should be matched to the patient's readiness for change.

- Diet management during pregnancy is essential for both mother and the child.
- Comprehensive nutritional advice in one sitting is useless.
- Social cognitive behavior therapy and motivational interviewing should be encouraged.
- A food diary should be maintained.

OBESITY

Weight should be addressed ideally in the prepregnancy period. Even a 5% reduction can reduce the metabolic impact of obesity. Prepregnancy obesity > 30 body mass index (BMI) kg/m^2 is the most important predictor of maternal weight gain, which can result in both maternal and fetal complications. Insulin sensitivity is reduced in pregnancy, and this reduction is greater in obese mothers. Elevated blood sugars, lipids, and low-grade inflammation can lead to metabolic syndrome, particularly in the obese. Diet and lifestyle changes upregulate gene and protein expression of insulin signaling. A calorie deficit of 500–1,000 calories in the prepregnancy period will reduce insulin resistance and hyperandrogenemia of polycystic ovarian syndrome, improving metabolic and reproductive outcomes. Close monitoring, motivational interviewing, a food diary, and regular diet and exercise interventions are beneficial in preventing excessive weight gain during pregnancy. Higher maternal BMI and gestational weight gain may be a risk factor for striae gravidarum, hidradenitis suppurativa, psoriasis, acanthosis nigricans, chronic venous insufficiency, etc. Although diet and exercise may be beneficial in preventing striae gravidarum, there is little data on this.

EXERCISE IN PREGNANCY

Exercise interventions should begin in the prepregnancy period with moderate intensity aerobic exercise of at least 30 minutes minimum 5 days a week, strenuous intensity aerobic physical activity of at least 20 minutes three times a week, and resistance training twice weekly on nonconsecutive days. It is essential to reduce sedentary behavior like prolonged sitting, preferably after a meal, reduces glucose spikes.

Exercise during pregnancy offers numerous benefits and can contribute to a healthier pregnancy, smoother labor, and quicker postpartum recovery.

- *Maternal health*:
    - Cardiovascular fitness
    - Weight management
    - Mood enhancement
    - Musculoskeletal health
    - Prevents constipation
- *Fetal health*:
    - Improved oxygen flow
    - Improves birth weight
    - Reduced risk of complications like preterm birth

Gestational diabetes mellitus is increasing; thus, exercise interventions during pregnancy are essential to improve glycemic control and overall well-being. Aerobic activity involving large muscle groups or body weight-based exercise prevents constipation and improves mental health during pregnancy.

Exercise interventions in pregnancy include the following:

- Any type of exercise of any length and frequency is beneficial.
- Previously active women can continue their exercise regimen.
- New exercise programs should be started after consulting a physician. 5–10 minutes of warm-up and cooling down should be done.
- Inactive women can begin with low-intensity aerobic exercises and strength training. Exercise can be started in multiple short sessions. Mild-to-moderate exercise should be done at least three times per week.
- Exercise that involves lying on the back and prolonged standing should be avoided.
- Plyometric exercises, hot yoga, hot Pilates, overhead lifts, contact sports, and activities with a risk of falling should be avoided.
- Non-weight-bearing exercises such as swimming and stationary cycling are better.
- High-intensity exercise increases heart rate by >90%, which should be avoided as it can affect blood flow to the fetus.
- Pelvic floor exercises during pregnancy and the postpartum period improve the strength of pelvic floor muscles.
- Pregnant women should consume plenty of fluids and use the correct clothing to dissipate heat.
- Pregnant women should stop exercising when they are tired.
- A physician should be consulted if there are any unusual symptoms.

Physical activity can be influenced by individual, social, and environmental factors such as lack of time, misinformation from others, social or cultural norms, and physical symptoms of pregnancy. These factors may have to be addressed for changing behavior. Pregnant women must be provided with instructions on safe exercise with regular monitoring and feedback.

- Type of exercises which are safe:
  - Aerobic—waking/swimming/stationary cycling
  - Strength training—light/moderate weight lifting and resistance bands
  - Flexibility and stretching—yoga and stretching exercises
  - Pelvic floor exercises—Kegel
- Overexertion/strenuous exertion/lying on back should be avoided.
- Warming up and cooling down should be done.
- Hydration to be maintained.

Yoga

Yoga dates back to >5,000 years. Yoga combines posture, flexibility, exercise, sounds, rhythm, meditation, and relaxation. Mind, body, and spirit are united to improve overall well-being. It promotes symmetry, coordination, endurance, and balance. It is beneficial for depression in nonpregnant adults and may improve mood and lower stress during pregnancy. It modulates the neuroendocrine axis and may improve parasympathetic activity. Prenatal yoga is gentle, and some poses are avoided or modified. Props may be needed for support. It reduces the aches and pains of pregnancy, improves sleep, and improves mothers' and children's bonding. Patients with depression may have low motivation to begin yoga. It is better practiced in groups to avoid social isolation and increase connection between expectant mothers. Yoga should be started under supervision and practiced safely to avoid injuries.

EXERCISE AND SKIN HEALTH DURING PREGNANCY

Exercise increases blood flow to skin hence improves glow of pregnancy. Pelvic floor exercises helps to decrease incontinence of urine which may occur during pregnancy hence reduce contact dermatitis. Also venous return is increased thus reducing incidence of varicosities in pregnancy.

MENTAL HEALTH AND STRESS MANAGEMENT DURING PREGNANCY

Women are more susceptible to depression than men, and the perinatal period is sensitive. Around one-fifth of women from developed countries experience at least one episode of major depressive disorder. For mild depression, psychological interventions such as cognitive behavior therapy and psychotherapy, exercise, and lifestyle changes are recommended. Moderate-to-severe depression requires pharmacotherapy and shared decision-making with the patient. Maternal depression causes changes in cortisol levels and has immunological effects. It can impact the child's hypothalamic-pituitary-adrenal (HPA) axis, physical growth, and brain development. Suicide is a leading cause of death in the postnatal period; thus, it is essential to identify depression and treat depression early. Depression leads to lower self-care and lower bonding with their children.

Patient may present with headache, irritability, and sleep disturbances. Many pregnant women report higher symptoms of stress, anxiety, and depression. During stress, the body reacts to real or perceived threats. Endocrine, immune, and nervous systems are activated in complex pathways. Stress can affect fertility and influence the outcomes of fertility treatments. Because of changing physiology, there is a shift toward a more sympathetic tone in pregnancy. Unmanaged stress in prenatal, perinatal, and early childhood has several biological and epigenetic effects. There can be intergenerational transmission of stress reactivity. Stress may aggravate many immunological dermatoses. Psychological health influences other parameters such as eating patterns, diet, and physical activity. Anxious and stressed patients may engage in stress eating, leading to visceral fat deposition. Stress disrupts sleep, which can worsen obstetric outcomes. Anxiety symptoms should be screened for in the first trimester and referred early. Regular tracking of mood and sleep is important in women with bipolar disorder. Stress is an inherent aspect of life and must be managed with process involvement and commitment. Socioeconomic factors can worsen stress. Regular exercise and yoga may combat the negative effects of stress and elevated cortisol. Patients need education on self-care, exercise, sleep, a healthy diet, and mindfulness.

Mindfulness-based cognitive behavior therapies are helpful in infertility treatment and in promoting overall wellness during pregnancy. Thoughts trigger other thoughts, and patients may spend hours engaged and confused in a chain of thoughts and worries. Mindfulness improves awareness and systemic thinking. Mindfulness can have "formal" and "informal" interventions. It helps pregnant women to accept changes in pregnancy and its challenges with a nonjudgmental attitude. Pregnant women may also use aromatherapy, music, and other complementary therapies to improve their well-being.

Pregnancy is a time of significant physical and emotional changes, which can lead to increased stress.

- *Sources of stress specific to pregnancy*: Health concerns, financial worries, relationship changes, and fears about labor and parenting.
- *Effect of stress on mother*:
    - Changes in cortisol level effects immunological, endocrine, and nervous system
    - Decreased fertility
    - Effects diet and physical activity
- *Effect of maternal stress on fetus*:
    - Low birth weight and preterm labor
    - *Long-term effects*: Behavioral and emotional problems in children

Management of pregnancy induced stress:

- Identify stressors and try to counsel patient
- Deep breathing exercises, muscle relaxation and contraction exercises/meditation/yoga/healthy lifestyle modification, and social support from family and friends

Sleep

Most women suffer from sleep problems during pregnancy. Short duration and poor quality sleep can lead to chronic fatigue, negatively affect birth weight, and increase cesarean rate and neonatal APGAR scores. Sleep and influence diet and diet can affect sleep. Sleep affects mood, impulse behavior, and emotions. Disturbed sleep is a significant risk factor for both mental health and general disorders. There can be an increased risk of suicide with poor sleep in the peripartum period. The patient may have disturbed sleep due to stress, increased frequency of micturition, fetal movements, and nightmares. Obstructive sleep apnea and restless leg syndrome are common during pregnancy. Patients with snoring should be evaluated for obstructive sleep apnea. Iron and folate should be screened in women with restless leg syndrome. Patients need to prioritize their seven to nine hours of sleep. Naps should be shifted to earlier in the day. Fluid intake should be reduced before bedtime. Regular exercise, yoga, mindfulness, and a high-fiber diet low in saturated fats and refined rice are beneficial. Multicomponent cognitive behavior therapy for insomnia is the first-line treatment for insomnia. Lack of awareness of interventions to promote sleep is highly prevalent. It includes sleep hygiene, addressing environmental factors such as noise, light, and temperature that may affect sleep, relaxation, sleep restriction (restricting the time spent in bed), cognitive restructuring of thoughts about sleep, stimulus control to reassociate sleep with bed, and establishing a regular sleep-wake schedule.

OTHER LIFESTYLE CHANGES

Pregnancy is associated with increased basal metabolic rate. There is increased sweating. There is more occlusion at intertriginous folds due to increased weight. This maceration may predispose females to fungal infections of skin. Pruritus may further damage the sin barrier facilitating infiltration by microorganisms. If possible, pregnant female should stay in an environment with ambient temperature and humidity. Also pregnant females should wear loose, breathable, and natural fiber clothing to prevent skin irritation and allow the skin to breathe.

Low sensitizing moisturizers and cosmetics should be used because some of the chemicals may be harmful to the fetus. Also compromised maternal skin barrier increases chances of contact dermatitis.

Hand and general hygiene should be maintained as there is increased predisposition for infections.

CONCLUSION

Comprehensive lifestyle modifications for maintaining dermatological health during pregnancy, including avoiding smoking and alcohol, managing environmental factors, choosing appropriate clothing, using safe personal care products, practicing good hygiene, staying hydrated, regular exercise, and balanced nutrition with supplements as and when required, ensuring quality sleep, and supporting mental well-being.

A summary for the common lifestyle interventions are summarized in **Figure 1.**

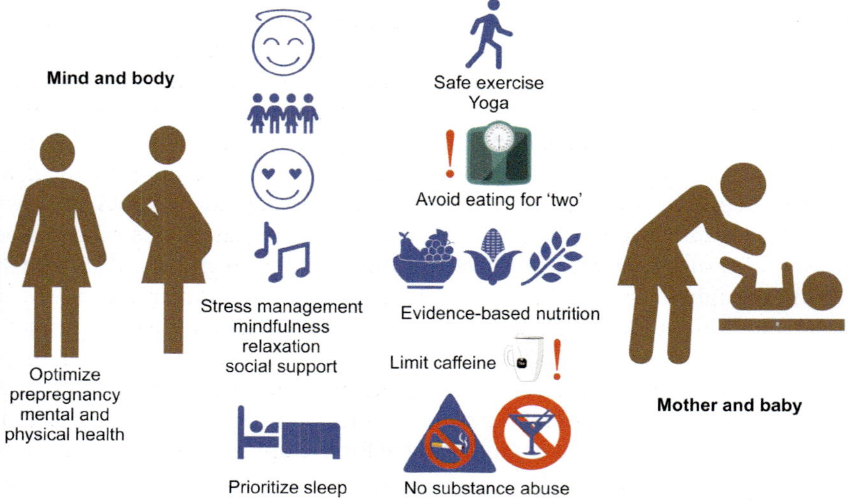

FIG. 1: Lifestyle interventions for dermatological conditions during pregnancy.

There is a paucity of data on lifestyle interventions for dermatological conditions during pregnancy, so dermatologists may have to follow general lifestyle recommendations until more specific research data is available. Guidelines change over time; thus, the websites of international associations and organizations are essential sources of up-to-date information. Pregnancy is a unique period where small changes can have a "butterfly effect" on future generations. Positive lifestyle interventions in a supportive and empathetic environment can transform several lives.

SUGGESTED READINGS

1. Vaquero-Abellan M, Marquez FG, Martínez PA. The importance of healthy lifestyles in helping achieve well-being. In: Vaamonde D, Hackney AC, Garcia-Manso JM (Eds). Fertility, Pregnancy, and Wellness. Amsterdam, Netherlands: Elsevier; 2022. pp. 1-19.
2. Martinhago CD, Furtado CL. Genetics and epigenetics of healthy gametes, conception, and pregnancy establishment: embryo, mtDNA, and disease. In: Vaamonde D, Hackney AC, Garcia-Manso JM (Eds). Fertility, Pregnancy, and Wellness. Amsterdam, Netherlands: Elsevier; 2022. pp. 73-89.
3. Vaamonde D, Algar-Santacruz C, Dillard DM. Epigenetic and biological consequences of unmanaged stress during prenatal, perinatal and early childhood periods. In: Vaamonde D, Hackney AC, Garcia-Manso JM (Eds). Fertility, Pregnancy, and Wellness. Amsterdam, Netherlands: Elsevier; 2022. pp. 193-207.
4. King JH, Kwan ST, Caudill MA. Improving pregnancy outcomes with one-carbon metabolic nutrients. In: Lammi-Keefe CJ, Couch SC, Kirwan JP (Eds). Handbook of Nutrition and Pregnancy. Cham: Springer International Publishing; 2018. pp. 133-61.
5. Adineh P, Amini S, Abolnezhadian F, Jafari F, Ebrahimian N. Nuts, vegetables, fruits, and protein dietary pattern during pregnancy is inversely associated with risk of childhood allergies: a case–control study. Sci Rep. 2024;14:842.
6. Aldhous MC, Hor K, Reynolds RM. Epigenetics and diet in pregnancy. In: Lammi-Keefe CJ, Couch SC, Kirwan JP (Eds). Handbook of Nutrition and Pregnancy. Cham: Springer International Publishing; 2018. pp. 163-81.
7. Hackney AC, Vaamonde D, Garcia-Manso JM. Nutrition and exercise intervention for female fertility. In: Vaamonde D, Hackney AC, Garcia-Manso JM (Eds). Fertility, pregnancy, and wellness. Amsterdam, Netherlands: Elsevier; 2022. pp. 149-59.
8. D'Anna R, Santamaria A. Myo-inositol supplementation in gestational diabetes. In: Rajendram R, Preedy VR, Patel VB (Eds). Nutrition and Diet in Maternal Diabetes. Cham: Springer International Publishing; 2018. pp. 229-35.
9. Barkoukis H. Management of obesity in pregnancy. In: Lammi-Keefe CJ, Couch SC, Kirwan JP (Eds). Handbook of Nutrition and Pregnancy. Cham: Springer International Publishing; 2018. pp. 185-99.
10. Gopman S, Leeman L, Wagner LK. Preeclampsia. In: Lammi-Keefe CJ, Couch SC, Kirwan JP (Eds). Handbook of Nutrition and Pregnancy. Cham: Springer International Publishing; 2018. pp. 221-9.
11. Trouva A, Diamanti Kandarakis E. Links between polycystic ovary syndrome and gestational diabetes mellitus. In: Rajendram R, Preedy VR, Patel VB (Eds). Nutrition and Diet in Maternal Diabetes. Cham: Springer International Publishing; 2018. pp. 189-206.
12. Mikkonen RS, Rodrigues-de-Souza DP, Ihalainen JK. Exercise and pregnancy. In: Vaamonde D, Hackney AC, Garcia-Manso JM (Eds). Fertility, Pregnancy, and Wellness. Amsterdam, Netherlands: Elsevier; 2022. pp. 319-41.

13. Atkinson L, Teychenne M. Psychological, social and behavioural changes during pregnancy: implications for physical activity and exercise. In: Santos-Rocha R (Ed). Exercise and Physical Activity During Pregnancy and Postpartum: Evidence-Based Guidelines. Cham: Springer International Publishing; 2022. pp. 21-5.
14. Tardin RM, Martínez PA, Bonow MP, Schuffner A. Mindfulness and yoga approach for fertility: the benefits of mindfulness in human reproduction treatments. In: Vaamonde D, Hackney AC, Garcia-Manso JM (Eds). Fertility, Pregnancy, and Wellness. Amsterdam, Netherlands: Elsevier; 2022. pp. 183-91.

CHAPTER 18

Vitiligo and Other Hypopigmentary Disorders in Pregnancy

Shivani Bansal, Himani Chawla

INTRODUCTION

The physiological process of pregnancy is characterized by distinct changes in the various functions of the body systems necessary to accommodate and nurture the placenta and fetus within the challenging maternal immune system environment. There are specific skin changes associated with pregnancy besides physiological skin changes.

Autoimmune diseases (ADs) encompass a wide range of disorders that stem from the dysregulation of the immune system. The specific pathogenic mechanisms are not yet fully elucidated. These disorders are more commonly seen in females than males and also in reproductive age groups. It is now widely accepted that different ADs exhibit distinct responses to pregnancy, with some showing improvement, others remaining stable or worsen.

VITILIGO

Vitiligo is a chronic acquired skin/mucosal disease of progressive melanocyte loss characterized by well-defined milky white macules/patches. The disease has a significant effect on a patient's quality of life. Vitiligo is classified based on distribution as nonsegmental or segmental. Nonsegmental form encompasses mucosal, acrofacial, generalized, mixed, and universal type. Segmental is subcategorized as unisegmental, bisegmental, and multisegmental.

Epidemiology

The global incidence of vitiligo varies with an average of 0.4–2%. In an Indian study, it was found to be 8.8%. This difference may be because vitiligo may be more visible in darker skin types. Otherwise, there is no ethnic, racial, or gender predilection. In 50% cases, disease manifests at under 20 years of age. Though a bimodal distribution is seen with the second peak occurring at mean 34 years.

Etiopathogenesis

The exact mechanism behind vitiligo is not fully understood. There is either a destruction of melanocytes or their functioning is lost. Nonetheless, it is widely accepted to have a multifactorial basis, with the autoimmune hypothesis being the most prominent **(Fig. 1)**. This hypothesis suggests that changes in humoral and cellular immunity lead to the destruction of melanocytes and the subsequent loss of pigmentation. Vitiligo can be associated with autoimmune conditions like thyroiditis, type I diabetes, alopecia areata, pernicious anemia, and connective tissue disorders. As a result, vitiligo is commonly connected with autoimmune disorders and similar states involving immune imbalances. The connection between vitiligo and pregnancy is not widely recognized.

Immunological Changes in Pregnancy and Vitiligo (Fig. 2)

- The Th1/Th17 cytokine profile is upregulated in the early trimester, making it a proinflammatory state.
- Hormones like progesterone, estrogen, and human chorionic gonadotropin (hCG) are upregulated during pregnancy's second and third trimester. These hormones also have an effect on innate and adaptive immunity.
- There is upregulation of Th2 cytokines like interleukin-2 (IL-2), -4, -5, -13 in the second and third trimester of pregnancy.

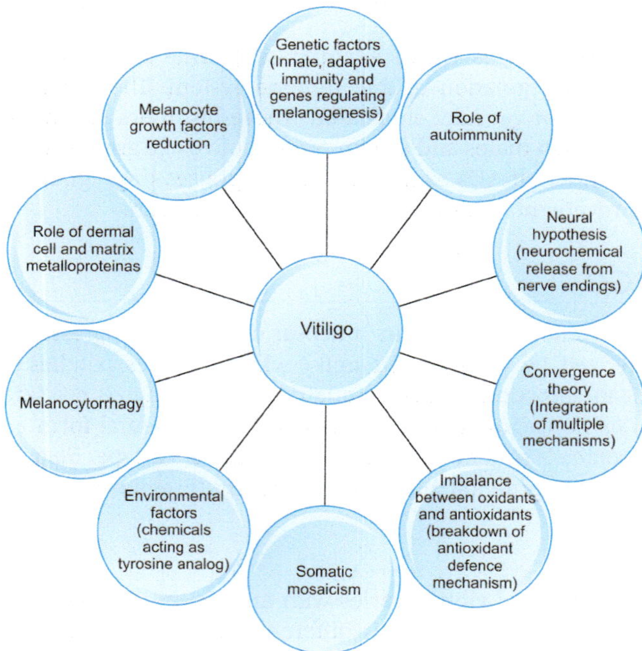

FIG. 1: Various etiological factors in vitiligo.

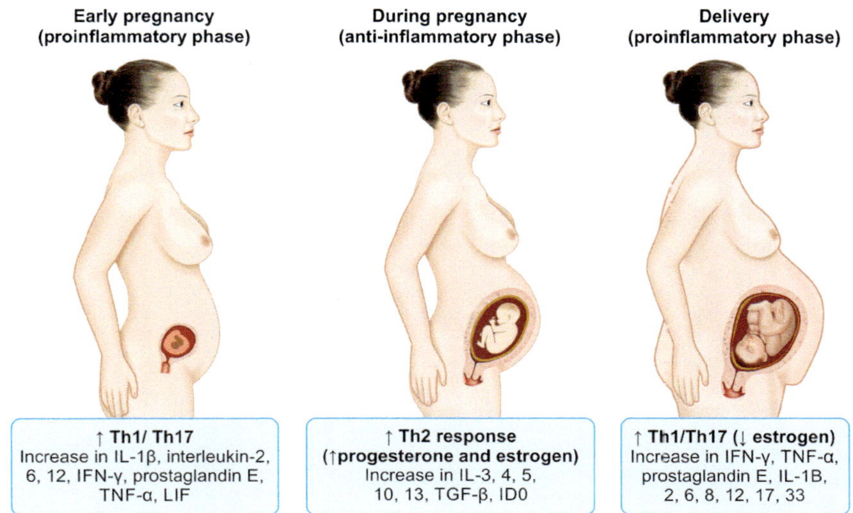

FIG. 2: A diagram depicting immunological changes in pregnancy.
(IFN: interferon; IL: interleukin; TGF: transforming growth factor; TNF: tumor necrosis factor)

- Uterine dendritic cells and decidual CD14+ monocytes also upregulate anti-inflammatory cytokine like IL-10, reducing the secretion of proinflammatory cytokines. Moreover, antibody formation is decreased by autoreactive B cells.
- Hence, autoimmune disorders having a Th1 profile will improve in pregnancy as compared to the Th2 profile, which will worsen.

During Delivery

Levels of hormones decrease, which in turn again result in a milieu of proinflammatory cytokine.

Immunological Changes in Vitiligo

- There is an increase in proinflammatory cytokines like IL-1, IL-6, IL-8, and IL-12 in vitiligo. Also, studies have shown low levels of IL-10 in active vitiligo and decrease in T regulatory cells **(Flowchart 1)**.
- A beneficial effect was proposed by pregnancy against the destruction of melanocytes and the resulting depigmented macules. This effect is mediated by increased levels of cortisol and IL-10, which are observed during pregnancy.

Effect of Pregnancy on Vitiligo

- As per the evidence, most cases exhibit stabilization or enhancement of vitiligo repigmentation during pregnancy, with only a minority of cases showing worsening disease.

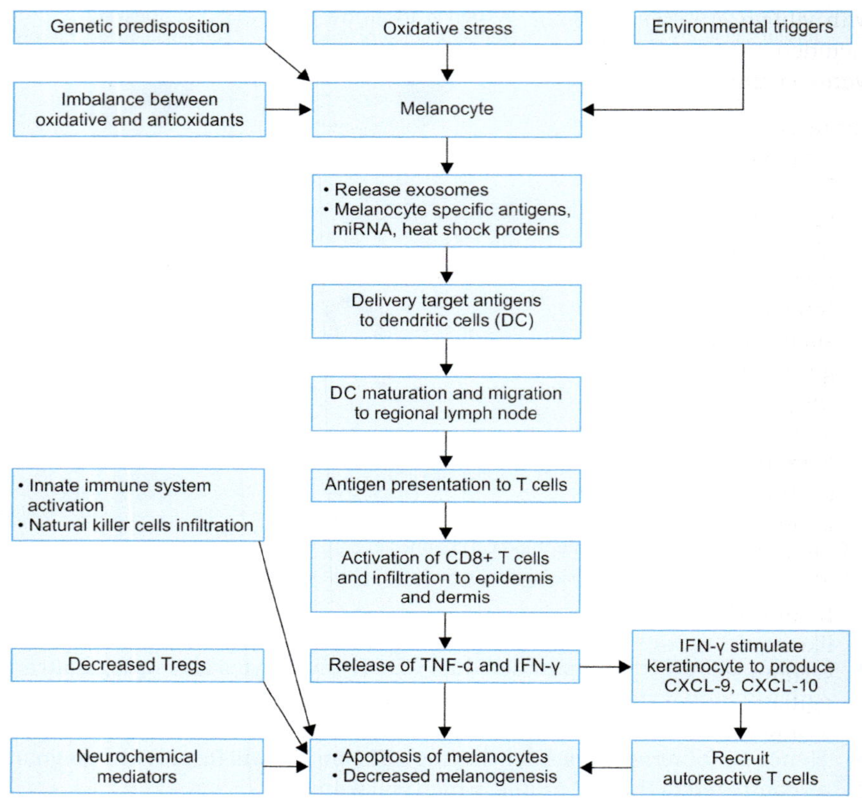

FLOWCHART 1: Interaction of various factors and immune cells in causing melanocyte damage. (IFN: interferon; TNF: tumor necrosis factor)

- A study by Nasca et al. revealed that 17.54% of cases experienced deterioration of the disease during pregnancy, while 66.66% showed no change or stability in their condition, and 12.8% reported improvement.
- Quite often patients stop using medicines leading to aggravation of disease.

Effect of Puerperium on Vitiligo

- Delatorre et al. observed that the course of vitiligo usually remained unchanged for 6 months after delivery.
- During the 6 months postpartum, 28.07% of patients experienced a worsening of their condition, 63.15% saw no change, 5.26% showed improvement, and 3.50% were unable to give the history of the disease's progression in one study.

Effect of Vitiligo on Pregnancy

There are very few large studies which have observed the impact of vitiligo on pregnancy. Park et al. in Korea retrospectively analyzed 4,738 pregnant patients with vitiligo. Another study in Taiwan by Hung et al. in a retrospective study included 1,096 number of pregnant patients with vitiligo and 4,384 pregnant women without vitiligo.

Various conclusions they drew from their study were:
- Women with vitiligo had an increased susceptibility to miscarriages, and lower rates of live births, with heightened risk being connected to a more severe form of the disease.
- Moreover, these women exhibit a significantly higher incidence of chronic hypertension and placenta previa compared to those without vitiligo.
- Interestingly, there were no significant variations in other obstetric risk factors such as preterm delivery, labor characteristics, preeclampsia/eclampsia, gestational diabetes, stillbirths, and intrauterine growth restriction between the groups.
- They also observed that patients who had received preconception systemic steroids had a reduced risk of abortion compared to those who did not take such treatment. So, treating vitiligo before conception decreases the risk of abortion.
- They also evaluated the risk of miscarriage with different systemic treatments. The risk was significantly lower in patients who received systemic steroids before conception compared to those who used other immunosuppressants like methotrexate. Additionally, the combination of phototherapy with other systemic agents further reduced the risk of miscarriage.
- Patients did not show any significant differences in terms of the cesarean section rate.

Effect of Vitiligo on Fetus

- There is an increased risk of prematurity and intrauterine growth retardation (IUGR) in the fetus of vitiligo mother with no increased risk of other fetal complications.
- *Congenital vitiligo*: Kambhampati et al. postulated that autoimmune process is responsible for development of congenital vitiligo starts in utero.
- As explained in **Figure 1 and Flowchart 1**, genetics plays an important role in vitiligo. But as other factors especially environmental triggers are essential. Thus, pregnant patients should be counseled appropriately depending on their history, that the risks exist but are low.
- Vitiligo may pose a higher risk for patients with specific methylenetetra-hydrofolate reductase (MTHFR) polymorphisms, which have been linked to shorter birth length and lower birth length for age. Screening for this polymorphism and providing vitamin B12 supplementation could help improve pregnancy outcomes in such cases.

Effect of Vitiligo on Fertility

Decreased ovarian reserve and low sperm count with decreased motility have been observed in patients of vitiligo.

Probable Reason for Vitiligo Leading to Adverse Pregnancy Outcome

- Autoimmunity in vitiligo is systemic rather than limited to skin or vitiligo patch only.
- In patients with recurrent abortions, Th1 pattern is seen. Vitiligo also shows a predominant Th1 activity.

There is conflicting data that few studies report no effect of vitiligo on pregnancy.

Reasons for improvement in vitiligo:

- Response of various autoimmune diseases to pregnancy is different. Some like rheumatoid arthritis may improve, others like systemic lupus erythematosus worsen while some may remain static. These variations are because of differences in pathophysiology.
- Accordingly, a protective effect exerted by pregnancy against the process of melanocyte destruction and subsequent skin depigmentation was postulated. Increased cortisol and IL-10, which normally occurred in pregnancy, could explain the associated disease improvement.

Disease Associations

- Individuals with vitiligo who have experienced a miscarriage are more likely to develop other autoimmune conditions such as systemic lupus erythematosus, Sjögren's syndrome, and rheumatoid arthritis, compared to those without vitiligo. There is also a somewhat increased risk of Hashimoto's thyroiditis, as noted in a few cases. The heightened risk to the fetus may be more closely linked to these ADs rather than vitiligo itself. In a review by Horev et al., involving 79 pregnant women with vitiligo, no fetal complications were observed.
- Meanwhile, no significant variances were observed in psoriasis and atopic dermatitis prevalence.

Management

The target of vitiligo treatment is disease stabilization and repigmentation. Currently, there is no FDA-approved treatment for vitiligo. All treatment modalities are off-line. In vitiligo patients, improved pregnancy outcomes can be achieved through early and appropriate disease control using systemic treatment before conception.

Still, when it comes to treatment options for vitiligo in pregnancy, options are limited, i.e., corticosteroids and phototherapy.

Topical Treatment

- Topical corticosteroids, topical calcineurin inhibitors, and topical vitamin D analogs such as calcipotriol and tacalcitol are pregnancy category C drugs.
- Prostaglandin F2 alpha analogs are pregnancy category D drugs.

- The pregnancy category status of basic fibroblast growth factor (bFGF)-derived peptide remains unknown.
- The use of topical corticosteroids is often associated with the complication of skin atrophy, which can be seen as even after 2 weeks after starting treatment.
- However, these negative effects can be significantly minimized by opting for a low-potency corticosteroid for a shorter duration, following an alternate day or weekend regimen, avoiding occlusive dressings, and discontinuing treatment once the desired effect is achieved.
- As prolonged treatment is required for extensive vitiligo, a regimen involving topical corticosteroids with intermittent breaks from the medication may serve as a suitable compromise.
- One study has shown the association between IUGR and the use of potent or highly potent topical corticosteroids but not with low-potent topical corticosteroids.
- Given the risk-benefit ratio, topical tacrolimus should not be used during pregnancy.
- Due to the adverse effects of topical calcipotriene in animal studies, it is also labeled as pregnancy category C. It should not be used in pregnancy.

Systemic Treatment

- It should be noted that the systemic medications used to treat vitiligo fall under category C or D pregnancy drugs, with the decision to continue their use during pregnancy being dependent on the unfavorable risk-benefit ratio associated with these drugs.
- Oral corticosteroids are pregnancy category C drugs.
- Commonly used drugs like azathioprine, mycophenolate mofetil (MMF), minocycline, cyclophosphamide, and JAK-STAT inhibitors are classified as category D pregnancy drugs and should not be used during pregnancy and lactation.
- Also, a washout period of 4–12 weeks is required for various immunosuppressives before conception.
- Ginkgo biloba is likely unsafe in pregnancy due to its teratogenic effects in animal studies and antiplatelet activity.
- Patients with vitiligo have lower levels of vitamin B12 than control. Hence, vitamin B12 supplementation should also be given to pregnant patients with vitiligo.
- Intravenous immunoglobulin (IVIg) and zinc, on the other hand, do not have any contraindications for use during pregnancy.
- The use of afamelanotide, an analog of the α-melanocyte-stimulating hormone, has not been studied in pregnant women.

Phototherapy

- Narrowband ultraviolet B (NB-UVB) phototherapy is generally regarded as a safe treatment option for pregnant women. However, the FDA has not assigned any pregnancy category to it.

- With regards to dosing, an initial UVB dose can be started from 0.2 to 0.3 J/cm^2 depending upon MED (minimal erythema dose). At each visit, dose increments of 10–20% of the previous well-tolerated dose should be done according to erythema.
- Research findings have suggested that patients undergoing long-term phototherapy may experience a reduction in serum folate levels.
- Insufficient folate levels are associated with a higher risk of neural tube defects (NTDs), and folic acid supplementation around the time of conception can prevent most NTDs; it is advisable to recommend folic acid supplements to female patients of childbearing age who are undergoing NB-UVB phototherapy.
- Before and after NB-UVB phototherapy sessions, patients should also be counseled to maintain hydration.
- Patients can also notice flare of their melasma.
- Psoralens and ultraviolet A (PUVA) therapy is contraindicated in pregnancy.

Cosmetic Camouflage

It can improve the quality of life in patients with facial vitiligo lesions. These products are considered safe unless they contain other ingredients known to be unsafe for pregnant women.

General Advice

Reassure in pregnant vitiligo patients that the condition has no harmful effects on the fetus and that the likelihood of passing vitiligo to the child is low.

OTHER HYPOPIGMENTARY DISORDERS

Pityriasis Versicolor

- An Italian study found a similar frequency of pityriasis versicolor in pregnant patients and the general population. However, a higher degree of colonization was observed at the end of pregnancy and postpartum.
- Treatment of pityriasis versicolor during pregnancy primarily involves using topical agents.
- Topical antifungals like ciclopirox and clotrimazole 1% (category B) are generally considered safe and effective for pregnant women.
- Topical miconazole, econazole, selenium sulfide shampoo, ketoconazole cream, and shampoo come under category C drug.
- Using oral fluconazole during the first trimester of pregnancy may be linked to adverse pregnancy outcomes.

Lichen Striatus

- Lichen striatus is an acquired linear inflammatory dermatosis, most commonly seen in children and less frequently in adults. It usually presents unilaterally and heals with hypopigmentation. There are few case reports of lichen striatus in pregnancy.

- Pregnancy can trigger an autoimmune response, leading to the appearance of an eruption.
- Topical steroids can be given as a treatment modality; otherwise, the disease is self-limiting in nature.

Progressive Macular Hypomelanosis

- It is a nonscaly condition characterized by hypopigmented macules primarily on the trunk, and it is more commonly observed in young women.
- In one case report, the patient had a sudden eruption of progressive macular hypomelanosis (PMH) in the 2nd month of pregnancy. So, hormonal etiology can be proposed.
- 10% benzoyl peroxide can be used for treatment.

Leprosy

- Pregnancy leads to a relative decrease in cellular immunity, which enables *Mycobacterium leprae* to proliferate.
- Lepromatous leprosy and relapse after treatment are more commonly observed during pregnancy due to the immunodeficient state of pregnant women.
- It can worsen during pregnancy and, if left untreated, can cause permanent damage to the skin, nerves, limbs, and eyes.
- There is an increased risk for premature birth and a small for gestational age infants. It is crucial to treat leprosy during pregnancy. Leprosy in pregnancy can be safely and effectively treated with multidrug therapy.

KEY POINTS

- In most cases, vitiligo repigmentation either stabilizes or improves during pregnancy, with only a minority of cases experiencing a worsening of the condition.
- Women with vitiligo showed an increased susceptibility to miscarriages, both spontaneous and otherwise, and had lower rates of live births. This heightened risk was associated with more severe forms of the disease.
- There is an increased risk of prematurity and intrauterine growth retardation (IUGR) in fetus of mothers with vitiligo.
- The treatment modalities include NB-UVB phototherapy and topical steroids. Folic acid supplementation should be given with phototherapy.
- Evidence about other hypopigmentary disorders in pregnancy is limited.

SUGGESTED READINGS

1. Abdelhafez MMA, Ahmed KAM, Ping Pang NT, Pg Baharuddin DM, Than WW, Kadir F, et al. Vitiligo and pregnancy: How do each affect the other? Ann Med Surg (Lond). 2021;70: 102833.
2. Webb KC, Lyon S, Nardone B, West DP, Kundu RV. Influence of Pregnancy on Vitiligo Activity. J Clin Aesthet Dermatol. 2016;9(12):21-5.
3. Delatorre G, de Oliveira CABM, Chaves TP, Linsingen RF Von, de Castro CCS. A study of the prognosis of vitiligo during pregnancy. Surg Cosmet Dermatol. 2013;5(1):37-9.

4. Hung CT, Huang HH, Wang CK, Chung CH, Tsao CH, Chien WC, et al. Pregnancy outcomes in women with vitiligo: A Taiwanese nationwide cohort study. PLoS One. 2021;16(3):e0248651.
5. Park KY, Kwon HJ, Wie JH, Lee HH, Cho SB, Kim BJ, et al. Pregnancy outcomes in patients with vitiligo: A nationwide population-based cohort study from Korea. J Am Acad Dermatol. 2018;79(5):836-42.
6. Horev A, Weintraub AY, Sergienko R, Wiznitzer A, Halevy S, Sheiner E. Pregnancy outcome in women with vitiligo. Int J Dermatol. 2011;50(9):1083-5.
7. Chen YT, Chen YJ, Hwang CY, Lin MW, Chen TJ, Chen CC, et al. Comorbidity profiles in association with vitiligo: a nationwide population-based study in Taiwan. J Eur Acad Dermatol Venereol. 2015;29:1362-69.
8. Nasca MR, Giuffrida G, Micali G. The Influence of Pregnancy on the Clinical Evolution and Prognosis of Pre-Existing Inflammatory and Autoimmune Skin Disorders and Their Management. Dermatology. 2021;237(5):771-85.
9. van Driessche F, Silverberg N. Management issues for vitiligo in children and pregnant women. In: Gupta S, Olsson MJ, Parsad D, Lim HW, Geel N, Pandya AG (Eds.). Vitiligo: Medical and surgical management. Hoboken, NJ: Wiley-Blackwell; 2018. pp. 427-38.
10. Chi CC, Mayon-White RT, Wojnarowska FT. Safety of topical corticosteroids in pregnancy: a population-based cohort study. J Invest Dermatol. 2011;131(4):884-91.

CHAPTER 19

Hair Disorders and Pregnancy

Kuldeep Verma, Mudita Gupta

INTRODUCTION

Pregnancy is a complex condition associated with various hormonal and immunological changes which directly or indirectly affect the hair growth cycle leading to various hair disorders observed during this phase.

HORMONAL CHANGES DURING PREGNANCY AFFECTING HAIR CYCLE

Progesterone

Progesterone is the main hormone throughout pregnancy. Primary source is corpus luteum for the initial 8 weeks followed by placenta and membranes of fetal decidua. A level of progesterone continues to increase throughout pregnancy to maintain the viability of fetus. Post pregnancy, levels falls to normal levels. Levels of progesterone are 4–6 times higher than the nonpregnancy state.

Progesterone has an influence on hair follicles by acting locally at the level of hair follicle as well as acting at the level of pituitary gland and indirectly affecting the hair follicles. Locally, it inhibits the 5-α reductase activity which decreases the conversion of testosterone to dihydrotestosterone (DHT). At the level of pituitary, it decreases the luteinizing hormone (LH) level, low level of LH inhibits the ovarian theca cells which cause decrease in androgen production. Low androgen helps in increasing the anagen phase and hair growth **(Flowchart 1)**.

Estrogen

Similar to progesterone, estrogen levels continue to rise throughout pregnancy. Source of estrogen for initial 8 weeks is ovaries, after 8 weeks, placenta is formed which remains as a primary source of hormone.

Estrogen acts at the level of estrogen receptors present in dermal papilla and alters the hair growth cycle. It also influences the metabolism of androgens decreasing androgen levels and decreasing hair growth.

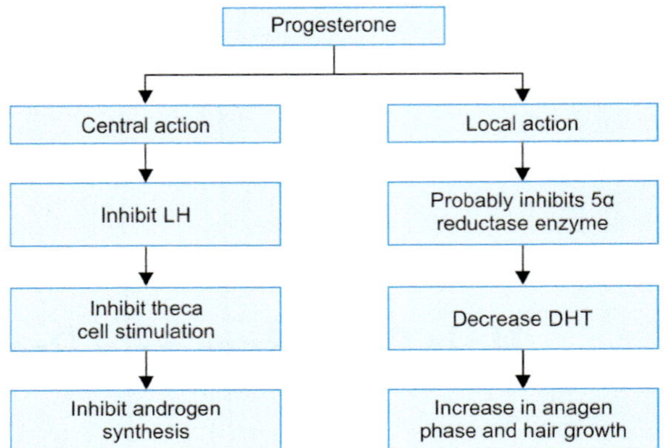

FLOWCHART 1: Mechanism of action of progesterone on hair.
(DHT: dihydrotestosterone; LH: luteinizing hormone)

Estrogen has also been shown to reduce the sensitivity of hair follicles to DHT.

KEY POINTS

- Estrogen levels continue to increase throughout pregnancy.
- It binds to estrogen receptors on hair follicles, thus altering hair cycle.
- It inhibits aromatase leading to decreased conversion of androgen to estrogen.

Prolactin

Prolactin (PRL) levels begin to rise early in pregnancy due to increased secretion from anterior pituitary. Levels continue to rise in each trimester which peaks in third trimester. After delivery, if breastfeeding is frequent, PRL levels remain elevated to support lactation.

Foitzik et al., in 2006, identified the presence of PRL receptors at the level of hair follicle outer root sheath, proximal inner root sheath, and matrix keratinocytes. Same study identified PRL in scalp keratinocytes.

Prolactin has inhibitory effect on hair growth phase causing inhibition of hair shaft elongation and induction of catagen phase. PRL also increases the levels of free testosterone and dehydroepiandrosterone sulfate (DHEAS) causing a decrease in the levels of sex hormone-binding globulin (SHBG) which is serum testosterone-estradiol-binding globulin.

After childbirth, increase in the level of PRL contributes to TE.

KEY POINTS

- Levels of PRL increase in the third trimester and peak in lactation.
- Act on prolactin receptor (PRLR) presents on hair follicles and causes inhibition of hair shaft elongation.
- PRL converts anagen hairs to catagen hairs prematurely.
- Increases free testosterone and DHEAS, and decreases SHBG.

Anterior Pituitary Hormones

There is a significant increase in the weight of anterior pituitary gland (more than twofold) in pregnancy because of the increase in the metabolic demand in the state. It leads to increase in the levels of hormones like adrenocorticotropic hormone (ACTH) and melanocyte-stimulating hormone (MSH). There is also an increase in the levels of steroid hormones like gonadotropins, corticotropin leading to increase in the levels of cortisol in the blood as well as at the level of hair follicles.

Cortisols have been shown to increase the anagen phase of the hair cycle leading to prolongation of anagen phase in pregnancy. Postpartum decrease in cortisol levels contributes to telogen effluvium (TE).

KEY POINTS

- There is an increase in the size of anterior pituitary gland in pregnancy.
- Increase in ACTH and MSH levels occurs which increases anagen phase in murine models.
- Postpartum decrease in cortisol levels contributes to TE.

Adrenal Gland

Adrenal gland hypertrophy leads to increased production of cortisol, aldosterone, and DHEAS.

Cortisol level begins to rise early in pregnancy due to increased corticotropin-releasing hormone (CRH) from placenta and level reaches at peak in third trimester. After childbirth, cortisol levels decrease to prepregnancy levels. There are various studies which have shown a positive relationship between raised cortisol level in pregnancy and hair cortisol concentrations (HCCs). HCC continues to rise in pregnancy and in postpartum period. Some studies have shown that HCC levels were 200% higher in the postpartum period than nonpregnant, nulliparous women.

Increase in the levels of HCC negatively affects the synthesis of hyaluronans and proteoglycans which are important modulators of hair follicle function. Premature degradation of these molecules alters the hair growth cycle leading to suppression of the anagen phase and triggering TE postpartum **(Flowchart 2)**.

Thyroid Gland

During pregnancy, there occurs a relative iodine deficiency which often leads to compensatory hypertrophy of the thyroid gland. It causes increase in the basal metabolic rate due to increased secretion of thyroid hormones.

Major action of thyroid hormones on hair follicles includes prolongation of the anagen phase, hair matrix stimulation, proliferation of keratinocytes, and alteration of intracellular keratin expression.

Density of the scalp hairs tends to increase during pregnancy because of the increase in hair shaft diameter. In a study done on 26 pregnant women by Lynfield et al., it was observed that the number of anagen hairs tends to increase in each trimester of pregnancy. It was found that the mean percentage of anagen hairs in

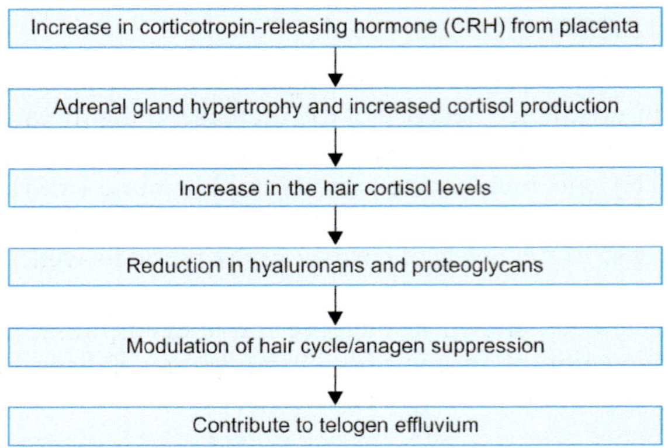

FLOWCHART 2: Pathomechanism of action of adrenal glands causing telogen effluvium.

first trimester was 85% which increased to 95% in second trimester. Mean increase in anagen hairs was maintained till 1st week after delivery. Probable reason of this change is decrease in conversion of anagen hairs to telogen hairs under the influence of hormones. An alternative explanation of increase in anagen hairs is because of increased shedding of telogen hairs. Increased androgen production from ovaries as well as from ACTH and cortisol secretion from anterior pituitary contributes to hirsutism.

PHYSIOLOGICAL HAIR CHANGES

Hirsutism

Hirsutism is the most common finding in pregnancy which is defined as increased hair growth in both normal and abnormal distribution. Common site of hirsutism includes face (especially over androgen sensitive region) followed by arms, legs, and back. Changes of hirsutism are common in early phases of pregnancy. The changes are more pronounced in women with a tendency toward male pattern hair distribution, or women with hormonal imbalance like polycystic ovary syndrome (PCOS). During the postpartum period, most of the fine hairs tend to shed but coarse and terminal hairs persist. In the subsequent pregnancies also, similar changes of hirsutism are common.

Increase in the levels of estrogen also contributes to hirsutism. Multiple studies have confirmed the presence of estrogen receptors at the level of hair follicles. Common sites include nuclei of outer root sheath, epithelial matrix, and dermal papilla cells. Predominant receptor is β-type estrogen receptor which is major steroid receptor expressed in human skin. Estrogen acts on these receptors causing prolongation of anagen phase leading to increase in the hair growth.

In few cases presenting with fetal malformation or stillbirth, abnormal hair growth and virilization are observed but mechanism of such findings remains unknown.

In pregnant females who have marked hirsutism, a proper workup is recommended to rule out virilizing tumors causing hair growth which include ovarian tumors, PCOS, lutein cyst tumors, etc.

Mainstay of treatment includes educating and reassuring patient about benign nature of disease and cosmetic treatment of unwanted hairs in postpartum period. Cosmetic treatment options include use of shaving, waxing, electrolysis, and laser epilation for temporary hair reduction. Diode laser treatment for hirsutism has become very popular in recent years because not only it is very effective and safe, it does provide a sustainable results. Ideal time to start lasers is only after delivery as not much studies are there which establish safety of lasers in pregnancy. As most of the hairs tend to shed post delivery, most dermatologists recommend a waiting time of at least 6 months post delivery.

KEY HIGHLIGHTS

- Hirsutism is the most common change defined as an abnormal hair growth over body under the influence of hormones mainly progesterone, estrogen, and cortisol.
- Marked hirsutism can be associated with virilizing tumors of ovaries and corpus luteum which needs to be excluded.
- Treatment consists of reassuring the patient by educating them. Various temporary hair removal methods can be used for management.
- Diode laser is a newer modality which gives sustainable results.

Telogen Effluvium

Telogen effluvium is defined as the increase in the shedding of telogen hairs in abnormally high amount. Common triggers include severe stress, infection, acute febrile illness, major surgery, trauma, and postpartum phase of pregnancy.

In the normal scalp, 80–85% of hairs are in anagen phase, 10–15% of hairs are in telogen, while 2–3% of hairs are in catagen phase. During pregnancy, as the anagen phase is prolonged, number of anagen hairs increase to over 90%. During labor, severe stress on the body precipitates majority of anagen hairs into the telogen hairs. Transition is further increased due to hormonal changes which occur in postpartum period. When the telogen hairs shed, it leads to severe hair loss which is termed as TE.

Prolongation of anagen phase is mainly because of hormonal fluctuations which occur during pregnancy which delays the conversion of anagen hairs to telogen hairs. In the postpartum period, as the hormones return to normal levels, there is temporary synchronization of hair cycle where majority of anagen hairs goes into the telogen phase and eventually shedding starts at 3–4 months postpartum. Telogen shedding generally lasts for 3–4 months but may last up to 1 year.

Recently, role of raised cortisol levels and decreased proteoglycan in hair follicle region has been shown to have a negative effect on hair cycle causing precipitation of majority of hairs from anagen to telogen phase in the postpartum period leading to TE.

Schiff and Kern conducted a study on 98 women in postpartum period suffering from TE. It was found that in majority of patients, hair loss was reported between 8 and 16 weeks postpartum. Almost 66% patients recovered in next 4–6 months. Area-wise distribution of hair loss was also studied in the study with anterior scalp involvement being the most common in 59.1% patients followed by diffuse scalp involvement in 20.4% patients and in 11.2% patients, only frontal region was involved.

In another study, it was found that number of telogen hairs increased to 30% at the end of 9 weeks postpartum. These telogen hairs were shed after 3–4 months causing TE. Other triggers of TE include stress during the delivery including surgical stress, emotional stress, labor pain, blood loss, and infections.

Telogen effluvium has an excellent prognosis. Role of education by a doctor is very important as the condition is extremely worrisome to few patients. Reassurance is the most important therapeutic modality.

Although complete recovery is common in TE, the hair may not be as abundant as it was as compared to prepregnancy, and women often complain of decreased density, changes in hair color, curliness, and altered hair texture. Because of this observation, there has been a search for safer treatment options which helps in complete recovery of anagen hairs after TE. One such treatment option is proteoglycan replacement therapy (PRT) which has been shown to prevent postpartum hair loss leading to early recovery from TE by causing anagen phase induction.

Proteoglycan replacement therapy was given to females in postpartum period suffering from TE. It was found that the hair count was increased by 35.7% approximately over a 6-month period with decrease in the number of vellus hairs causing the overall increase in hair number. Thus, telogen–anagen ratio was replaced helping in fast recovery. PRT is a good anagen-inducing therapy which can be used as a prophylactic or as a part of treatment in postpartum TE where proteoglycans levels are reduced as a natural function of pregnancy as well as due to raised cortisol levels during peripartum period.

If TE persists for >1 year then other causes of hair loss should be considered which include female pattern hair loss, iron deficiency anemia, pernicious anemia, low vitamin D levels, or abnormal thyroid function. Rare causes include Sheehan's syndrome which occurs due to decrease in the blood supply to pituitary gland causing hypopituitarism and Chiari–Frommel syndrome which is caused due to persistent hyperprolactinemia.

KEY HIGHLIGHTS

- Telogen effluvium is defined as shedding of telogen hairs in the postpartum period.
- It occurs because of prolongation of anagen phase in pregnancy under the influence of hormones. Post delivery, synchronization of hair cycle occurs with increase in the telogen hairs leading to TE.
- Major trigger for TE is raised cortisol levels and decreased proteoglycan in hair follicle region causing precipitation of majority of hairs from anagen to telogen phase in the postpartum period leading to TE.
- Excellent prognosis with majority of cases recovering in 6 months
- PRT is an effective anagen-inducing agent which can be used for early recovery in patients with TE.

Male Pattern Baldness and Hypotrichosis

These are uncommon findings in pregnancy and usually observed in third trimester. Clinically, it presents with mild frontotemporal recession or with diffuse thinning of hairs. Prognosis is good with spontaneous recovery in most of the patients but uncommonly complete recovery does not occur. Exact cause of these changes is unknown but high cortisol level inhibiting gonadotropins might play a role.

MISCELLANEOUS CAUSES AFFECTING HAIRS IN PREGNANCY

Nutritional Causes

Density and number of hairs in any individual directly correlate with nutritional status, hence a balanced amount of proteins, calories, trace elements, and vitamins is necessary to maintain the hair follicles.

Common nutritional deficiencies include iron, protein, vitamin B12, zinc, folic acid, omega-3 fatty acids, biotin (vitamin B7), and vitamin D.

Incidence of Various Pre-existing Diseases Affecting Hairs in Pregnancy

Incidence of female pattern hair loss decreases in pregnancy because of anagen phase prolongation under hormonal influence.

Incidence of seborrheic capitis in pregnancy is not well documented. In some patients, there is flare of seborrheic dermatitis while in other group there is improvement.

Hormonal changes during pregnancy can potentially exacerbate the condition due to increased sebum production and alteration of skin flora while immunosuppressive effects might cause improvement in some of the patients.

Incidence of autoimmune diseases like alopecia areata, lichen planopilaris, discoid lupus erythematosus, etc. decreases during pregnancy because of the immunosuppressive state of pregnancy and high cortisol levels. Exact incidence of various autoimmune diseases affecting hair in pregnancy is unknown. During pregnancy, the immune system is modulated to tolerate the fetus, which might explain why some women with preexisting alopecia areata experience an improvement in their condition during pregnancy. However, postpartum hormonal shifts and return to prepregnancy immune state can trigger a relapse or onset of diseases in some women.

Incidence of scalp infections/infestations during pregnancy increases during pregnancy because of immunosuppressive state and hormonal influence creating a favorable environment for organism to grow. With good scalp hygiene, there is no specific increase in the incidence of scalp infections/infestations.

SAFETY OF VARIOUS COSMECEUTICALS PRODUCTS TO BE USED IN HAIRS DURING PREGNANCY

Use of hair color during the pregnancy and its negative impact on fetus are often a cause of concern for the pregnant females. Various studies have proved that most of the chemicals are absorbed in a very less amount from the scalp skin, hence cannot reach systemic circulation causing any harm to a developing fetus.

There are five categories of hair dyes available in the market: (i) gradual hair coloring, (ii) vegetable dyes, (iii) temporary dyes, (iv) semipermanent dyes, and (v) permanent dyes. Hair chemicals have been used for various purposes like giving colors to hairs, for altering the natural shape of hair in the form of straightening or curling.

Common chemicals which are used in hair colors especially permanent hair colors include paraphenylenediamine (PPD), oleic acid, sodium hydroxide, ammonium hydroxide, propylene glycol, and isopropyl alcohol, resorcinol, Toluene-2,5-diamine sulfate, sodium sulfite, and 3-aminophenol.

Common chemicals used as hair straightening agents, hair relaxing, or bleaching agent include ammonium thioglycolate, ammonium hydroxide, sodium hydroxide, guanidine hydroxide, petroleum, and hydrogen peroxide.

There has been a concern with use of chemical hair dyes in pregnancy. Studies by Jiaang et al. have shown that there was increase in the incidence of low-birth weight babies in females who had exposure to hair dye while other studies have shown no risk to fetus with hair dye use. Most probable explanation is that hair dyes are absorbed in a very limited amount systematically, unless there is breach in the scalp skin in the form of burn or abscess. Therefore, risk of chemicals reaching the placenta and harming fetus is very unlikely.

A case–control study on 525 pregnant black women was conducted by Blackmore-Prince et al. who were using hair chemicals for straightening or curling of hairs. It was found that hair chemicals were safe with no increased risk of low-birth weight or preterm delivery.

Similarly, a case–control study on 5,944 black women was conducted by Rosenberg et al. who were using hair relaxers. It also found no increased risk of preterm deliveries in these women.

When considering safety of shampoos in pregnancy, it is important to look at the ingredients they contain and avoid those with potentially harmful chemicals.

The following is the list of safe ingredients which can be preferred in pregnancy:
- *Cocamidopropyl betaine*: Mild surfactant derived from coconut oil, often used in place of harsher sulfates
- *Decyl glucoside*: Plant-derived surfactant
- *Sodium cocoyl isethionate*: Source is coconut oil and acts as mild surfactant aloe vera plant-derived
- Glycerin
- Panthenol (vitamin B5)
- Shea butter
- Natural oils like Jojoba oil, coconut oil, and Argan oil

The following is the list of ingredients to be avoided in pregnancy:
- Sulfates (sodium lauryl sulfate, sodium laureth sulfate)
- Parabens (methylparaben and propylparaben)
- Phthalates
- Formaldehyde and formaldehyde-releasing agents like DMDM hydantoin
- Synthetic fragrances
- Triclosan

SUGGESTED READINGS

1. Ingber A. Obstetric Dermatology: A Practical Guide. New York City: Springer; 2009.
2. Lynfield YL. Effect of pregnancy on the human hair cycle. J Invest Dermatol. 1960;35:323-7.
3. Grymowicz M, Rudnicka E, Podfigurna A, Napierala P, Smolarczyk R, Smolarczyk K, et al. Hormonal Effects on Hair Follicles. Int J Mol Sci. 2020;21(15):5342.
4. Wong RC, Ellis CN. Physiologic skin changes in pregnancy. J Am Acad Dermatol 1984;10: 929-40.
5. Black M. Obstetric and Gynecologic Dermatology. London: Mosby; 2001.
6. Jiang C, Hou Q, Huang Y, Ye J, Qin X, Zhang Y, et al. The effect of pre-pregnancy hair dye exposure on infant birth weight: a nested case-control study. BMC Pregnancy Childbirth. 2018;18(1):144.
7. Thom E. Pregnancy and the hair growth cycle: anagen induction against hair growth disruption using Nourkrin® with Marilex®, a proteoglycan replacement therapy. J Cosmet Dermatol. 2017;16(3):421-7.

CHAPTER 20

Nail Disorders and Pregnancy

Vishal Pal, Chander Grover

INTRODUCTION

Pregnancy is a state of altered immunologic, metabolic, endocrine, and vascular changes that make the pregnant woman susceptible to physiologic and pathologic changes in the skin and its appendages, including nails. This chapter gives an insight into the various nail changes that occur during pregnancy **(Box 1)**. In order to understand these nail changes, it is pertinent to understand the nail growth dynamics and physiology of nail growth.

ANATOMY AND PHYSIOLOGY OF THE NAIL UNIT

The nail unit is a specialized keratinous appendage composed of the nail plate, nail folds (one proximal and two lateral), nail bed, eponychium (cuticle) and hyponychium. Nail plate is a hard, semitransparent, and slightly convex structure made of anucleated keratinocytes. Ventral surface of the nail plate has longitudinal ridges that correspond to reciprocal grooves in the nail bed, making the attachment firm. The dorsal surface is relatively smooth. The proximal nail fold is a double layer of skin that covers the proximal part of the nail and protects it from trauma, solvents, and infectious agents. The ventral layer of the proximal nail fold is a continuation of the nail matrix, also known as the dorsal matrix.

BOX 1 Nail changes during pregnancy.

- Increased growth rate of nail
- Increased nail plate thickness
- *Most common nail changes*: Leukonychia (true) and onychocryptosis
- *Well-documented nail changes*: Leukonychia, onychocryptosis, Beau's line, longitudinal melanonychia, koilonychia, and onychoschizia
- *Less frequent nail changes*: Subungual hyperkeratosis, distal onycholysis, and nail brittleness

Eponychium is a thin layer of cornified epithelium that adheres to the nail at the edge of the proximal nail fold, effectively sealing off this space. Any damage to the cuticle due to inflammation of the nail fold can also disturb the underlying matrix and alter nail plate production.

The nail plate rests upon the nail bed (75–85%) and nail matrix (15–25%). The half-moon-shaped lunula demarcates the abrupt junction between the nail matrix and bed. The nail bed has a peculiar arrangement of capillaries running longitudinally and arranged in rows. This rich vasculature explains the pink appearance of the nail plate. The direction of nail growth is guided by multiple factors, including the underlying bone (phalanx) and the shape of the nail folds. The lateral nail folds contain the nail plate from both sides, contributing to its transverse curvature. The shape of proximal nail fold and arrangement of matrix rete ridges leads to the emerging nail grow obliquely from its point of origin.

The nail plate consists of "hard" hair-type keratins embedded in a matrix of sulfur-rich, high-cysteine, and high-glycine/tyrosine proteins. The growth rate of fingernails is physiologically faster than that of the toenail. The average growth rate of fingernails is 0.1 mm/day and toenails is 0.03 mm/day. Numerous factors including age, sex, and disease states affect the rate of growth of nails.

STRUCTURAL NAIL CHANGES IN PREGNANCY

Broadly, pregnancy is associated with thicker and healthier looking nails. However, some specific structural nail changes which alter the formation of nail are seen in pregnancy. These are summarized as follows:

- *Nail growth rate*: Earlier studies had reported the growth rate of nails to be faster in pregnant women. This was explained on the basis of increased estrogen and progesterone levels associated with pregnancy. These hormones increase the vascular endothelial growth factor (VEGF) synthesis that promotes vascularization. Increased VEGF then leads to an increase in peripheral blood flow that appears to stimulate a faster nail growth rate. However, a recent study using advanced nail growth measurement with a digital caliper (accuracy of 0.01 mm) concluded that pregnancy is not significantly associated with a faster growth rate of nails.
- *Nail plate thickness*: The nail plate thickness has been reported to be more in pregnant females, again attributable to increased levels of estrogen and progesterone.
- *Other structural changes*: Ponnapula et al. carried out an evaluation of nail changes in the lower extremity during pregnancy. They found coarsening of the nail texture and lamellar peeling from the free edge of the nail as common findings.

MORPHOLOGICAL NAIL CHANGES IN PREGNANCY

Changes in nail morphology have been reported to be more common in pregnancy, with a prevalence of up to 62.8% in pregnant females. The most common nail findings in pregnant women are leukonychia and onychocryptosis **(Box 1)**.

- *Leukonychia*: Pregnancy has been associated with true leukonychia **(Figs. 1 and 2)**. A study by Erpolat on 312 pregnant females found that almost two-thirds of patients had nail changes. Leukonychia was the most common nail alteration affecting up to one-fourth of the patients. Another study from Lahore also reported leukonychia to be the most common nail change in pregnant females, seen in up to 15% of women. Among the three types of leukonychia (true, apparent, and pseudoleukonychia); true leukonychia is characterized by abnormal nail matrix keratinization. Possible cause could be elevated estrogen levels in pregnancy, with an increased blood flow, causing matrix dysfunction and delayed keratin maturation with keratohyalin granule retention.

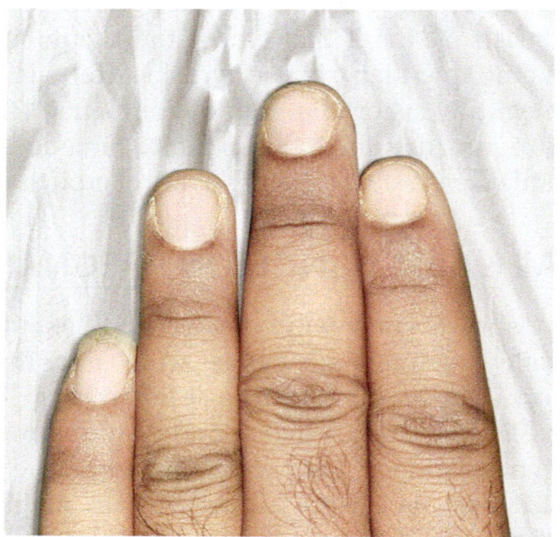

FIG. 1: Punctate leukonychia involving the ring fingernail in a 24-year-old pregnant lady.

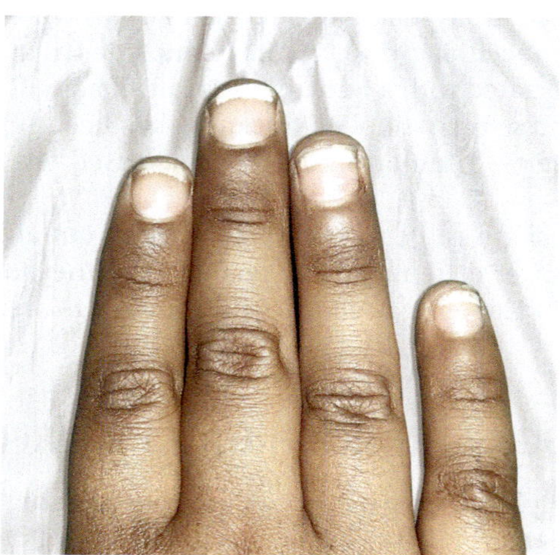

FIG. 2: Transverse leukonychia involving multiple fingernails.

- *Onychocryptosis (ingrown toenail)*: Ingrown toenail has been observed in up to 12.3% of pregnant women **(Figs. 3 and 4)**. During pregnancy, the mechanical pressure from excessive pedal edema has been implicated as a causative factor causing a higher incidence of ingrown toenail. This is further compounded by ill-fitting footwear. In these cases, patients should be advised regarding wearing appropriate sized shoes, and avoiding ill-fitting or tight shoes. Nails should be properly trimmed, cutting straight across rather than in a curved fashion.
- *Beau's lines*: These are transverse grooves in the nail plate, running parallel to the lunula **(Fig. 5)**. They are caused by an insult to the nail matrix which leads to temporary impairment of nail plate formation. Matushansky et al.

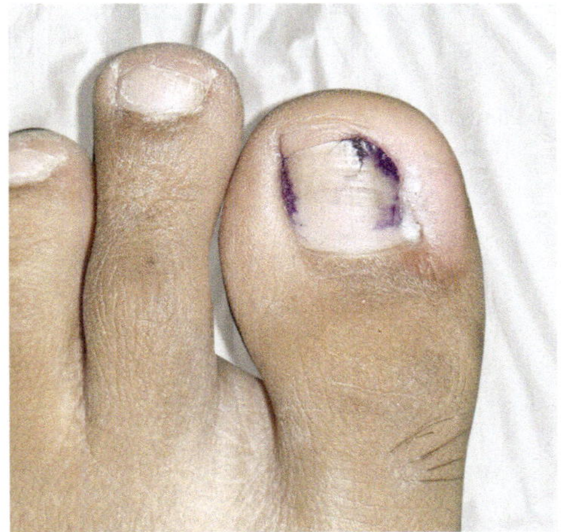

FIG. 3: Ingrown nail with inflammation in the posterior part of lateral nail fold.

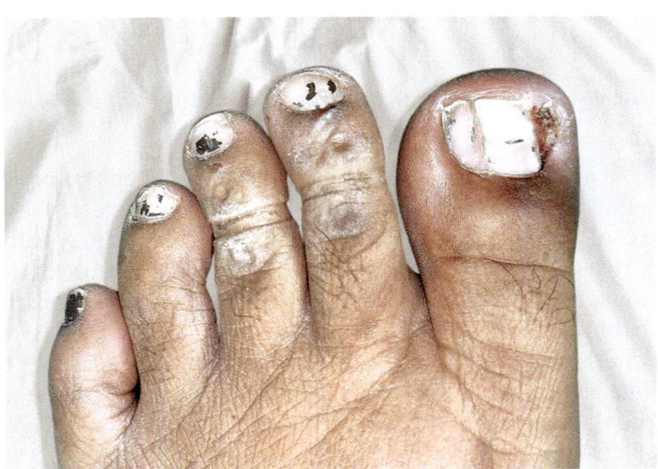

FIG. 4: Ingrown nail with extensive granulation tissue.

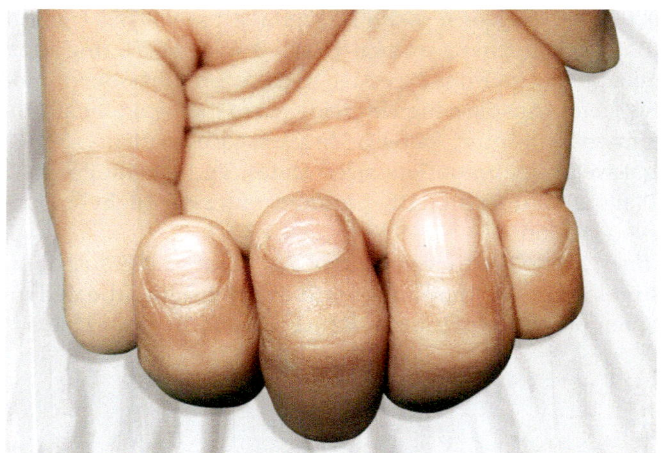

FIG. 5: Beau's lines involving the medial two fingernails.

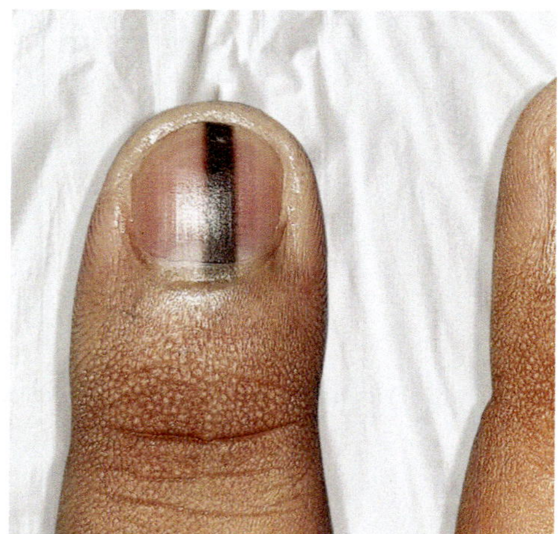

FIG. 6: A preexisting longitudinal pigmented band becoming darker and thicker with pregnancy.

reported that 8.2% of pregnant women developed Beau's line; whereas an Indian study reported Beau's line in 15% of pregnant females. These lines may develop even after delivery as it is a stressful event which may halt nail matrix activity. Measuring the distance of Beau's line from the proximal nail plate and dividing by the growth rate of the nail can tell us the approximate time of nail matrix insult.

- *Longitudinal melanonychia (LM)*: Melanonychia is a result of melanin deposition within the nail matrix. LM is characterized by the presence of longitudinal, demarcated pigmented bands on the nail unit **(Fig. 6)**. Studies by Erpolat, Matushansky and Sharma et al. reported LM in 3.2%, 8.2%, and 8% of pregnant women respectively. LM can present before, during, and after pregnancy. In women with LM, the number of streaks or width of the bands tends to increase with pregnancy. This is due to the effect of pregnancy-related hormones, especially estrogen, causing its progression. LM may also spontaneously regress or gradually disappear postpartum, due to a decrease in the hormone levels. In patients with multiple nails involved, LM is generally benign. In patients with single nail involvement, where a positive Hutchinson's sign is seen (spread of pigment into the skin and soft tissue surrounding the nail plate), further evaluation is warranted irrespective of the stage of pregnancy, as the sign is considered almost pathognomonic of subungual melanoma.

- *Koilonychia (spoon nails)*: Koilonychia is classically seen in iron deficiency anemia **(Fig. 7)**. Pregnancy is a state of increased nutritional requirements and iron deficiency is common in pregnant females. Erpolat et al. reported koilonychia in 1.9% of pregnant females, though a higher incidence (8.5%) was reported from Pakistan.
- *Onychoschizia*: It is characterized by the splitting of the distal nail plate into layers at the free edge. Onychoschizia is considered a manifestation of increased brittleness of nails. It is seen in up to 10% of pregnant females. Increased growth rate and softening of nails during pregnancy are responsible for onychoschizia.
- *Other nail changes*: Subungual hyperkeratosis, distal onycholysis, and nail brittleness may be seen in pregnant females. However, these changes are less frequent and any increased incidence over nonpregnant females is inconclusive. These changes may appear during the first trimester with onycholysis being reported in up to 4.5%, brittle nails in up to 8%, and subungual hyperkeratosis in up to 6.5% of pregnant females. However, a questionnaire based survey of 73 pregnant females found that 86% had no changes with respect to nail brittleness, while 13.7% had decreased nail brittleness (less breakage) during pregnancy. Nail brittleness may occur due to acceleration in nail growth and softening of the nail plate during pregnancy. The presence of these changes should also prompt exclusion of other causes including

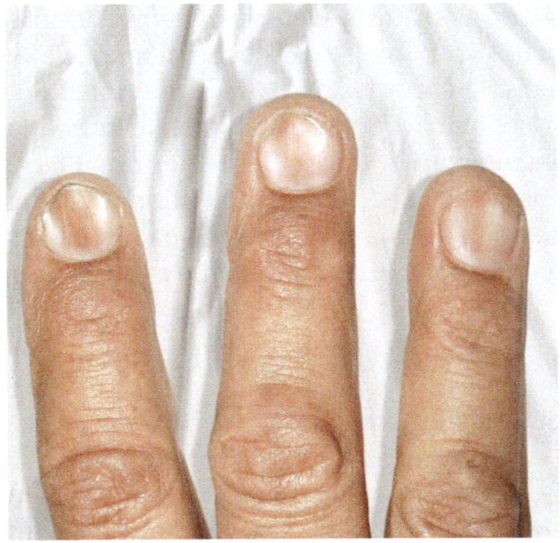

FIG. 7: Severe koilonychia or spoon-shaped nails with pre-existing LM in a pregnant patient with severe anemia.

psoriasis, lichen planus, and onychomycosis. Chromonychia, nail pitting, and splinter hemorrhage have also been reported in pregnant females. However, these findings were reported as incidental and statistically not significant in one out of 92 pregnant females.

NAIL AS A TOOL TO MEASURE HORMONE LEVELS

The nail acts as a true window to systemic disease, by not just showing morphological changes, but also reflecting the systemic milieu. Nail clippings are a noninvasive way of monitoring levels of many metabolites in the body, thus facilitating their easier detection. A study measured nail cortisol levels in 30 healthy women during pregnancy and 12 months postpartum. It was observed that cortisol levels in fingernail clippings were elevated around childbirth and peak levels were detected at 2 months postpartum. The authors also found variations in fingernail cortisol levels with parity. Primiparas exhibited higher fingernail cortisol levels after childbirth. This study highlighted that nail cortisol levels might be a useful tool for monitoring cortisol variations in pregnant women, and also act as a retrospective index of hormone production.

OCCUPATIONAL HAZARDS IN PREGNANCY

Nail grooming and aesthetics is a multibillion dollar industry. It is already immensely popular in the west and picking up in the developing countries as well. Nail technicians or nail salon workers are exposed to various nail care products that often contain ingredients such as toluene, formaldehyde, acetone, acetonitrile, ethyl and methyl methacrylate, phthalates, and other substances. These are not only hazardous to the health of the workers and users, but also have a detrimental effect on pregnancy. Nail changes known in this population occur due to prolonged exposure to the chemicals, and include chronic paronychia, allergic contact dermatitis, Beau's lines, and brittle nails. Additionally, they are known to be associated with birth defects. A population-based study found that offspring of females working as nail technicians have an increased risk of congenital heart defects (Odds ratio: 2.7–3.5) and neural tube defects (Odds ratio: 2.6). It is strongly advised that worker should wash their hand with a moisturizer-based sanitizer, apply moisturizer before and after providing services to clients, use sterile instruments, and seek medical attention at the earliest. No specific regulatory advice related to pregnancy; however, could be found. However, it can be safely assumed that the precautions should be adhered to strictly.

NAIL PROCEDURES DURING PREGNANCY

It is suggested that nail-related procedures are better avoided during pregnancy as most nail changes are transient. As discussed earlier, these changes may arise due to changes in posture, increased weight, or hormonal impact on nail thickness and growth. However, higher severity grades of onychocryptosis may necessitate surgical intervention. Though there is no absolute contraindication to performing nail surgery during pregnancy, it is advisable to avoid surgical interventions during the first and third trimesters. Use of phenol should be absolutely avoided during chemical matricectomy. This precaution is advisable both for the patient as well as the operator.

DRUG SAFETY DURING PREGNANCY

Among the various therapeutic agents required for management of nail disorders during pregnancy, the safety should be particularly weighed and drug safety recommendations should be followed. The Pregnancy safety categories assigned to the drugs for various nail related complaints, likely to be used during pregnancy, are summarized in **Table 1**.

TABLE 1: Pregnancy category recommendations for drug safety.

Drug category	Drug name	Pregnancy category*
Anesthetic agents	Lignocaine	B
	Bupivacaine	C
Topical drugs		
Anti-inflammatory	Corticosteroids	C
	Tacrolimus and pimecrolimus	C
	Calcipotriol	C
	Coal tar	C
	Tazarotene	X
Antifungals	Ciclopirox olamine 8% nail lacquer	B
	Efinaconazole 10% lotion	C
	Amorolfine 5% nail lacquer	C
Antibiotics	Mupirocin	B
	Clindamycin	B
	Neomycin	B
Systemic drugs		
Antifungals	Terbinafine	B
	Itraconazole	C
	Fluconazole	C
	Griseofulvin	C
Anti-inflammatory	Corticosteroids	C
	Acitretin	X
	Methotrexate	X
	Azathioprine	D
	Apremilast	C
	Secukinumab	B
	Tofacitinib	C
	Anti-tumor necrosis factor (TNF)-α inhibitors	B

Continued

Continued

Drug category	Drug name	Pregnancy category*
Antipruritics	Chlorpheniramine	B
	Hydroxyzine	C
	Cetirizine	B
	Fexofenadine	C
	Loratadine	B
Antibiotics	Penicillin	B
	Tetracycline	D
	Cephalosporins	B
	Aminoglycosides	D
	Fluoroquinolones	C
	Sulfonamides	C

*Pregnancy category—A: No risk in human studies; B: No risk in animal studies; C: Risk cannot be ruled out; D: Evidence of risk; X: Contraindicated.

NAIL CARE DURING PREGNANCY

As can be seen, nail changes during pregnancy are mostly minor and can be minimized by taking adequate care during pregnancy. **Box 2** summarizes the precautions or instructions which can be shared with pregnant females to ensure good nail health during this crucial period.

BOX 2 Nail care instructions during pregnancy.

- Keep nails clean and apply moisturizer daily
- Keep nails short. Soaking for 10–20 minutes before cutting helps prevent onychoschizia
- Avoid tight-fitting shoes and cone heeled sandals
- Avoid nail products which contain formaldehyde, toluene, dibutylphenol, xylene, ethyl tosylamide, triphenyl phosphate, and acetone
- Manicure and pedicure may be performed but should be done by professional using sterile instruments
- Avoid pushing back of cuticle or trimming

CONCLUSION

Nail changes in pregnancy have not been studied in much detail or very systematically. Most of the nail changes in pregnant females are transient and do not require any treatment. However, these changes may cause cosmetic concerns and psychosocial impact. Clinicians should be aware regarding the spectrum of nail changes, and their progression. Reassurance, promotion of good nail care and avoiding application of nail sensitizers needs to be advised. Onychocryptosis may be transient and wearing appropriate footwear and proper cutting of nails can help. Further controlled studies involving larger number of pregnant ladies are required to give us in-depth knowledge about these changes.

KEY POINTS

- Pregnancy is associated with an increased growth rate as well as thickness of the nail plate.
- Majority of the nail changes associated with pregnancy are transient and resolve spontaneously during postpartum period, not requiring any treatment.
- Leukonychia and onychocryptosis are the most common nail changes associated with pregnancy.

SUGGESTED READINGS

1. Matushansky J, Wang Y, Chang MJ, Thomas C, Hockstein S, Lipner SR. Nail Changes during Pregnancy: A Cross-sectional Survey of Patients at an Academic Center. Skin Appendage Disord. 2023;9(1):27-9.
2. Erpolat S, Eser A, Kaygusuz I, Balci H, Kosus A, Kosus N. Nail alterations during pregnancy: a clinical study. Int J Dermatol. 2016;55(10):1172-5.
3. Siegel MR, Rocheleau CM, Broadwater K, Santiago-Colón A, Johnson CY, Herdt ML, et al; National Birth Defects Prevention Study. Maternal occupation as a nail technician or hairdresser during pregnancy and birth defects, National Birth Defects Prevention Study, 1997-2011. Occup Environ Med. 2022;79(1):17-23.
4. Reilly IN, Ousey J, Blandford T. (2022). A literature review of the use of phenol for nail matrix ablation on pregnant and breastfeeding patients: implications for safe use. [online] Available from https://internationalfootankle.org/journal/index.php/JIFAF/article/view/25. [Last accessed January, 2025].
5. Izawa S, Kawasaki M, Sugaya N, Nomura S. Time-course changes in fingernail cortisol levels during pregnancy and postpartum. Sci Rep. 2024;14:1145.
6. Tyagi M, Singal A. Nail cosmetics: What a dermatologist should know! Indian J Dermatol Venereol Leprol. 2024;90:178-85.
7. Ikram S, Malik A, Suhail M. Physiological skin changes during pregnancy. J Pak Assoc Dermatol. 2018;28(2):219-23.
8. Ohta R. Deformed nail from stress related to childbearing. J Gen Fam Med. 2019;21(1):29.

CHAPTER 21

Genodermatoses and Pregnancy

Vishal Pal, Deepika Pandhi

INTRODUCTION

Genodermatoses are hereditary conditions characterized by genetically mediated abnormalities affecting the skin and its appendages. More than 500 distinct Mendelian skin disorders were reported in Online Mendelian Inheritance in Man (OMIM) database. Genodermatoses are broadly divided into (1) single gene disorders (also known as monogenic or Mendelian traits); (2) chromosomal disorders; and (3) complex traits.

EPIDEMIOLOGY

True incidence and prevalence of genodermatoses are difficult to estimate because of rarity of the diseases. However, multiple studies in hospital-based setting have been conducted giving a rough estimate of how prevalent these diseases are in the population. An Indian study conducted by Puttur et al. over a period of 1 year found a total of 105 cases of genodermatoses including neurofibromatosis (NF)—18, tuberous sclerosis complex (TSC)—12, ichthyosis vulgaris—9, ectodermal dysplasia—7, lamellar ichthyosis and Darier's disease—5 each, and congenital ichthyosiform erythroderma—4. They also reported cases of inherited hair disorder, inherited immunodeficiencies, metabolic disorders, and disorder of pigmentation. Another study by Sameen et al. in a Muslim majority population over a period of 2 years included 128 cases of genodermatoses, with the most common diseases being ichthyosis vulgaris—16, Lamellar ichthyosis—8, focal palmoplantar keratoderma (PPK)—7, TSC—6, NF—5, xeroderma pigmentosa (XP)—4, and porphyria [congenital erythropoietic porphyria (CEP) and erythropoietic protoporphyria (EPP)]—5. A retrospective study by Velázquez-Ávila et al. from Cuba conducted over 40 years, found the prevalence of genodermatoses was 46.51 per 1 lakh population. The highest incidence and prevalence were of neurofibromatosis type 1 (NF1), classical Ehlers-Danlos syndrome, and Ichthyosis vulgaris. Another nationwide study from Sweden by Zagoras et al. found that the most common disease to be: Ichthyoses (25%), porokeratosis

(17%), PPK (13%), epidermolysis bullosa (EB) group (7%); Darier's disease (6%), Hailey–Hailey disease (4%) and Gorlin syndrome (3%). Explaining each and individual genodermatoses is beyond the scope of this chapter therefore, we are describing the common genodermatoses and their effect on pregnancy **(Table 1)**.

PRENATAL DIAGNOSIS

As early as 1956, Fuchs and Rils analyzed fetal cells from amniotic fluid to determine the fetal gender, therefore paving the way for the prenatal diagnosis of hereditary condition. The first prenatal test was performed on fetal skin biopsy in 1980 and was examined by light microscopy and transmission electron microscope. Bullous congenital ichthyosiform erythroderma and junctional EB were the first conditions successfully diagnosed using this technique. The essence of prenatal diagnosis is to detect or exclusion of an inherited condition or congenital defect in utero. The prenatal diagnosis helps the parent at risk of having an affected child to opt for an abortion or to continue the pregnancy and to help them to prepare psychological as well as financially. Prenatal diagnosis also anticipates the medical problem that can occur during pregnancy and delivery and prepare the obstetrician accordingly **(Boxes 1 and 2)**.

Indication for prenatal diagnosis includes:
- If parents are affected or a known carrier of genetic disease
- If there is a history of previous affected pregnancy
- If there is a family history of inherited skin disorder

Prenatal diagnosis tests are broadly divided into two types.

Invasive Prenatal Diagnosis Technique

Fetal Skin Biopsy

The first test for the prenatal diagnosis was performed in 1980s. It is an invasive test done under ultrasound guidance and fetal skin tissue of 1–2 mm is removed using the biopsy forceps. The commonly used sites are back, buttocks, and chest. It is commonly performed at 15–22 weeks of gestation after the morphological and biochemical development of fetal skin. However, the exact timing of doing this test depends on the particular skin disease **(Table 2)**. It is useful when causative gene is unknown or specific mutation is not identified in causative gene or equivocal/unsatisfactory results of deoxyribonucleic acid (DNA)-based tests have been obtained. The major drawback is the timing of the test and long waiting period of the test result. Further, if the result confirms the presence of genetic abnormalities then terminating pregnancy is challenging. It is associated with 1–3% risk of fetal loss. Other complications are amniotic fluid leakage and fetal scarring.

Amniocentesis

It is a DNA-based prenatal diagnosis test uses fetal cell for analysis of any genetic or structural abnormalities. It is suggested when there is a family member who is affected or a previously impacted offspring. Parental and affected member DNA samples are necessary to detect the pathogenic mutation and rule out

TABLE 1: Common genodermatoses and their effect on pregnancy.

Disease	Preconception	Antenatal	Intrapartum	Postpartum
Neurofibromatosis type 1 (NF1) (OMIM-162200)	Assess for hypertension, precocious puberty, developmental delay, learning disabilities, seizure, and scoliosis	• Spontaneous abortion, cerebrovascular complications, preeclampsia, placental abruption, fetal growth restriction, and preterm labor can occur • Cutaneous NF may increase in size, malignant transformation and recur in subsequent pregnancy	• Vaginal delivery—safe and preferred • Patient at increased risk for cesarean delivery due to fetal malpresentation and obstructing pelvic neurofibromas • Kyphoscoliosis may present a technical challenge for spinal anesthesia for labor and delivery	New-onset neurofibromas may regress. Breastfeeding should not be withheld and be encouraged. Increased rates of postpartum depression
Neurofibromatosis type 2 (NF2) (OMIM-101000)	• Dermatological, ophthalmological, and neurological examination • Auditory testing • MRI brain	Meningiomas and vestibular schwannomas may grow and symptomatically worsen significantly in the third trimester and may cause increased intracranial pressure (ICP) and obstructive hydrocephalus if large enough	Cesarean section does not prevent neurologic event with known intracranial or spinal cord pathology. However, delivery using epidural anesthesia, delayed pushing, and assisted second stage should be advised to minimize the use of Valsalva maneuver. These efforts blunt physiologic hemodynamic changes and prevent increase in intracranial pressure	Same as NF1. Breastfeeding should not be withheld and be encouraged. Increased rates of postpartum depression and suicide
Tuberous sclerosis complex (TSC) (OMIM TSC1-191100 TSC2-613254)	Assessment for hypertension, renal function, MRI brain and spine	Renal angiomyolipoma (AML) can present as retroperitoneal hemorrhage associated with either growth or rupture. Acute renal failure, new or worsening of lung, lymphangioleiomyomatosis can cause respiratory symptom. Preterm labor, preeclampsia, amniotic fluid abnormalities, fetal growth restriction, and placental abruption more common in patient with TSC-associated renal disease	Patient with renal AMLs may be at increased risk of bleeding therefore, cesarean delivery should be preferred	Vigilant monitoring for postpartum depression and psychosis as patients are at a high risk for worsening of mental health. Everolimus can be given in patient who is breast feeding. Rhabdomyomas can be seen in fetus leading to dysrhythmias and hydrops

Continued

Continued

Disease	Preconception	Antenatal	Intrapartum	Postpartum
Von Hippel–Lindau syndrome (OMIM-193300)	• Neurology, ophthalmology, and urological examination • Surgical removal of pheochromocytomas should be performed before conception	• Hemangioma can increase in size • If blood pressure (BP) is elevated, evaluate for an adrenal mass • Patient presents with headache, sweating, tachycardia, and paroxysmal hypertension • Perform plasma or a 24-hour urine collection for metanephrine and catecholamines • If abnormal values are detected, an MRI is recommended	Vaginal delivery can be done as cesarean section does not prevent neurologic event with known intracranial or spinal cord pathology	Patient has increased risk of anxiety and depression. Therefore, close postpartum monitoring and support is advised to tackle the depression
Sturge–Weber syndrome (OMIM-185300)	Achieve seizure control on a stable medication regimen Start high-dose folic acid supplementation regardless of anticonvulsant use	Monitor patient for gestational hypertension, continue antiepileptics, and add aspirin for prevention of strokes and seizures	Not a contraindication for vaginal delivery	High risk for worsening of mental health as incidence of psychiatric morbidity is up to 50%
Epidermolysis bullosa (EB) (OMIM-131900)	Antisecretory/mucosal protectant prophylaxis is required	Lubricant or emollient should be applied to gloves and the patient's skin before examination, measuring BP, use of cuffs or tourniquets and while doing ultrasonography (USG). Nonadhesive tape should be used and padding applied under BP cuffs or tourniquets	Vaginal birth should be the preferred mode of delivery for women with all EB subtypes as vaginal birth does not appear to increase the risk of subsequent vaginal scarring or stenosis. Avoid vaginal birth if there are extensive EB-related genital blistering/wounds, or vaginal stenosis, avoid prolonged pressure/immobility and back rubbing	Breastfeeding should be promoted. Physician should assist the mother with positioning of the baby and adequate latching on to the areola, which may reduce subsequent blistering. Lubricated nipple shields may be useful

Continued

Continued

Disease	Preconception	Antenatal	Intrapartum	Postpartum
Klippel–Trénaunay syndrome (KTS) (OMIM-149000)	• Capillary malformations, venous malformations or varicose veins, and hypertrophy of bone and soft tissue • Two of the above three features need to be present	• Increased venous stasis, stroke volume, and lower extremity edema exacerbate KTS manifestations • Increased risk of thrombophlebitis, ulceration, cellulitis, and pulmonary embolism • Abdominal varices have to be looked into • Rule out anemia and coagulation abnormality	If varices of external genitalia then cesarean needs to be done	Increased risk of thromboembolism
Hereditary hemorrhagic telangiectasia (OMIM-187300)	Multiple arteriovenous malformations	• Increased episodes of nasal bleeds • Development of new mucocutaneous telangiectasia • Increased risk of bleeding from pulmonary arteriovenous malformations (AVMs) and right to left shunt • Screening for pulmonary, cerebral and spinal AVM should be done	• Increased risk of rupture of cerebral AVM • Spinal AVM if not excluded local anesthesia to be avoided • A course of antibiotics to be given prophylactically • Prolonged second stage of labor to be avoided	
Pseudoxanthoma elasticum (OMIM-264800)	Ocular, cardiovascular, and cutaneous examination	• Continue monitoring for cardiac and renal function, BP, changes in the retina, and any signs or symptoms suggestive of gastrointestinal bleeding • Initiate adequate medicine for the control of BP because it reduces the risk of bleeding	Vaginal delivery is not contraindicated. Epidural anesthesia is recommended because it induces relative hypotension, thereby decreasing the risk of cerebral bleeding, facilitates instrumental delivery, allowing a shorter second stage and thus decreasing pushing	

Continued

Continued

Disease	Preconception	Antenatal	Intrapartum	Postpartum
Marfan syndrome (OMIM-154700)	• Cardiovascular examination by transthoracic and transesophageal echocardiogram or by CT or MRI for assessment of both the ascending as well as the descending aorta • Patient should go undergo aortic root replacement prior to pregnancy • Prophylactic use of β-blockers • BP should be controlled	• Marfan syndrome with no dilation of the aorta • Monthly echocardiographic evaluation for the size of the aorta each trimester and prior to delivery • Aortic root dilatation (>4.0 cm), progressive dilatation during pregnancy or a history of surgery for aortic dilatation or dissection prior to pregnancy • Echocardiographic examination every 4–6 weeks	• No cardiovascular involvement or stable minimal aortic dilatation (4.0 cm) • Vaginal delivery • Epidural anesthesia to minimize pain and keep BP under check • Forceps or vacuum to shorten the second stage of labor • C-section for obstetrical indications, with aortic dilatation 4.0 cm or with progressive dilatation of aorta during pregnancy	• Continue monitoring for aortic dissection • There are 50% chances that the child will also have Marfan syndrome
Ehlers–Danlos syndrome type 4 (OMIM-130500)	Increased mobility of joints		• Uterine rupture or vasculature rupture • Preterm rupture of membrane	• Postpartum bleeding • Delayed wound healing

BOX 1 Point to be noted while doing genetic counseling.

- The parents are advised about:
    - Course, treatment, and prognosis of the genetically inherited disease present in the family
    - Risk of inheritance of that disease during each pregnancy
    - Methods to have a normal child
- Physician should estimate the risk of a fetus being affected by a genetic disease
- Proper consent should be taken from the parents before doing investigation
- Counseling should be nondirective and counselor should facilitate informed decision-making
- Parents should also be counseled about the terminating the pregnancy if the test results are positive for a genetic disease

BOX 2 General recommendations for pregnancy care for patients with neurocutaneous disorders.

- Early establishment of multidisciplinary care
- Discussion of preimplantation genetic testing for monogenic disorder and antenatal diagnosis
- Consider central nervous system (CNS) imaging and fetal ultrasonography (USG) for structural abnormality
- Individual obstetrician should carefully consider the specific needs of their patients and individualized intra- and postpartum care
- Contraceptive counseling for patients to facilitate careful planning of future pregnancies

TABLE 2: Period of gestation at which fetal skin biopsy should be performed.

Disease	Timing of fetal skin biopsy
Epidermolysis bullosa	16–17 weeks
Albinism	18–20 weeks
X-linked hypohidrotic ectodermal dysplasia	20 weeks
Lamellar ichthyosis, and Sjögren–Larsson syndrome	20–22 week
Harlequin ichthyosis	22 weeks

circumstances such as de novo mutations, uniparental disomy, and germline mosaicism. It is performed at 15–20 weeks of gestation. Under ultrasound guidance, a needle is inserted transabdominally through uterus and 15 mL of amniotic fluid is aspirated which contains fetal cells. Risk of fetal loss is 0.5%.

Chorionic Villi Sample

Similar to amniocentesis, it is also DNA-based prenatal diagnosis test uses fetal cell. Under the guidance of USG sample of the placental tissue is obtained either transcervically or transabdominally. It is performed in the 11–12th week of pregnancy. The risk of fetal loss is 1% and it may be associated with cramping, vaginal bleeding, infection, and amniotic fluid leakage. Transcervical chorionic villi sampling is associated with increases incidence of infantile hemangiomas, that too threefold higher than following amniocentesis.

Preimplantation Genetic Diagnosis

This is an alternative to postconception diagnostic procedure in which embryo obtained after in vitro fertilization (IVF) are tested for the genetic disorder before implantation, thereby ensuring only embryos free of the disorder are placed in the uterus. This obviates the necessity of terminating a pregnancy, as abortion may be seen ethically reprehensible and linked to substantial psychological and physical illness. This procedure is advantageous for patients who are at risk of passing on a serious genetic condition to their children. DNA can be acquired during three specific stages of embryonic development: Polar body biopsy, day 3 cleavage stage biopsy of a single blastomere, and day 5 blastocyst stage trophectoderm biopsy. In instances of maternal inheritance, it is possible to biopsy the polar body, which contains a set of 23 maternal chromosomes. The risk of incorrectly transferring an afflicted fetus that is classified as normal is roughly 2% for autosomal recessive disorders and 11% for autosomal dominant disorders. Limitations encompass the excessive expense of the operation, restricted availability, misdiagnosis, and lower pregnancy rates. Even after the confirmation of pregnancy, numerous people still need to undergo further prenatal tests. Approximately 50% of patients who had clinical pregnancies following pre-implantation genetic diagnosis underwent an amniocentesis, according to a comprehensive study conducted by Gutierrez-Mateo et al.

Noninvasive Prenatal Diagnosis Technique

Fetal Cell in Maternal Circulation

Nucleated fetal cells were isolated from maternal circulation in 1960s. Various types of fetal cells have been separated from the mother's bloodstream, such as nucleated red blood cells, trophoblasts, mesenchymal stem cells, and hematopoietic stem cells that express the CD34 antigen. According to a study conducted by Krabchi K et al., it was estimated that there are only two to six fetal cells per milliliter of maternal blood between the 18 and 22nd week of pregnancy, making them extremely uncommon. Furthermore, the ultimate level of purity of fetal cells is typically diminished due to frequent contamination with maternal cells.

Fetal DNA and Messenger Ribonucleic Acid (mRNA) in Maternal Blood

Presence of male fetal DNA in maternal plasma was first described by Lo et al. in 1977 using polymerase chain reaction (PCR) amplification of Y-specific sequences in the circulation of women carrying male fetuses. Maternal blood was found to contain fetal mRNA 3 years later. Cell-free fetal DNA (cffDNA) primarily originates from the placenta, with a lesser portion potentially coming from hematopoietic stem cells and direct transfer between the fetus and the mother. Fetal DNA comprises around 3% of the overall DNA found in maternal plasma and is composed of small pieces, each measuring <200 base pairs. The optimal timeframe to do this test is between 4 and 10 weeks. The challenges in this context involve isolating the genome of the fetus from the interfering background of maternal DNA. Additionally, the presence of maternal DNA can obscure the identification of the maternal allele in the cffDNA, making it challenging to distinguish between an individual who carries both affected

TABLE 3: Role of ultrasonography (USG) in genodermatoses.

Disease	USG findings
Epidermolysis bullosa	Presence of pyloric atresia, ureteral stenosis, arthrogryposis, and nose or ear deformities and snowflake sign in the amniotic cavity of fetal skin sloughing in junctional epidermolysis bullosa (JEB) with pyloric atresia
Harlequin ichthyosis	Echogenic amniotic fluid, large joint contractures, digital contractures, and facial dysmorphism such as flat face and wide mouth with thickened lips
Noonan syndrome	Short stature, congenital heart defects, and webbed neck with characteristic faces
Tuberous sclerosis complex	Cardiac rhabdomyomas is the earliest and most common (66%) marker

and unaffected alleles from the father, and an individual who only carries the unaffected paternal allele.

Mid-trimester Maternal Serum Screening

It is often indicated for screening of the neural tube defects, trisomy 21, and trisomy 18 during the second trimester of pregnancy but it may also be useful for the identification of X-linked ichthyosis. This test is performed in 15–20 weeks of gestation. It is available either as triple (alpha-fetoprotein, human gonadotropin, and unconjugated estriol) or quad screen (addition of inhibin A). Steroid sulfatase deficiency is the most common cause for very low levels of unconjugated estradiol seen in X-linked ichthyosis. This occurs due to defective steroidogenesis due to deficiency of steroid sulfatase in the placenta. If the diagnosis of X-linked ichthyosis is suspected from screening of an abnormal maternal serum, further prenatal testing via amniocentesis or chorionic villus sampling is warranted.

Ultrasonography

USG cannot detect morphological abnormalities associated with the fetal skin disease as these are microscopic hence it has no direct role in prenatal diagnosis. It can visualize better fetal details after 18–20 weeks and it is useful in detecting abnormalities in the absence of any given family history **(Table 3)**.

BIOCHEMICAL DIAGNOSIS OF GENODERMATOSES

Over the past two decades, tools for the genomic diagnosis have evolved rapidly, resulting in incredibly improved diagnostic rates. Genetic testing laboratories have progressed from using Sanger sequencing and karyotype analysis to employing next-generation sequencing (NGS)-based tests and chromosomal microarrays. Biochemical tests are divided into two major types; cytogenetics and molecular genetics.

Cytogenetics (Karyotyping)

It is the detection of the number and composition of metaphase chromosomes based on the examination in light microscope. This is the first test if we are suspecting patients with a suspecting aneuploidy (trisomy's or sex chromosome aneuploidy) or family history of a rearrangement (translocation or inversion). Limitation of this test is failure to detect large structural change <5 Mb.

Molecular Genetics

It emerged in the late 1980s with the advancement of fluorescence in situ hybridization (FISH). The capacity to identify the presence or absence of distinct sections of DNA creates ambiguity between cytogenetic and molecular (DNA-based) genetic testing. It can also detect structural changes between 50 kb and 1 Mb. Various tests of molecular genetics are:

- *Chromosomal microarray analysis (CMA)*:
  - Single-nucleotide polymorphisms (SNPs) arrays: SNPs are variations in DNA that commonly occur in normal populations. SNP probes can identify differences in the allele ratio, facilitating the detection of low-level mosaicism. SNP array can detect a changes range between 10 and 100 kb. They are best utilized for identification of regions of homozygosity and low-level mosaicism.
  - *Array comparative genomic hybridization (aCGH)*: aCGH is useful for gene-level copy number variants (CNVs). aCGH uses larger oligonucleotide probes as compared to SNP, therefore, capable of capturing any unique sequence in the genome.

  The major drawback of CMA is its inability to detect inversions, insertions, or balanced translocations because there is no net loss in material and no visualization of chromosomes.
- *Multiple ligation-dependent probe amplification (MLPA)*: It is a semiquantitative technique. In MLPA sequence-specific probe pairs are hybridized to the target region of DNA, ligated, and amplified. This makes a stuffer sequence of a specific length for each target region allowing identification of the multiplexed targets. Commercial kits are available.
- *Sanger sequencing*: Considered the "gold standard" for sequence determination. It can detect even a change of single blood pressure (BP). However, its unable to detect deletion, duplication, or structural genome rearrangements.
- *NGS panels*: NGS provides the capability to identify and analyze both sequence variants and structural variants, such as deletions, duplications, inversions, translocations, and other genetic abnormalities.
- *Targeted gene panels*: Perform genetic profiling on a select set of genes to identify any genetic variations that may increase the risk or cause diseases. Targeted panels typically examine a range of 2–500 genes. Targeted gene panels offer significant benefits over exome sequencing (ES), including increased sequencing depth and complete coverage of genes.
- *Whole-genome sequencing (WGS)*: The whole genome containing both coding and noncoding regions is sequenced without prior selection. Now the emphasis is toward WES due to its lower costs, need for greater speed and ease in data handling. Various private laboratories offer this test all across India with a price, ranges from 75,000 to 1 lakh rupees.

- *Whole-exome sequencing* (WES): The part of the genome encoding the proteins is called exonic regions and collection of all of the exons is known as the exome. It comprises around 1–2% of the genome. These regions can be selectively targeted thus reducing the amount of sequencing. The diagnostic yield of ES varies between 10 and over 50%. Cost of this test ranges from ₹20,000 to 25,000.
- *Repeat-primed PCR (RP-PCR)*: A single PCR reaction utilizes three primers. The amplification of the entire region is achieved by using two primers located outside the repeat, while a third chimeric primer is used to anneal to the repeating region and generate multiple amplicons.

GENETIC COUNSELING

Genetic counseling in genodermatoses is essential for diagnosing inherited skin disorders, assessing familial risks, and guiding management and reproductive decisions. Conditions like epidermolysis bullosa, xeroderma pigmentosum, ichthyoses, and neurofibromatosis often require genetic testing to confirm mutations and determine inheritance patterns. Counseling helps families understand the condition's progression, recurrence risks, and available interventions, including prenatal and preimplantation genetic testing. It also provides emotional support, addressing the psychological impact of these conditions and connecting families with resources and support networks. By integrating genetic counseling with dermatological care, affected individuals and their families can make informed decisions and receive comprehensive care.

CONCLUSION

Genodermatoses are rare diseases and pregnant females with genodermatoses need specific monitoring and care. The incidence and prevalence of genodermatoses is under-reported because of ethical concerns with pregnancy and nonavailability of genetic testing laboratory, as well as high price of the genetic test. This chapter briefly summarizes the details of a few genetic laboratories in India providing genetic testing **(Box 3)**.

BOX 3 List of laboratories doing genetic testing.

North zone:
- Sir Ganga Ram Hospital, Center of Medical Genetics, New Delhi
- Sanjay Gandhi Postgraduate Institute of Medical Sciences, Lucknow
- All India Institute of Medical Sciences, New Delhi

West zone:
- Center for Genetic Diagnosis, Deenanath Mangeshkar Hospital and Research Center, Pune
- Navi Mumbai Institute of Research in Mental and Neurological Handicap (Nirman), Mumbai

South zone:
- Center for Cellular and Molecular Biology, Molecular Diagnostics Division, Hyderabad
- Center for Human Genetics, Bengaluru
- Christian Medical College and Hospital, Vellore

SUGGESTED READINGS

1. Bayart CB, Brandling-Bennett HA. Congenital and hereditary disorders of the skin. In: Gleason CA, Juul SE (Eds). Avery's Diseases of the Newborn, 10th edition. Amsterdam, Netherlands: Elsevier; 2018. pp. 1475-94.
2. Puttur N, Kapoor A, Lakhey K, Reddy A, Malik N, Deokar S. Investigating the Prevalence, Gender Predilection, and Inheritance Patterns of Genodermatoses: A Tertiary Hospital Study. Cureus. 2024;16(6):e62455.
3. Idler J, Turkoglu O, Patek K, Stuart S, Taskin B, Sivaswamy L, et al. Neurocutaneous Disorders in Pregnancy. Obstet Gynecol Surv. 2023;78(10):606-19.
4. Greenblatt DT, Pillay E, Snelson K, Saad R, Torres Pradilla M, Widhiati S, et al. Recommendations on pregnancy, childbirth and aftercare in epidermolysis bullosa: a consensus-based guideline. Br J Dermatol. 2022;186(4):620-32.
5. Camacho M, Rengel C, López-Herrero E, Carrillo JL, Eslava AJ, Valdivielso P. Approach to the management of pregnancy in patients with pseudoxanthoma elasticum: a review. J Obstet Gynaecol. 2016;36(8):1061-6.
6. Goland S, Barakat M, Khatri N, Elkayam U. Pregnancy in Marfan syndrome: maternal and foetal risk and recommendations for patient assessment and management. Cardiol Rev. 2009;17(6):253-62.
7. Gautam M, Ali F. Prenatal diagnosis in dermatology. Indian J Paediatr Dermatol. 2021;22(4): 293-300.
8. Luu M, Cantatore-Francis JL, Glick SA. Prenatal diagnosis of genodermatoses: current scope and future capabilities. Int J Dermatol. 2010;49(4):353-61.
9. Ramot Y. Intrauterine diagnosis of genodermatoses. Curr Dermatol Rep. 2013;2:243-8.
10. Ashton GH, Eady RA, McGrath JA. Prenatal diagnosis for inherited skin diseases. Clin Dermatol. 2000;18:643-8.
11. Fassihi H, Eady RA, Mellerio JE, Ashton GH, Dopping-Hepenstal PJ, Denyer JE, et al. Prenatal diagnosis for severe inherited skin disorders: 25 years' experience. Br J Dermatol. 2006;154:106-13.
12. Verlinsky Y, Rechitsky S, Verlinsky O, Ivachnenko V, Lifchez A, Kaplan B, et al. Prepregnancy testing for single-gene disorders by polar body analysis. Genet Test. 1999;3:185-90.
13. Krabchi K, Gros-Louis F, Yan J, Bronsard M, Massé J, Forest JC, et al. Quantification of all foetal nucleated cells in maternal blood between the 18th and 22nd weeks of pregnancy using molecular cytogenetic techniques. Clin Genet. 2001;60(2):145-50.
14. Watanabe T, Fujimori K, Kato K, Nomura Y, Onogi S, Sato A. Prenatal diagnosis for placental steroid salfatase deficiency with fluorescence in situ hybridization: a case of X-linked ichthyosis. J Obstet Gynaecol Res. 2003;29:427-30.
15. Lalonde E, Rentas S, Lin F, Dulik MC, Skraban CM, Spinner NB. Genomic Diagnosis for Pediatric Disorders: Revolution and Evolution. Front Pediatr. 2020;8:373.

CHAPTER 22

Orodental Care in Pregnancy

Preeti Garg, Sanjeev Gupta

"Pregnancy is a time to cherish
As this is an experience you always relish
Take care of the little soul and you
As God has given you an important duty to do"

INTRODUCTION

Pregnancy is an important period in a woman's life as at this time the female is nurturing another life in her. So this period is filled of multiple emotions such as the person becomes overwhelmed, can have anxiety, fear, and sometimes depression. On one side the person is all excited as she is going to give birth but sometimes it is also associated with depression and emotional turmoil as the female starts to think that this will change her life and she will become bound to a bundle of responsibilities and would lose herself in the process. During this unique period of pregnancy, the body of expecting mother undergoes a lot of complex physiological and hormonal changes. These changes can also manifest as adverse effects in the oral cavity.

The common saying goes that "mouth is the mirror of the body" which suggests that oral health is considered an integral part of general health, so the oral problems encountered in pregnancy should be promptly addressed. Hence, pregnancy and postpartum periods are very important to guide a female to adopt a healthy lifestyle and motivating them to follow new and better rules is higher than other times.

In addition to all the physiological changes that a female comes across during pregnancy, these also show major reflection and may adversely affect the oral cavity and fetal outcome too.

PHYSIOLOGICAL MATERNAL CHANGES

During pregnancy endocrine, hematological, respiratory, and cardiovascular alterations take place with the placenta becoming an active endocrine organ that starts secreting: Chorionic gonadotropin, estrogen, and progesterone. These are important for the viability of both the placenta and the developing fetus. In pregnancy, the cardiac output increases by 20–40%, and blood volume increases by 30% to meet the requirements of the growing fetus. There is an increase in the metabolic rate which increases maternal respiratory rate too.

ORAL CONDITIONS IN PREGNANCY

The oral conditions commonly seen during pregnancy include dental caries, gingivitis, tooth movement, halitosis, gingival polyps, pregnancy tumor/epulis gravidarum (pyogenic granuloma), gingival hyperplasia, enamel erosions, teeth abrasions, periodontitis, xerostomia, and tooth loss.

- Numerous microbial symbionts or normal microbiomes of the oral cavity are altered in pregnancy due to hormonal changes
- Dysbiosis and altered immune response are the main reasons for oral conditions in pregnancy

DENTAL CARIES AND ENAMEL EROSIONS

Dental caries is the demineralization of the hard tissues of the tooth structure. The association of pregnancy to dental caries is not very significant, but as there is increase in energy need and food cravings, so dietary intake is increased. This increase in the dietary carbohydrates gets fermented by oral microbes into acid thus increasing the chances of a pregnant woman to have an increased risk of dental caries.

Morning sickness or vomiting is present in about 70% of the pregnancies which start between 4 and 8 weeks and continue till 14–16 weeks. If long-term vomiting condition persists (hyperemesis gravidarum) can cause erosion of enamel of maternal teeth. Moreover, there are changes seen in the composition of maternal saliva during late pregnancy which can also temporarily predispose the maternal teeth to dental caries and erosion. During pregnancy there is increased salivary lipid peroxidation (LPO) and total sialic acid (TSA) levels and reduced human beta-defensins.

In pregnant females, the oral cavity gets exposed to exacerbated gastric acid reflux, especially in the third trimester due to upward pressure of the gravid uterus and a lax esophageal sphincter which causes erosion of dental enamel surfaces.

There is also a fear of getting dental treatment and sometimes unawareness is also the basic cause which leads to an increase of demineralization of the tooth structure leading to an increase in decayed, missing due to caries, and filled teeth (DMFT) index during pregnancy.

Risk factors for dental caries/dental erosion:
- Increased and frequent carbohydrate act as substrate for oral bacteria
- Morning sickness
- Gastric reflux
- Altered salivary composition
- Decreased tendency for oral hygiene
- Avoiding dental treatment

PERIODONTAL DISEASES RELATED TO PREGNANCY

The diseases of periodontal tissues are described as chronic inflammatory, and a noncommunicable widely present infectious condition affecting the gums and supporting tissues. Periodontal diseases are supposed to be the 11th most prevalent of the diseases in the world. The periodontal tissues of a pregnant female are more susceptible to various internal and external factors promoting an increase in inflammatory responses.

Pregnancy Gingivitis

Gingivitis is the most common finding in the oral cavity during pregnancy, affecting about 75% of all pregnancies in which there is edema, erythema, hyperplasia, and increased bleeding from gingiva. These gingival inflammatory changes are more frequent during the first trimester, i.e., seen in 2nd to 3rd week and persist or may increase during the second trimester and 3rd trimester and usually regress after parturition. The mechanism for this increased response during pregnancy is elevated estrogen and progesterone levels. Various effects of hormonal changes are:
- Sex hormone causes a depression in the neutrophil chemotaxis, their phagocytosis activity, and T cell and antibody response.
- Estrogen reduces the preventive function of gingival tissue by enhancing the epithelial glycogen and cellular proliferation of the blood vessels present in the gingiva and decreasing the gingival keratinization levels.
- As compared to normal levels of progesterone, a change in progesterone levels in pregnancy leads to more gingival crevicular blood flow, more vascular permeability of the vascular membrane, gingival edema, and gingival bleeding.
- Further there is a decrease in the gingival repair ability due to alteration in the rate and pattern of collagen production and decreased rate of proliferation of the fibroblasts caused by altered level of progesterone.
- There is a relative deficiency in the folate level, which increases the inflammatory destruction and inhibits the repair of the oral tissues.
- There is an increased concentration of periodontopathic bacteria like *Prevotella intermedia* which substitutes vitamin K with progesterone and estrogen due to altered sex hormones during pregnancy causing an effect on gingival health.

So during pregnancy, an altered periodontal tissue structure with dilating blood vessels caused by changes in hormonal levels may cause painful inflammation to

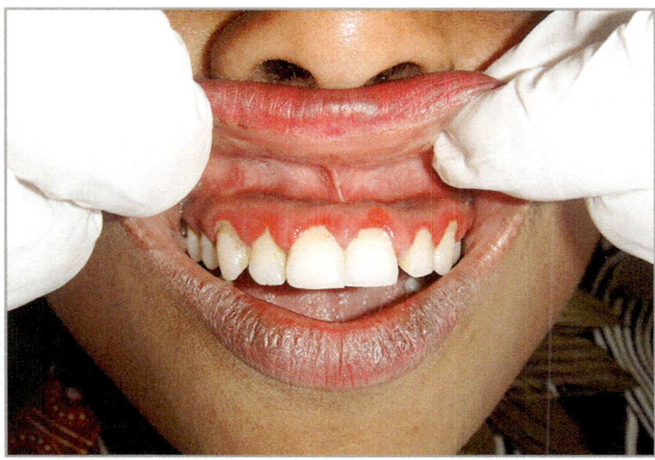

FIG. 1: Gingivitis in pregnancy.

even the slightest layer of biofilm present, so a preexisting gingivitis condition flares up in the pregnancy period **(Fig. 1)**.

- Gingivitis maximum in the third trimester
- Prepregnancy gingivitis further increases the risk

Changes predisposing to pregnancy gingivitis are:

- Immune alteration
- Increased concentration and activity of *Porphyromonas gingivalis*, *Prevotella intermedia*, *Fusobacterium nucleatum*, etc.
- Increased epithelial glycogen
- Increased blood vessels, their permeability, and blood flow
- Decreased gingival keratinization and fibroblasts
- Folate deficiency

CHANGES IN OVERALL MICROBIAL BALANCE DURING PREGNANCY

Porphyromonas gingivalis, *Fusobacterium nucleatum*, *Prevotella intermedia*, *Treponema denticola*, and *Campylobacter rectus* are the various bacteria which increase in pregnancy oral mucosa. Increased levels of opportunistic fungi (*Candida albicans*) can also be there. Beneficial bacteria such as *Streptococcus sanguinis and Streptococcus mitis* decrease during pregnancy. *Lactobacillus* species and *Veillonella* species also show altered concentration in oral mucosa during pregnancy.

ORAL DYSBIOSIS AND EFFECTS ON MATERNAL AND FETAL HEALTH (FLOWCHART 1)

Dysbiosis stimulates proinflammatory cytokines and increases oxidative stress leading to adverse pregnancy outcomes.

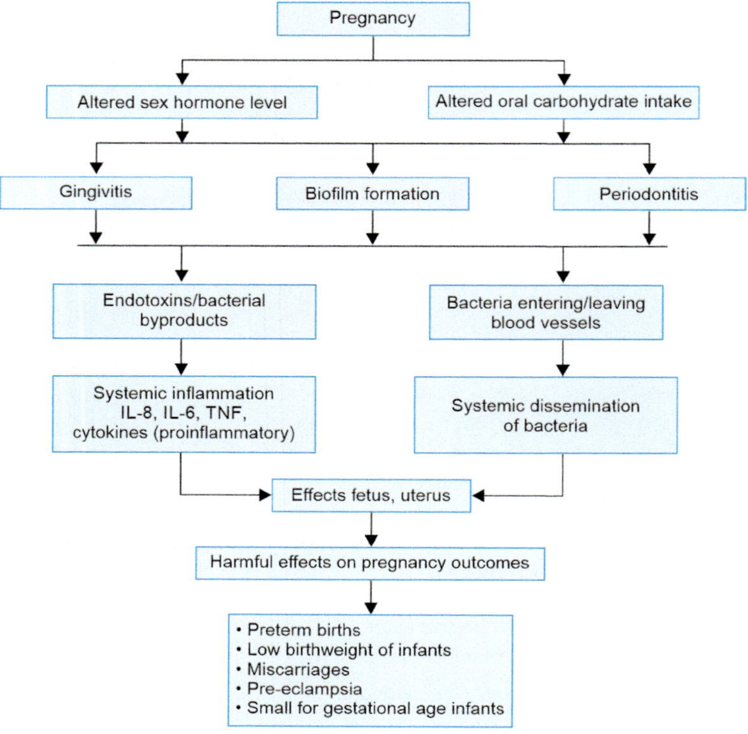

FLOWCHART 1: Oral dysbiosis and materno-fetal effects.
(IL: interleukin; TNF: tumor necrosis factor)

Effects on Maternal Health

- *Increased risk of periodontal disease*: Dysbiosis can lead to gingivitis or periodontitis, which are common in pregnancy. Chronic inflammation in the gums may exacerbate systemic inflammation, potentially influencing overall health.
- *Systemic inflammation*: Damage endothelium can trigger a systemic inflammatory response. This inflammation has been linked to conditions such as preeclampsia and gestational diabetes.

Effects on Pregnancy Outcomes

- *Preterm birth*: Inflammatory mediators produced in response to oral infections can cross into the placenta, leading to early labor.
- *Low birth weight*: The systemic inflammation caused by oral dysbiosis may interfere with normal fetal growth, leading to low birth weight.
- *Preeclampsia*: As seen with bacteria like *Porphyromonas gingivalis*, oral dysbiosis can contribute to endothelial dysfunction and placental damage, increasing the risk of preeclampsia.

- *Fetal growth restriction*: Growth retardation of the fetus and death can occur insufficient remodeling of the uterine spiral artery due to stimulation of apoptosis and the inhibition of invasiveness of extrachorionic trophoblast cells caused by *P. gingivalis.*
- *Miscarriage*: Severe dysbiosis and periodontal disease have been linked to an increased risk of miscarriage due to the heightened inflammatory response and potential infection of the placenta.

GINGIVAL ENLARGEMENT

Gingival enlargement also called as gingival hyperplasia is an overgrowth in the gum tissues **(Fig. 2)**. One of the causative factors for these enlargements is hormonal changes occurring in the body such as during pregnancy, puberty, or menstrual periods. During second and third trimester of pregnancy, the increase in the gingival response to local irritants caused by elevated levels of progesterone can lead to gingival enlargement.

PERIODONTITIS

Periodontitis is a destructive inflammation of periodontium due to bacterial infiltration and it is manifested as the gums are pulled away from the teeth and the supporting gum tissues get destroyed. Periodontitis is the presence of at least four teeth with probing depth of at least 4 mm and clinical attachment loss of at least 2 mm and bleeding on probing at 35% or more teeth sites. There is a toxin produced by the bacteria thus creating pocket formation that can become infected later on. This will lead to elevated inflammatory markers such as prostaglandin E_2 (PGE_2) and interleukins (IL-6 and IL-8) and these are found in the amniotic fluid (according to a few studies) and can lead to preterm birth **(Fig. 3)**.

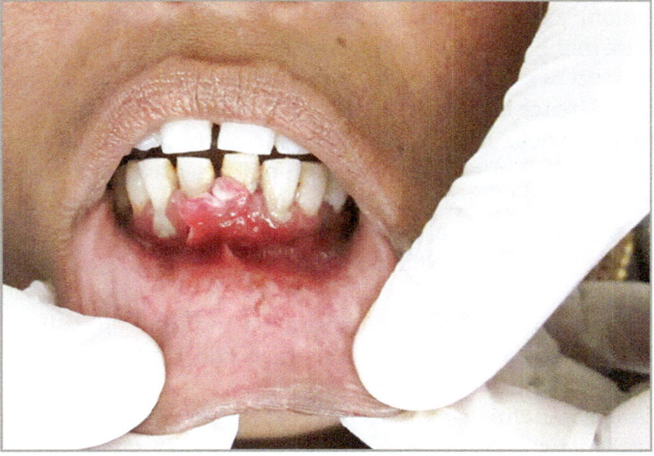

FIG. 2: Gingival enlargement in pregnancy.

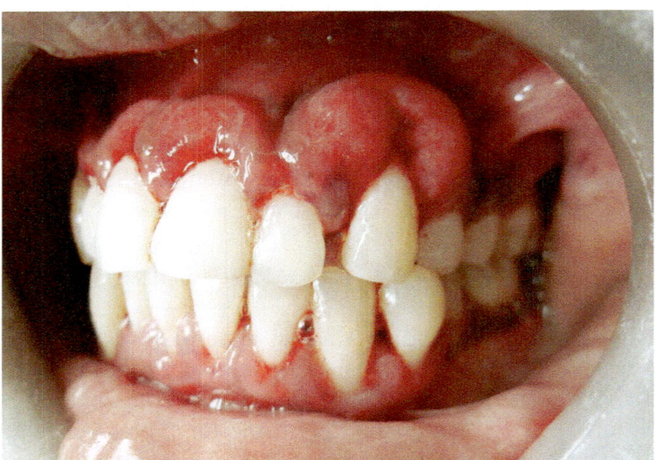

FIG. 3: Periodontitis in pregnancy.

According to the literature, the condition of periodontitis varies between 0.6 and 47%. This condition prevalence is also dependent on several other factors which are as follows:

- *Sociodemographic factors:*
    - Age: Age plays an important role in the prevalence of periodontal disease or health. In younger pregnant females, periodontal diseases increase due to a lack of oral health education and preventive care exposures. In old-age female pregnancies, periodontal problems are usually due to neglect in oral health care.
    - Socioeconomic status: The lower the socioeconomic background, the more prevalent the periodontal problems. These may be due to lesser ability to afford preventive treatments, lower education/literacy level for maintaining health, and may be due to limited access to dental care facilities.
    - Education: Lower education levels in pregnant females make them unaware to the importance of health literacy. Various studies suggest that higher level of education of the person, better is the preventive measures taken and hence better oral health.
    - Ethnicity: Various research publications have shown that certain ethnic groups exhibit higher rates of periodontal disease, which may be a combination of certain factors such as genetic predisposition, socioeconomic conditions, and cultural beliefs (like a common belief is that brushing should not be done for 40 days postpartum as it can lead to loosening of teeth).
    - Health care access: Financial constraints and geographic limitations are the barriers to healthcare access which can lead to more periodontal problems and subsequent complications.
- *Iron deficiency*: Anemia is one of the most important reasons which lead to adverse pregnancy outcomes. So if iron supplementation medication are not been regularly taken can cause iron deficiency anemia which can in turn

affect the periodontal health as this can lead to production of reactive oxygen species thus disturbing the host defense mechanism in general.

- *Smoking*: Recent studies have highlighted the role of smoking which has a direct effect on changing the oral microbioflora. Smoking leads to a decrease in the levels of oral flora of the beneficial species which lead to pathogen rich biofilm formation within 24 hours in the oral tissues, causing cluster anchors of the harmful microbiome in pregnant females.

A few studies suggest that there is an increased rate of cesarean section in women bearing low gestational age infants with such neonates having a higher risk to have birth trauma.

- Periodontitis if not given appropriate treatment at the right time can affect the course and outcome of pregnancy
- So discrete and isolated inflammatory signs of periodontitis should be taken care of immediately

PREGNANCY ORAL TUMOR (EPULIS GRAVIDARUM)

A single tumor like growth of gingival tissue enlargement can be seen in about 5% of the pregnancies and are known as pregnancy granuloma/epulis gravidarum/ pregnancy tumor. It occurs during second or third trimester and usually indistinguishable from pyogenic granuloma. The cause of this is presence of gingivitis (vascular lesion) with recurrent local irritation due to trauma. There is presence of nodular clinical mass, may be sessile or pedunculated and is painless. The lesion grows rapidly but seldom increases to >2 cm in diameter and even on gentle manipulation there is evident bleeding or hemorrhage seen. Management is usually to keep it under observation as surgical removal during pregnancy causes its recurrence. It usually regresses after delivery (the mechanism for regression of pregnancy tumor postpartum is still unclear) but if persist, postpartum surgical excision is of choice **(Fig. 4)**.

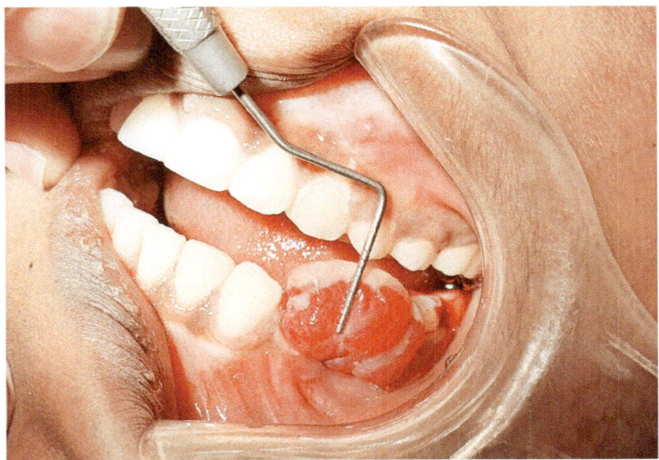

FIG. 4: Epulis gravidarum in pregnancy.

Loose (Mobile) Teeth

In pregnant females, generalized tooth mobility can be seen which can be attributed to the gingival diseases and the degree of disturbances in the attachment apparatus (i.e., the ligaments and the bone supporting the tooth structure). Most of the studies have concluded with the fact that no permanent loss of teeth has been seen during pregnancy.

Xerostomia

There may be temporary dryness of mouth experienced by pregnant females which may be caused due to the hormonal level changes. Another cause leading to xerostomia can be the increased dietary intake of sugary food items. This is one of the most important reasons to increase the caries in pregnant females. Management of xerostomia in pregnant female should include more consumption of water and use of sugar-free candy so as to maintain the mineralization of teeth and reduce the risk of caries.

OTHER MATERNAL ILLNESSES AFFECTING FETAL DENTAL APPARATUS

There are a number of infections and other pathologies of pregnancy which can affect fetal dental structures **(Table 1)**.

TABLE 1: Maternal illnesses affecting dental structures of human offsprings.

Maternal conditions	Dental effects on children
Infections:	
• *Cytomegalovirus* • Human immunodeficiency virus (HIV) • Rubella • Syphilis	• Enamel hypoplasia • Increase in caries • Enamel hypoplasia • Enamel hypoplasia
Pregnancy-related events:	
• Toxemia of pregnancy • Breech • Prolonged delivery/labor • Rh factor incompatibility	• Enamel hypoplasia • Enamel hypoplasia • Enamel hypoplasia • Tooth staining
Maternal systemic illness:	
• Diabetes mellitus • Hydantoin intake • Tetracycline intake • Alcohol abuse • Maternal hyperthermia	• Enamel hypoplasia • Cleft lip/cleft palate • Tooth staining • Maxillary hypoplasia • Cleft lip/cleft palate

DENTAL CONSIDERATIONS IN PREGNANCY

Screening of Oral Cavity in Pregnancy

All pregnant females should be screened and assessed for their dental hygiene habits, their access to dental care, the level of fluoridated water available and the existing oral problems, and the degree of disease. It is stated that dental care can be given in all the trimesters of pregnancy, but our approach remains conservative as pregnancy is a finite process. Visits to dental care centers can be done in any trimester prenatal visits give us a number of opportunities to help with oral health promotion intervention. There is transition of *HEENT to HEENOT* (head, eyes, ears, nose, oral, and throat) examination counseling for all patients extending from preconception to the postpartum period.

Advice and Education of Pregnant Females

Pregnancy is an ideal period as it provides a unique opportunity to motivate a person to follow a healthy lifestyle and new rules. The pregnant female is more receptive and ready for change so delivering oral health prevention information and education benefits two individuals at the same time, i.e., the mother and the child. The most powerful tool is educating women about how her own oral health can have an effect on the developing child. They are advised to follow good practices such as regular exercise, having a balanced diet to control weight and oral health, avoiding alcohol and smoking, eat healthy food, and minimizing sugar consumption.

Oral Hygiene Measures to be Followed during Pregnancy

- Use of fluoridated toothpaste twice a day, use of dental floss, and interdental cleaner are encouraged.
- *To help in the reduction of harmful bacteria multiplication*:
  - Use of alcohol-free mouth rinse daily
  - Chew xylitol-containing gums like mints
- *To stop acid attack on the tooth surface after vomiting*: In a cup of water add one teaspoon of baking soda to rinse the oral cavity after vomiting (person should be advised not to brush the teeth immediately after vomiting as it increases the erosive effects of the elevated acid level in the mouth).

Treatment Considerations

- The first trimester is a period of organogenesis so this is the most sensitive period. So this period is avoided for elective procedures as the medication use can lead to teratogenic effects in the developing embryo.
- After the first trimester, usually the patient is evaluated for oral prophylaxis treatment procedure.
- All the nondeferrable treatments could be undertaken in the latter period of second trimester when organogenesis is complete and the size of the developing embryo is not large enough to hinder the mother.

- Restoration procedures can be performed in second trimester with use of best practices such as rubber dam and rinsing of remnant restorative material.
- Scaling and root planning procedures are also carried out in the second trimester and can prevent adverse pregnancy outcomes.
- Treatment should be avoided in the middle or end of the third trimester of pregnancy as there will be positional discomfort and the fetus will impinge on the inferior vena cava causing *supine hypotensive syndrome/inferior vena cava compression syndrome.*

- Non deferrable treatment to be carried out in the second trimester
- Propping the women to her left side, keeping the visits at comfortable time and short and repositioning often helps to complete the procedure with ease

DIAGNOSIS/RADIOGRAPHS

The use of radiographs should be avoided in pregnancy, especially during first trimester of pregnancy. If radiographs must be done, minimum images required for the examination should be done using lead shielding in the form of a lead abdominal apron and thyroid collar.

Sedation and Anesthesia

No fetal or maternal harm are seen using local anesthesia but still, they are to be used judicially. Nitrous oxide use should be limited to the problems where topical or local anesthesia fail to work (limited duration of use to <30 minutes, preferably in the second trimester, use of 50% oxygen and avoid repeated exposures).

Medication in Pregnancy

The first 3 months of pregnancy are a period of embryogenesis or organogenesis. So elective dental procedures, radiological examination, and medicinal treatment should be avoided as certain drugs have teratogenic effects or can affect the growing fetus in certain ways. The prescription of any medicine should also be considered if there are certain comorbid conditions are present such as diabetes, hypertension, bleeding disorders, and cardiac and pulmonary diseases **(Table 2)**.

To conclude, we should take oral health as a part of our systemic health only and during pregnancy we should start taking all the essential measures from preconception period to keep our oral cavity free of pathogenic outburst of microflora. We should visit dental care centers preconceptions and should properly follow the instructions given by dental healthcare giver to avoid unprecedented events to occur during such an important phase of life. It is the responsibility of the gynecologists and the medical healthcare givers to guide pregnant women nicely about the importance of maintaining proper dental health. If we follow all the precautionary measures, we can benefit two people from various complex discomforts.

TABLE 2: Safety of medicines used in dental care of pregnant patients.

Pregnancy category / Drug	Category A (No risk to fetus in animal or human studies)	Category B (Safe to the fetus in an animal model without human safe data or vice versa)	Category C (Risk to fetus in animal studies and no human safety studies present)	Category D and X (Risk to human fetus data available)
Analgesic	-	Meperidine, paracetamol/ acetaminophen	Codeine, diflunisal, and rofecoxib	Aspirin and NSAIDs*
Antimicrobial	-	Azithromycin, cefadroxil cefuroxime, cephalexin, clindamycin, erythromycin metronidazole, and penicillin	Aciclovir, ciprofloxacin, and fluconazole	Doxycycline, minocycline, and tetracycline
Local anesthetics	-	Lidocaine	Bupivacaine and mepivacaine	-
Sedatives	-	Promethazine	-	Benzodiazepines
Others	-			

*NSAIDs: Nonsteroidal anti-inflammatory drugs.

SUGGESTED READINGS

1. Bobetsis YA, Barros SP, Offenbacher S. Exploring the relationship between periodontal disease and pregnancy complications. J Am Dent Assoc. 2006;137(Suppl):7S-13S.
2. Fardini Y, Chung P, Dumm R, Joshi N, Han YW. Transmission of diverse oral bacteria to murine placenta: evidence for the oral microbiome as a potential source of intrauterine infection. Infect Immun. 2010;78:1789-96.
3. Gaffield ML, Gilbert BJ, Malvitz DM, Romaguera R. Oral health during pregnancy: an analysis of information collected by the pregnancy risk assessment monitoring system. J Am Dent Assoc. 2001;132(7):1009-16.
4. Madinos PN, Bobetsis GA, Kinane DF. Is periodontitis associated with an increased risk of coronary heart disease and preterm and/or low birth weight births? J Clin Periodontol. 2002;29(Suppl 3):22-36.
5. Anderson ME, Johnson DC, Batal AH. Sudden Infant Death Syndrome and Prenatal Maternal Smoking: Risk Attributed in the Back to Sleep Era. BMC Med. 2005;3:4.
6. Bhalla S, Kaur K, Mahmood A, Mahmood S. Postnatal development of alcohol dehydrogenase in liver and intestine of rats exposed to ethanol in utero. Indian J Med Res. 2005;121:39-45.
7. Christensen LB, Jeppe-Jensen D, Petersen PE. Self-reported gingival conditions and self-care in the oral health of Danish women during pregnancy. J Clin Periodontol. 2003;30:949-53.

CHAPTER 23

Dermatologic Surgery and Aesthetic Treatments during Pregnancy

Chaithra Shenoy, Varsha R Koti, Madura C

INTRODUCTION

The incidence of women seeking procedures during pregnancy is on the rise. The ambiguity in the matters of safety of most of the procedures is due to lack of randomized controlled trial and is based on anecdotal case reports and case series. The question is generally raised when the procedure has been inadvertently performed on the female before she is aware of the pregnancy.

Melasma and other pigmentation, striae, acne and hirsutism are common occurrence in a pregnant female owing to the physiological change in the hormones. These might be a cause of distress in an otherwise healthy patient who expected the "glow of pregnancy". Hypervascular and immune-compromised state in pregnancy might increase the size of viral dermatological diseases, especially genital warts, warranting their removal before delivery. The reasons for seeking procedures during pregnancy may be myriad but human controlled trials are lacking due to obvious ethical concerns.

The pregnant patients seeking cosmetic and dermatological procedures should be thoroughly counseled.

The points to be highlighted are:

- Risk-benefit ratio of the procedure. Even theoretical risks need to be explained.
- Alternative options, if available
- Is it a physiological change, likely to be reversed postdelivery
- Known complications, if any
- Lack of evidences for safety, if there, should be explained.
- The urgency of the procedure or ability to wait till delivery.

The procedures can be classified as essential and elective. The essential procedures can be further classified into urgent and nonurgent.

Suspicion of pregnancy associated melanoma and clinical or dermoscopic signs of melanoma in a dysplastic nevi are indications for urgent intervention namely biopsy and further wide local excision as feasible are done, irrespective of the duration of pregnancy.

A particularly friable or aggressive pyogenic granuloma would have to be treated as an urgent procedure; otherwise this "pregnancy tumor" can be expected to spontaneously resolve postdelivery. Cryotherapy, electrocautery of the base, and carbon dioxide (CO_2) laser ablation are the modalities available while treating a pregnant female. Rarely these might warrant a surgical excision in especially oral invasive type.

Treatment of genital warts or condyloma acuminata is termed "essential and nonurgent", as to prevent juvenile-onset recurrent respiratory papillomatosis (JORRP). Cryotherapy was the preferred modality in the first and second trimester, whereas laser ablation was preferred in the third trimester particularly when extensive as per the systematic review done by Sugai et al.

Treatment of acne and hirsutism occurring because of acne can be deemed "elective".

PROCEDURE WISE CATEGORIZATION AND THEIR RECOMMENDATION DURING PREGNANCY (TABLE 1)

Intralesional Corticosteroid Injections

Triamcinolone acetate is known to cross the placental barrier. Though there are anecdotal reports of retrobulbar and intravitreal injection of triamcinolone in pregnant women without any fetal compromise or congenital abnormality. The usage as intralesional injection in alopecia areata and keloids is avoided unless benefit weighs more than the risk associated.

Electrocautery and Various Ablative Lasers

Electrocautery is known to be safe for usage in pregnant mother. CO_2 laser is very tissue specific and does not penetrate the depth of tissue. Hence, safety profile is very good for ablation of nevi, pyogenic granuloma, and warts, if necessary.

TABLE 1: Dermatological procedures and their safety recommendations in pregnancy.

Procedures	Recommendations in pregnancy
Cryotherapy	Safe
Fractional ablative lasers—CO_2 laser, Er:YAG	Safe
Chemical peels	• Glycolic acid and lactic acid peels—safe • Phenol, trichloroacetic acid and Jessner's peel—avoided in pregnancy
Laser hair removal	No recommendations—to be avoided
Fillers—HA	No data available
Botulinum toxin	No recommendations—avoided in pregnancy
Platelet-rich plasma	Not recommended for cosmetic indications

(Er:YAG: erbium-doped yttrium aluminum garnet; HA: hyaluronic acid)

Particulate and total volatile organic matters are higher in the ablative laser settings.

- *Chemical exposure*: Electrocautery plumes can contain toxic chemicals such as benzene, hydrogen cyanide, and formaldehyde, which may be harmful, if inhaled. These chemicals can be toxic, mutagenic, or carcinogenic. These tiny particles may also cause cardiac anomaly in fetus.
- *Infectious agents*: The smoke may carry viable cellular material, including viruses and bacteria, potentially increasing the risk of infection, especially human papilloma virus.
- *Respiratory issues*: Inhalation of surgical smoke can lead to respiratory irritation and other pulmonary problems, which might be more pronounced in pregnant women due to changes in their respiratory system.
- *Nausea and dizziness*: Exposure to the plume can cause symptoms such as nausea and dizziness, which can be particularly uncomfortable during pregnancy.

The plumes from the procedure have to managed by using a smoke evacuator to prevent alveolar damage and carcinogenic exposure to the mother as well as the operator.

Cryotherapy

It has a long safety record in pregnancy. For warts and pyogenic granuloma, this is the first line of treatment, especially in first and second trimester as the need for local anesthesia is not there.

Chemical Peel

Acne in pregnancy is more of inflammatory than the noninflammatory comedonal type. Maternal androgen levels spike results in increased sebum production leading to the bothersome acne. The treatment options are limited due to withdrawal of oral and topical retinoids during gestation. Glycolic acid (GA) is category N—meaning it is not rated. Safety of GA in pregnancy has been proven over the years and its action as exfoliant improves the follicular hyperkeratosis. Lactic acid is another peel with a long proven efficacy. Salicylic acid peels are widely used in treatment of acne because of lipophilic nature and due to its keratolytic potential. Usage of salicylic acid on intact skin and smaller areas has negligible absorption into the blood circulation making it safe for use in pregnancy. Likewise trichloroacetic acid peel used in dermatology has been found to be safe. Although the usage of chemical peel in pregnancy is widespread, the randomized controlled studies are lacking in pregnancy. The literature regarding the safety of peels other than mentioned earlier is grossly lacking.

Laser Hair Reduction

Hirsutism is a common symptom expressed by pregnant females due to increased circulating maternal androgens. Abdomen, lower back, and upper lip areas were most likely to develop increased hair growth which was likely to subside postdelivery needing no active intervention. Non-laser hair removal methods are recommended for them during the period of gestation. It is prudent to avoid lasers for hair reduction cause selective damage and have not been found to cause any side effect during pregnancy. But hirsutism being only a cosmetic concern it can be restarted postdelivery owing to lack of adequate data.

Neuromodulators

Anecdotal reports of botulinum toxin injections received before the diagnosis of pregnancy are published with favorable fetal outcome. Case reports of higher dose of botulinum toxin for the treatment of cervical dystonia, migraine, and achalasia during pregnancy are available. A study by Brin et al. evaluated 913 pregnancies with exposure to onabotulinum toxin in prenatal or first trimester with 2.6% having fetal defects which are similar to the general population. Having said this, these articles at the current time must serve as a tool for counseling inadvertent first trimester injections before pregnancy detection and not as permission to inject toxins for cosmetic concerns till proven safety is demonstrated in literature.

Dermal Fillers

Hyaluronic acid (HA) used in most fillers in India is very similar to natural structure of HA found in the human skin and the changes of inflammatory reaction are low even in general population. The compelling evidence regarding the safety profile of fillers in pregnancy is unavailable. Theoretically pregnancy is a hypercoagulable and hypervascular state with altered immune status. The chances on inadvertent intra-arterial injections and increased chances of bruising and hematoma are a possibility. Lidocaine present in most HA-based filler may enter the circulation in a pregnant woman.

Platelet-rich Plasma and Other Autologous Preparation

Although intrauterine platelet-rich plasma (PRP) is known to improve the implantation chances and birth outcome, PRP for hair and facial rejuvenation are not recommended in pregnancy. The improvement in hair growth as well as diameter and skin quality due to increased vascularity and maternal hormones during the gestational period mainly reduces the number of patients who seek these therapies. Varied injectables are not recommended in pregnancy for cosmetic indications to prevent inadvertent introduction into maternal body and also to not create unnecessary pain as studies have shown that pain threshold is reduced when compared to nonpregnant state.

DERMATOLOGICAL SURGERIES

Timing of Surgical Procedure

Avoid nonemergency surgeries during first trimester (risk of spontaneous abortion) and third trimester (risk of premature birth). Plan to perform necessary procedures either in second trimester or in postpartum period.

Patient Preparation

Complete medical history including history of hypertension, diabetes, or heart condition. Any history of vaginal spotting and recent contractions need to be consulted with obstetrician. Vitals to be monitored including the signs of pre-eclampsia. Monitoring fetal heart rate is important to detect early signs of fetal distress during the procedure. Hence, it is necessary for an anesthetist to monitor the mother and fetus throughout the procedure.

Planning the Surgery

Refer to **Table 2**.

Indications of Dermatological Surgeries Performed during Pregnancy (Table 3)

- *Biopsy*: Tumors like basal cell carcinoma, verrucous carcinoma on the lip, protuberant dermatofibrosarcoma, human papillomavirus (HPV) lesions and

TABLE 2: Planning dermatologic surgery in pregnancy.

Steps of surgery	To be preferred in pregnancy	To be avoided in pregnancy
Positioning of the patient	The left lateral position is preferred as the expanded uterus in supine positioning poses risk for inferior vena cava compression	Supine position. The symptoms of vena cava compression (dizziness, tachycardia, and sweating) can mimic lidocaine toxicity and therefore need to be differentiated by the surgeon. Supine position may lead to uterine hypoxia
Antiseptics	Alcohol (should be allowed to dry completely before starting the procedure) and chlorhexidine	• Povidone absorption through mucous membrane can cause fetal hypothyroidism • Hexachlorophene to be avoided
Anesthesia	• Lidocaine and prilocaine • Use small volumes, as it can cross placental barrier and great volumes can cause fetal cardiac or central nervous system toxicity • Sedation in very anxious patient. Needs evaluation by obstetrician and anesthetic monitoring • Lidocaine with epinephrine is a pregnancy category B medication. It is advantageous in its vasoconstrictive effects, reduction of peak serum lidocaine levels, and decreased placental transfer to the fetus	• Avoid usage on conjunctiva and mucous membrane increased absorption. Prilocaine cream can cause methemoglobinemia • Benzocaine causes methemoglobinemia • Bupivacaine and mepivacaine—risk of toxicity and fetal bradycardia • Allergic reactions due to sensitivity to the anesthetics of the ester group → production of para-aminobenzoic acid • Higher epinephrine doses → uterine artery spasm

Continued

Continued

Steps of surgery	To be preferred in pregnancy	To be avoided in pregnancy
Surgical incision	Along relaxed skin tension lines or if uncertain circular	
Sutures	• Dehiscence is more common in pregnancy due to slow cicatrization process • Slow absorbing buried sutures with increased strength and knot security are preferable, especially on the abdomen and breasts • Removal of the stitches in stages could reduce the dehiscence in areas of great tension. Suture removal should be done intermittently	
Perioperative antibiotics	• Penicillin derivatives cephalosporins and clindamycin • Erythromycin nonestolate and azithromycin are safe alternatives for patients with an allergy to penicillin	• Erythromycin estolate → risk of cholestatic jaundice • Clindamycin → liver function abnormalities • Sulfonamides taken in third trimester → neonatal hyperbilirubinemia with kernicterus • Fluoroquinolones → cartilage defects • Tetracycline → defects in dental enamel • Aminoglycosides → fetal ototoxicity • Chloramphenicol → gray baby syndrome and neonatal death
Postoperative analgesia	• Acetaminophen—category B, recommended doses for a limited period. Its prolonged or high dosage-associated with hemolytic anemia as well as fetal and maternal renal toxicity • Opiates—for short in intense pain, however the cost/benefit analysis to be evaluated	Ibuprofen and salicylates—interfere in the platelets function and increase the risk of bleeding and postpartum hemorrhage, avoided in third trimester. Can close arterial duct and delay onset of labor

vascular tumors like pyogenic granuloma, glomus tumors, and hemangioendothelioma presents with accelerated growth during pregnancy due to various growth factors and gestational hormones. Benign nevi can appear more dark or increase in size during pregnancy and a change in appearance of any pigmented nevi has a suspicion of melanoma. Incisional or excisional biopsy should not be delayed in such conditions and further management with wide local excision to be performed after confirmation. The risk posed

TABLE 3: Dermatologic surgeries which should be performed and those to be avoided.

Dermatological surgeries can be performed during pregnancy	Dermatological surgeries avoided in pregnancy
• Biopsy—skin, nail, and hair • Impacted nose or ear ring • Cysts and benign growths • *Abscess*: Incision and drainage • Ingrown toe nail—grade 2 or 3—use CO_2 laser for ablation • Inflamed skin tags	• Ear lobe tears • Keloid surgery • Acne scar surgery • Vitiligo surgeries • Sclerotherapy • Liposuction and autologous fat transfer • Hair transplantation

by not conducting a procedure, even an excisional biopsy, is greater than the potential.

- *Keloid*: Increase in the size or recurrence of keloid during pregnancy is observed which is attributed to hormonal surge. There is a lack of consensus regarding surgical excision and intralesional steroid injection. Conservative measures such as pressure garments and scar massaging can be continued during pregnancy.
- *Ear lobe tears*: Repairs being a cosmetic procedure can wait until delivery.
- Impacted ear or nose ring removal can be performed under local anesthesia.
- *Skin tags*: Shave excision with secondary intention healing or simple excision and closure can be performed for giant acrochordon or at areas of friction causing recurrent inflammation and infection.
- *Nail surgery*: Nail alterations occurring in pregnancy are benign and do not require treatment. However, in case of ingrown toe nail—grade 2 and 3 can be operated for partial nail avulsion with matricectomy using CO_2 ablation/radiofrequency, as phenol usage is contraindicated in pregnancy.
- *Nail biopsy*: This should be planned for suspected Bowen's disease or squamous cell carcinoma or nail melanoma—histopathological analysis with nail unit biopsy is mandatory. Nail melanoma presenting with longitudinal melanonychia, which is irregular in width and color and Hutchinson's sign, nail plate destruction, bleeding or rapid enlargement, and needs immediate intervention. Further complete surgical removal with adequate margins according to Breslow thickness and sentinel lymph node biopsy is performed.
- *Acne scars*: Acne flare is observed during pregnancy due to hormonal changes, further leading to scaring. Acne scar surgeries can be performed in postpartum period when inflammatory acne lesions settle down.
- *Vitiligo surgery*: The disease stability in pregnancy is unpredictable and hence surgery is not advised.

- *Hair transplantation*: During pregnancy, there is a prolonged anagen phase due to effects of progesterone, increases hair shaft diameter, and inhibits androgen secretion leading to anagen maintenance. Hair transplantation is avoided until postpartum period.
- *Liposuction and autologous fat transplantation*: It is not recommended during pregnancy as it can compromise the nutritional requirement of fetus. There is also a risk for fat embolism and occlusion.
- *Sclerotherapy*: There is paucity of data over the safety of its use in pregnancy. Though there are few studies showed it being a safe procedure with no complications.

Complications of Surgery

- Wound dehiscence
- Infections
- Keloid and hypertrophic scars
- Postinflammatory hyperpigmentation
- *Bleeding*: Cardiac output and volume of circulating blood is increased leading to hemodilution during pregnancy along with a decrease in peripheral vascular resistance. As maternal hypotension could rapidly compromise the uterine blood flow, the pregnant woman's blood pressure should be carefully monitored during surgical procedures. An aggregation of platelets in late pregnancy, combined with the reduced vascular resistance and the increased production of coagulation factors, may elevate the risk of thromboembolic events, especially in long-lasting procedures. High changes of acute perioperative bleeding due to hemodilution with cardiovascular alterations can be threatening to pregnant woman as uterine perfusion can be compromised.
- Aortocaval compression
- *Maternal complications*: Preeclampsia, premature rupture of membranes, and preterm labor
- *Fetal complications*: Fetal distress and morbidity

KEY POINTS

- Dermatologic surgery and aesthetic treatments during pregnancy should prioritize the safety of both the mother and the fetus, avoiding procedures with potential risks like teratogenic effects or systemic absorption.
- Noninvasive treatments such as mild chemical peels or topical therapies are often considered safer options during pregnancy. Avoid lasers, deep peels, or aggressive interventions.
- Elective aesthetic treatments, including Botox, fillers, and major cosmetic surgeries, should typically be postponed until after pregnancy to minimize risks.
- Close consultation with obstetricians and dermatologists is essential to evaluate the safety and necessity of any procedure during pregnancy.

SUGGESTED READINGS

1. Lee KC, Korgavkar K, Dufresne RG Jr, Higgins HW 2nd. Safety of cosmetic dermatologic procedures during pregnancy. Dermatol Surg. 2013;39(11):1573-86.
2. Trivedi MK, Kroumpouzos G, Murase JE. A review of the safety of cosmetic procedures during pregnancy and lactation. Int J Womens Dermatol. 2017;3(1):6-10.
3. Garg AM, Mysore V. Dermatologic and Cosmetic Procedures in Pregnancy. J Cutan Aesthet Surg. 2022;15(2):108-17.
4. Sugai S, Nishijima K, Enomoto T. Management of Condyloma Acuminata in Pregnancy: A Review. Sex Transm Dis. 2021;48(6):403-9.
5. Gontijo G, Gualberto GV, Madureira NA. Dermatologic surgery and cosmetic procedures during pregnancy: A systematic review. Surg Cosmet Dermatol. 2010;2:39-45.
6. Sweeney SM, Maloney ME. Pregnancy and Dermatologic Surgery. Dermatol Clin. 2006;24(2):205-14.
7. Ibrahim NE, Shaharan S, Dheansa B. Adverse Effects of Pregnancy on Keloids and Hypertrophic Scars. Cureus. 2020;12(12):e12154.

CHAPTER 24

Dermatological Drugs Safe in Pregnancy and Lactation: Topical and Systemic

Ankur Talwar, Kshama Talwar

INTRODUCTION

Doctors often encounter pregnant or breastfeeding women seeking advice on skin disorders. Dermatologists and other specialists must know of drugs are safe during pregnancy. The USA Food and Drug Administration (FDA) had introduced the different categories of drugs which are safe in pregnancy and lactation long back more than three decades **(Table 1)**. However, the generalizations of the old category system (i.e., A, B, C, D, and X), coupled with the lack of safety data leads to assessments of risks versus benefits difficult. Consequently, the United States FDA introduced a novel regulation called the Pregnancy and Lactation Labeling Rule (PLLR) in the year 2015. The new format includes three sections: Pregnancy, lactation, and a new section on the reproductive potential in men and women. The PLLR also includes information on contraception recommendations, pregnancy testing, and information on infertility **(Table 2)**.

TABLE 1: Previous pregnancy risk categories.

Pregnancy category	Description
A	There is no indication of any risk in human studies (studies with pregnant females have shown no risk to the fetus during the first trimester)
B	No evidence of risk in animal studies (there are no adequate studies in humans, but animal studies did not demonstrate a risk to the fetus)
C	Risk cannot be ruled out. There are no satisfactory studies in pregnant women, but animal studies demonstrated a risk to the fetus; potential benefits of the drug may outweigh the risks
D	Evidence of risk (studies in pregnant women have demonstrated a risk to the fetus; potential benefits of the drug may outweigh the risks)
X	Contraindicated (studies in pregnant women have demonstrated a risk to the fetus, and/or human or animal studies have shown fetal abnormalities; risks of the drug outweigh the potential benefits)

TABLE 2: Pregnancy and Lactation Labeling Rule (PLLR).

Pregnancy (including labor and delivery)	Lactation	Females and males of reproductive potential
• Pregnancy exposure registry • Risk summary • Clinical considerations • Data	• Risk summary • Clinical considerations • Data	• Pregnancy testing • Contraception • Infertility

TOPICAL ANTI-INFLAMMATORY AGENTS

Topical Corticosteroids

A 2015 Cochrane review of 5 cohort and 9 case-controlled studies concluded that topical corticosteroids, irrespective of potency do not lead to increased risks of fetal malformations or anomalies. However, there appears an association between the use of very potent topical corticosteroids and low birth weights, particularly when cumulative dose is very high throughout pregnancy. Mild-to-moderate potency topical corticosteroids are preferred according to general consensus, and usage should be limited to a short duration. Maximum duration for which moderate and high potency topical steroids can be applied for maximum 12 weeks and very high potent if essential can be used for maximum 3 weeks.

Calcineurin Inhibitors

Topical tacrolimus has not been extensively studied in pregnancy, so data is extrapolated from systemic tacrolimus use. There is increasing evidence of successful pregnancies with systemic tacrolimus, although maternal and fetal complications are increased. When used topically, calcineurin inhibitors are usually poorly absorbed systemically because their molecular size prevents effective penetration. Therefore, topical use on small surfaces is deemed permissible, especially when no alternatives exist.

Calcipotriene

After application on a psoriatic plaque, about 6% of calcipotriene is absorbed systemically while 5% is absorbed if applied on normal skin. Animal studies have shown an increased incidence of skeletal abnormalities; however, there are no studies on safety during human pregnancies. Use of calcipotriene in the recommended dosage range (>100 g/week of a 0.005% solution) does not lead to a disturbance in calcium homeostasis. Since there are no studies on safety in human pregnancies, when no alternatives exist, topical use on small surfaces is permissible.

Crisaborole

There is no available data with the use of crisaborole in pregnant women. Animal reproduction studies have shown no adverse developmental effects with the oral administration of crisaborole in pregnant rats and rabbits. There is no information available on the presence of crisaborole in human milk.

Coal Tar

Animal studies using high dose coal tar have shown increased risk of birth defects. However, on the contrary, several studies in humans have not shown any adverse effects with the use of coal tar. A large study did not reveal significant increase in spontaneous abortions or fetal abnormalities with the use of coal tar. Due to concerns raised by animal studies, many authorities have recommended avoiding coal tar products in pregnancy, although accidental use does not require any action.

ANTIFUNGAL AGENTS

Topical Azoles

Because there is a shortage of well-conducted trials, several topical azoles are classified as category C, whereas some more thoroughly examined compounds are classified as category B. Nevertheless, research has demonstrated that topical azoles have negligible systemic absorption, making them suitable for prescription during any trimester of pregnancy. A retrospective cohort research of pregnant women who were exposed to vaginal azoles found no significant correlation between the usage of these medications and the occurrence of congenital abnormalities or abortions.

Terbinafine

No embryo-fetotoxicity was shown in rabbits and rats during oral reproduction studies, even when they were given doses up to 23 times higher than the maximum advised for humans. Similarly, a nationwide cohort research that used a registry and lasted for 20 years did not discover any significant connections between terbinafine and negative outcomes during pregnancy. It is classified as the FDA pregnancy category B and is widely regarded as the safest oral antifungal drug, especially during the first trimester of pregnancy.

ANTIACNE AGENTS

Topical Retinoids (Tretinoin and Adapalene), Category C

The safety studies regarding adapalene and tretinoin are limited. Initial case reports suggested that the use of topical tretinoin during pregnancy resulted in ear, cerebral, and cardiac malformations that are typically associated with the use of systemic retinoids in pregnancy. However, larger studies evaluated subsequently have not found an increased risk of retinoid embryopathy or other major birth defects with the topical use of tretinoin. Although some studies recommend its use in pregnancy, especially after first trimester, the general consensus is to avoid its use during pregnancy.

Topical Tazarotene, Topical Isotretinoin, Category X

Topical isotretinoin is absolutely contraindicated in pregnancy in view of ample data showing increased pregnancy loss in first trimester and numerous birth defects. Tazarotene is a topical retinoid and some animal studies have reported adverse effects, so it is classified as pregnancy category X and should be strictly avoided during pregnancy. In addition, before prescribing tazarotene to any young women of childbearing agė, a pregnancy test should be ordered 2 weeks before starting medication.

Benzoyl Peroxide, Category C

Benzoyl peroxide is classified as pregnancy category C. Approximately 5% of topical formulation is absorbed systemically, and is metabolized into benzoic acid, which is a food additive. Since it has a rapid renal clearance, no systemic toxicity is expected, and therefore the risk of congenital malformations is theoretically minimal. Consequently, benzoyl peroxide is considered safe during pregnancy.

Azelaic Acid, Category B

Azelaic acid is classified as pregnancy category B drug. Animal studies have shown no teratogenicity, but human studies do not exist. When applied topically, about 4% of azelaic acid is absorbed systemically. It is advised to be used on small skin surfaces and preferably not in first trimester.

Salicylic Acid

Salicylic acid is classified as pregnancy category C drug. There are no human studies of topical salicylic acid use during pregnancy, though malformations have been reported in rat embryos from systemic salicylic acid and aspirin administration during pregnancy. The general consensus is that risk during pregnancy is low if use is restricted to local areas for a limited duration.

Topical Antibiotics

Topical antibiotics have been used for the treatment of acne since long time with topical erythromycin and clindamycin the two most commonly prescribed agents. Both topical erythromycin and clindamycin are classified as pregnancy category B. Short-term use of these agents is safe during pregnancy. In light of the association between *Clostridium difficile* diarrhea with topical clindamycin, it is advised to be used with caution in patients with a history of gastrointestinal disease.

Topical Dapsone

It is classified as pregnancy category C drug. High doses in animal studies have not shown any teratogenic effects. The use of topical dapsone during pregnancy has not been associated with an increased risk of fetal malformations. However, caution should be exercised, since it is a relatively new molecule and the lack of controlled human studies evaluating its safety during pregnancy. The consensus is that it should be prescribed in pregnancy when the benefits clearly outweigh the risks.

OTHER TOPICAL DRUGS

Minoxidil

Concentrations of minoxidil in the serum following topical application are far below therapeutic levels in adults. However, there have been case reports of cardiac, neurodevelopmental, gastrointestinal, and limb malformations with topical use of minoxidil. Since there are no conclusive studies to prove its safety, minoxidil is not recommended during pregnancy.

Hydroquinone

The use of hydroquinone is not recommended during pregnancy, although the available data suggests low risk. Topical use of hydroquinone results in 35–45% systemic absorption. High potency exposure of topical hydroquinone in rats did not lead to increased rates of malformation. In another study, hydroquinone did not increase risk of malformations, prematurity, or low birth weight.

BOTULINUM TOXIN A

In general, cosmetic treatments, such as botulinum toxin A injection, should be avoided during pregnancy, even though there are limited data to suggest that the risk to the fetus is low. In various studies, doses up to 1,200 units of botulinum toxin have been used for various medical indications without adverse effects.

Topical Antivirals

Liquid nitrogen is considered safe and is recommended as a first-line treatment for warts. Trichloroacetic acid is considered a second-line therapy for condylomata acuminata. Data for the use imiquimod for genital warts are limited, but teratogenicity has not been demonstrated in studies. Podophyllin is pregnancy class X and is to be strictly avoided in pregnancy.

Permethrin

Permethrin, topical sulfur, benzyl benzoate, and crotamiton are all considered safe for scabies therapy in pregnancy. There are ample data to support their use in pregnancy.

Lidocaine and Adrenaline

Both lidocaine and adrenaline are considered safe in small amounts for local anesthesia. Both the agents cross the placenta; animal reproductive studies

TABLE 3: Safety of topical drugs in pregnancy.

Topical medication	Pregnancy category	Comments
Corticosteroids*	C	Utilize corticosteroids of mild-to-moderate potency. Avoid using high-potency steroids as they provide a risk of causing low birth weight in newborns
Tacrolimus*	C	There is a lack of extensive human data on the safety of this product. However, it is generally deemed safe when applied topically to limited areas
Pimecrolimus*	C	There is limited human data and it is better avoided due to lack of data with its usage in pregnancy
Calcipotriene*	C	Limited information about the effects of the drug on humans. However, studies conducted on animals have shown negative effects, but there have been no reports of abnormalities in humans. Likely considered safe to use
Tazarotene*	X	Absolutely contraindication in pregnancy
Tretinoin*	C	Limited information about the effects of the drug on humans, animal data indicates teratogenic risk. Avoid use during pregnancy
Adapalene*	C	Limited information about the effects of the drug on humans, animal data suggest problems related to bones. Avoid use in first trimester
Benzoyl peroxide*	C	Limited use permitted
Salicylic acid*	C	Avoid excessive use, particularly during the third trimester, since it may lead to the closure of the ductus arteriosus
Azelaic acid*	B	Refrain from using during the initial 3 months of pregnancy, and only apply to limited regions of the skin
Minoxidil*	C	Refrain from using during pregnancy as there have been cases of fetal abnormalities

*In any topical formulation like ointment/cream/gel/lotion, etc.

of lidocaine reveal no evidence of harm to the fetus. In dermatologic surgery, the benefits of using small controlled amounts of adrenaline seem to outweigh potential risks **(Table 3)**.

ORAL DRUGS IN PREGNANCY

Immunosuppressants and Anti-inflammatory Drugs

Oral Steroids

Prednisone, a nonfluorinated corticosteroid, is the preferred choice because placental enzymes limit passage to the embryo. Oral prednisone and prednisolone when prescribed at low doses (10–15 mg/day) are tolerable during pregnancy due to the presence of inactivating placental enzymes which limit their fetal transmission. Studies note a three-fold increased risk of orofacial clefts 4 weeks before conception to 12 weeks after conception with the use of oral steroids; since lip formation occurs during weeks 5–7 and palate formation during weeks 8–12. The absolute risk is low. Other studies concluded that administration of high-dose oral corticosteroids during pregnancy was linked to stunted fetal growth, low birth weight, and suppression of the body's natural corticosteroid synthesis [due to permanent changes occurring in fetal hypothalamic–pituitary–adrenal (HPA) axis when 11β-hydroxysteroid dehydrogenase 2 is deficient]. HPA axis suppression may lead to a condition called early life programming when susceptibility to infections increases, altered neurological, cardiac, or metabolic diseases occurs. The consensus is to use the lowest effective steroid dose and avoid usage during first trimester when hard palate of the fetus is forming. Recent studies, however, have not shown increased risk of cleft deformities.

Azathioprine

The main risks associated with azathioprine use during pregnancy are preterm and low birth weight infants. Sporadic anomalies and hematologic toxicities have also been reported with the use of azathioprine. There is ample safety data available supporting the use of azathioprine in organ transplant patients, auto-immune bowel disease, and rheumatic disease. There is no clear-cut pattern of congenital malformation reported with azathioprine. To prevent the development of hematological toxicity in newborns, a consensus to halve the dose at 32 weeks of gestation if the mother's leukocyte count are >1 standard deviation below the mean is recommended. Azathioprine is categorized as a category D drug and should only be considered if the benefits significantly outweigh the listed hazards. There is a rise in thiopurine Smethyltransferase activity due to hormonal changes in pregnancy. This leads to a decrease in 6-thioguanine nucleotide (6-TGN) with increase 6-methylmercaptopurine (6-MMP). It is recommended to maintain treatment with azathioprine if patient already on azathioprine before pregnancy. But the initiation of this drug during pregnancy usually discouraged because the onset of action is slow and risk of bone marrow suppression and pancreatitis in the initiation phase may be seen. Azathioprine should be discontinued 2 days prior to conception.

Cyclophosphamide

Cyclophosphamide hinders the process of cell division and has been found to cause birth defects in both animals and humans based on scientific research. It is under category D drug and should only be considered if the advantages significantly surpass the hazards. There are some reports of safety after the second trimester of pregnancy. It is contraindicated during lactation. Ideally cyclophosphamide should be stopped 3 months prior to conception.

Mycophenolate Mofetil

Mycophenolate mofetil (MMF) was reclassified from class C to D drug in 2007 by the FDA in response to postmarketing studies indicating potential increased risk of first trimester miscarriage, microtia, external auditory canal atresia, cleft lip/palate, heart, esophagus, kidney, and central nervous system (CNS) abnormalities. The current consensus is that MMF should not be used in pregnancy, and women should use nonhormonal contraception until 6 weeks after stopping therapy. Pregnancy test should be done prior to starting mycophenolate.

Cyclosporine

Several case reports have shown the administration of cyclosporine during pregnancy for kidney transplant, and the majority of these cases did not show an increased occurrence of congenital abnormalities. Animal studies have demonstrated a higher rate of death. However, certain studies have indicated a higher occurrence of premature birth and impaired fetal growth. Cyclosporine is lipid soluble so has a high volume of distribution and also metabolism. P-glycoprotein pumps out the drug from trophoblast, hence restricting the fetal exposure. Cyclosporine is classified as a category C drug and is administered to pregnant women only when the advantages clearly surpass the possible hazards.

Methotrexate

Methotrexate is classified as a category X drug, meaning it is absolutely contraindicated for usage in pregnant women. Methotrexate is linked to a heightened risk of miscarriage, micrognathia, and developmental retardation, limb abnormalities, intrauterine growth retardation, and mental retardation. Methotrexate has to be stopped 1 month before conception by mother and 3 months by father.

Apremilast

A phosphodiesterase inhibitor used in various inflammatory dermatoses has no teratogenic effects in animals. There are reports of dose-dependent increased risk of abortion and decreased birth weight in animals. Adequate and well-controlled studies with apremilast are lacking in pregnant women. There are no current recommendations on PDE4 inhibitor drug safety during pregnancy and therefore should be avoided during pregnancy.

Dapsone

Available studies on dapsone do not indicate major fetotoxicity or congenital anomalies. Glucose-6-phosphate dehydrogenase (G6PD) levels should be ideally measured in all cases before initiating therapy because of the risk of maternal anemia. Neonatal hyperbilirubinemia and hemolytic anemia have also been attributed to gestational exposure to dapsone.

Hydroxychloroquine

Hydroxychloroquine (HCQ) is considered a first-line therapy for pregnant mothers with active lupus, and studies have not found the maternal use of HCQ to increase the risk of congenital abnormalities. Published studies continue to support the safety of HCQ during pregnancy.

Intravenous Immunoglobulin

Limited studies have shown intravenous immunoglobulin (IVIg) to be a safe therapy for pemphigus and pemphigoid gestationalis. A study of anti-Ro/La1 pregnant women concluded that the use of IVIg was safe during pregnancy and was effective in preventing recurrent neonatal lupus. IVIg crosses the human placenta in significant amounts only after 32 weeks of gestation and is not embryotoxic **(Table 4)**.

Antiacne Drugs

Oral Antibiotics

Erythromycin is a macrolide in pregnancy category B. This drug cross the placenta poorly. Erythromycin is generally considered safe during any stage of pregnancy. It was considered the antibiotic of choice for inflammatory acne in pregnant women. However, long-term use of the drug (>6 weeks) has not been studied. Importantly, erythromycin estolate is contraindicated in pregnancy because of drug-related maternal hepatotoxicity.

Azithromycin is another macrolide antibiotic that is the FDA category B. Animal studies have shown that azithromycin crosses the placenta without causing negative effects to the fetus. Azithromycin is generally considered compatible with pregnancy but has less available safety data than erythromycin.

TABLE 4: Immunosuppressants and anti-inflammatory drugs category in pregnancy.

Oral medication	Pregnancy category	Comments
Corticosteroids	C	• Low dose prednisolone (15 mg/day) not harmful • High dose may cause cleft lip if used in first trimester and hypothalamic–pituitary–adrenal (HPA) axis suppression in the fetus
Azathioprine	D/C	Can cause fetal anomalies and hematological toxicities in animals but has shown no effect on human fetus
Cyclophosphamide	D	Is teratogenic and can cause preterm labor and abortion
Mycophenolate mofetil	D	Increased risk of congenital anomalies of lip, palate, skeletal, heart, esophagus, and kidney
Cyclosporine	C	Prematurity and intrauterine growth retardation
Methotrexate	X	Teratogenic risk, mental retardation, growth retardation, and abortion
Apremilast	D	
Dapsone	C	Maternal anemia, neonatal hemolytic anemia, and hyperbilirubinemia
Hydroxychloroquine	C	In animal fetus neurological and hearing defects. No effect on human fetus
Intravenous immunoglobulin	B	Is recommended in various autoimmune conditions in a dose of 2 g/kg over 5 days

Amoxicillin is categorized as the FDA pregnancy category B. The use of this drug during the initial stages of pregnancy may elevate the likelihood of developing oral clefts.

Cephalexin belongs to first-generation cephalosporin and is considered a pregnancy category B drug. Cephalexin has not been associated with fetal defects in animal studies, with inadequate controlled data from human subjects.

Tetracyclines are classified under pregnancy category D drug. Animal studies have shown evidence of embryotoxicity and fetotoxicity, including toxic effects on fetal teeth and bone. Tetracycline antibiotics are actively deposited in teeth and bones. In teeth the deposition of the drug is permanent, causing the deciduous teeth of children exposed to the medication after the 20th week of gestation to become yellow, darkening with time. Deposition in bones has been suggested to result in a reversible decrease in fetal size and to inhibit fibula growth. As a result, tetracyclines should be avoided during pregnancy, especially after the first trimester **(Table 5)**.

Oral Retinoids

The teratogenic effects of isotretinoin are well known. Isotretinoin is absolutely contraindicated during pregnancy. They are classified as the FDA pregnancy category X drug. Isotretinoin leads to malformations involving the craniofacial area, CNS, cardiovascular system (CVS), thymus, and parathyroid glands.

Zinc

Zinc provides a safe option for pregnant patients with acne. Zinc sulfate is the FDA pregnancy category C drug. Normal dose is 11–12 mg/day. Animal studies and human studies treated for acne have not revealed increased risks of fetal abnormalities, and the risk of fetal harm at doses <75 mg/day is very less. Higher supplementation with zinc leads to copper deficiency.

TABLE 5: Oral antibiotics drug safety category in pregnancy.

Oral antibiotic	Pregnancy category	Comments
Erythromycin	B	Erythromycin sulfate is safe during pregnancy but erythromycin estolate may cause hepatotoxicity
Azithromycin	B	Safe during pregnancy
Amoxicillin	B	May increase risk of cleft palate
Cephalexin	B	Safe during pregnancy
Tetracycline	D	Toxic effect on fetal teeth and bone, especially if used after second trimester
Sulfamethoxazole-trimethoprim	C	• Teratogenic in animals • Should be avoided in first trimester. May lead to neural tube and cardiac defects. • In third trimester may lead to hyperbilirubinemia

Oral Antifungal Agents

Systemic Azoles

Fluconazole administration during pregnancy has been linked to occurrences of spontaneous abortions, congenital heart disease, as well as craniofacial and rib skeletal abnormalities. A cohort study found that the usage of oral fluconazole during the first trimester of pregnancy was linked to the development of musculoskeletal abnormalities. Several further research support the same risk of birth abnormalities. Fluconazole was found to have a substantial association with tetralogy of Fallot, according to another study. A recent meta-analysis and systematic review study found that the overall risk of prenatal malformations is not statistically significant. However, it is important to carefully analyze limb deformities and heart anomalies. The danger of birth abnormalities appears to be dependent on the dosage, with a total dosage of up to 150 mg being deemed relatively safer. The new FDA recommendations classify the use of 150 mg of fluconazole as category C, whereas doses beyond 150 mg are categorized as category D drug.

The use of itraconazole during the first trimester has been assessed in several extensive trials. A prospective study was conducted to evaluate the effects of itraconazole exposure during pregnancy on fetal development. The study found no evidence of an elevated risk of fetal deformity, even when daily dosages ranging from 50 to 800 mg were administered for a duration of 1–90 days. A further, more limited trial including 206 women found that itraconazole was linked to abortions, whether they were spontaneous or induced, but not to fetal abnormalities. A new meta-analysis examining the potential for prenatal abnormalities resulting from exposure to itraconazole found no significant correlation. However, the study recommended thorough investigation of eye problems in individuals exposed to itraconazole.

Oral Ketoconazole

Animal studies have demonstrated that oral ketoconazole is teratogenic and is linked to a range of musculoskeletal abnormalities. Currently, oral formulations are not advised for the treatment of fungal infections.

Voriconazole, a recently tested treatment for "resistant dermatophytosis", has been found to be teratogenic in rodents, even at low dosages. This means that it can cause anomalies in the skeletal and visceral systems of the rodents. Due to insufficient human data, this substance is classified as pregnancy category D drug and should be completely avoided during pregnancy.

Terbinafine

No embryo-fetotoxicity was shown in rabbits and rats during animal experiments, even when given doses up to 23 times higher than the maximum permitted dose for humans. Andersson et al. conducted a significant study on the utilization of terbinafine during pregnancy, which confirms the safety of terbinafine. The

TABLE 6: Oral antifungals safety category in pregnancy.

Oral antifungal	Pregnancy category
Fluconazole 150 mg	C
Fluconazole 400 mg	D
Itraconazole	C
Ketoconazole	C
Voriconazole	D
Terbinafine	B

medicine is classified as the FDA pregnancy category B and is widely regarded as the safest oral antifungal during the first trimester of pregnancy **(Table 6)**.

Systemic Antipruritics

First-generation antihistamines are usually preferred over second-generation antihistamines because of the preponderance of safety data. Chlorpheniramine, a first-generation antihistamine, is categorized as a category B drug and has shown no teratogenic risk in tests involving humans or animals. Due to the extensive safety evidence available, it is typically considered the primary antihistamine treatment for pregnant individuals who do not have relief from topical medicines.

Promethazine and dimethindene, two more first-generation antihistamines, lack adequate safety data. Promethazine is classed as a category C drug, indicating that it may have potential risks for pregnant women. On the other hand, dimethindene has not been assigned any specific category. Avoid using hydroxyzine during the first trimester of pregnancy due to its association with a slightly elevated risk (5.8%) of congenital abnormalities.

Among second-generation antihistamines, loratadine remains the first choice and cetirizine the second choice of drug. Loratadine is pregnancy category B. Fexofenadine and desloratadine are classified as category C. Mast cell stabilizers like oral sodium cromoglycate is category B drug.

Retinoids

Acitretin

It is categorized as a drug of category X. The risk of fetal abnormalities is 25 times greater in pregnant individuals who have been exposed compared to the general population. Possible consequences include microtia/anotia, micrognathia, and cleft palate. It takes around 2 months for the body to completely remove acitretin and its metabolites. Nevertheless, when alcohol is consumed while undergoing treatment, acitretin is transformed into etretinate, which subsequently exhibits an extended half-life of 168 days. This can result in the teratogenic impact persisting for up to 3 years. Consequently, it is recommended that female patients abstain from consuming alcohol while undergoing acitretin therapy and for a minimum of 2 months after stopping the treatment.

Alitretinoin

This drug is classified as a pregnancy category D drug and is specifically recommended for treating chronic hand eczema. It has teratogenic properties and can lead to fetal abnormalities when used during pregnancy. Women of reproductive age who are administered alitretinoin must utilize a minimum of two contraceptive methods for a duration of at least 1 month before to commencing therapy, throughout the course of treatment, and for an additional 1 month after completing treatment.

Antibiotics

In addition to antibiotics described earlier under antiacne drugs, safety of other common antibiotics as discussed here.

Cephalosporins

No problems were identified in fetus when cephalosporins were used during second and third trimesters in general. Older cephalosporins are usually preferred because of greater safety data. It is category B drug and is considered safe during the pregnancy.

Sulfamethoxazole–Trimethoprim

This drug crosses placenta and has been reported to be teratogenic in animals and humans. Cleft palate, neural tube defects, cardiac, and urinary tract defects may be seen if this drug is given in first trimester. In third trimester, it may lead to increase of unconjugated bilirubin due to competition for protein binding.

Beta-lactamases (Penicillin G, V, Amoxicillin, Ampicillin, and Cloxacillin)

These are considered the antibiotic of choice during pregnancy. These are category B and are considered safe during pregnancy. Cephalexin, cloxacillin, cefazolin, and amoxicillin/clavulanic acid are beta-lactamase antibiotics that are effective in treating staphylococcal infections. These antibiotics fall under category B drug and are considered safe for usage during pregnancy.

Fluoroquinolones

Generally avoided during pregnancy and lactation because these are found to be toxic to developing cartilage in animal studies, but not found in human studies. Accidental administration of these drugs should not be indication for abortion.

Clindamycin

Clindamycin is a category B drug and is considered to be a safer systemic alternative treatment for pregnant females with cellulitis who are allergic to beta lactamases.

OTHER IMPORTANT DRUGS

Clofazimine

It has been found to be safe for both mother and child. Leprosy may get exacerbated during pregnancy, so standard multidrug therapy should be continued during all trimesters of pregnancy.

Rifampicin

It can be continued in all trimesters of pregnancy.

Acyclovir

It is a category B drug and is supposed to be safe during pregnancy. No reported association with adverse fetal effects has been found in human studies.

Valacyclovir

It is a prodrug of acyclovir. Guidelines for use in pregnancy are same as for acyclovir.

Famciclovir

Limited data is available. Use when potential benefit clearly outweighs fetal risk in human pregnancy. Acyclovir and valacyclovir are preferred choices in pregnancy.

Tofacitinib

Limited data is available. Manufacturer label suggests avoiding use in pregnant women. While there are no definitive clinical studies monitoring their use during pregnancy, consensus is that Janus kinase (JAK) inhibitors should be avoided during pregnancy and should be discontinued 2–6 weeks prior to conception. These recommendations are based upon preclinical studies demonstrating in utero JAK inhibitor exposure led to (1) reduced fetal weight and survival and (2) teratogenicity leading to cardiovascular and skeletal malformations.

It is yet unknown if tofacitinib is secreted in breast milk. Manufacturer label does not recommend breastfeeding during treatment and for at least 18–36 hours after last dose of tofacitinib.

Thalidomide

It is a category X drug. It may cause severe birth defects or embryo-fetal death. Women are advised to strictly avoid pregnancy 4 weeks prior to starting the drug, during the treatment, and >4 weeks after therapy is discontinued.

Finasteride and Dutasteride

It is contraindicated in pregnancy. Pregnant women are advised to avoid direct contact with crushed or broken finasteride tablets. In addition, pregnant women are advised to avoid contact with semen from male partners on finasteride treatment, even though it has been shown that women are exposed to only a negligible amount of finasteride in their male partner's semen. It is a DHT blocker and may lead to feminization of a male fetus.

Ivermectin

Topical permethrin is the preferred treatment for pregnant individuals with scabies. It falls under category B and is considered safe to use during pregnancy. Ivermectin is classified as a category C drug and it is advisable to avoid its use during pregnancy. In animals it has been found to be teratogenic. In humans there is no evidence of teratogenicity; however, its safety is also not well documented. The difference in animals and humans is because of P-glycoprotein of placenta and blood-brain barrier. P-glycoprotein is responsible for efflux of ivermectin at placenta and blood-brain barrier, thus preventing drug toxicity to fetus and to brain. In humans placental P-glycoprotein wanes with progress of gestation while in animals it keeps on increasing. But the blood-brain barrier along with its P-glycoprotein in humans becomes functional as early as 8 weeks.

BIOLOGICS

Biologics are immunoglobulin G (IgG) monoclonal antibodies which can be recognized and transmitted across the placenta into fetal circulation by neonatal Fc receptors on the placental surface. Since the placental development predominantly occurs during the first trimester of pregnancy, fetal exposure to circulating maternal antibodies are minimal in the first trimester and subsequently increases throughout the second and third trimester and peaks near parturition. Due to the risk of neonatal immunosuppression, a risk benefit analysis must be done prior to use in second and third trimester to limit maternal-fetal transmission of biologics during parturition. It is important to remember that neonates with in utero exposure to biologics should avoid live-attenuated vaccinations during the first 6–12 months of life.

- Biologics gain access to fetus through Fc receptors.
- Minimal effect to fetus in first trimester.
- Immunosuppression occurring in next two trimesters is doubtful.
- Live vaccines have to be voided in the infant for 6–12 months.

Tumor Necrosis Factor-alpha Inhibitors

Multiple studies have shown adalimumab and infliximab use is safe during pregnancy. However, the consensus is that if the mother's disease course is stable with a low risk of flare, discontinuation of biologics at 20 weeks of pregnancy is recommended to allow for infant vaccination scheduling. If biologic discontinuation cannot happen before such timeline, adalimumab and infliximab antibody levels can persist up to 2–7 months postnatally. However, studies have not shown associations between exposure to tumor necrosis factor-alpha (TNF-α) inhibitors and increased rates of childhood infections, growth failure, or vaccination adverse reactions. But live vaccines should be avoided for 6 months if these drugs are given till end of second trimester and for 1 year if till term.

Etanercept: While etanercept can be transmitted through the placenta, it has a lower rate of transmission when compared to adalimumab and infliximab. Many large-scale studies have not found any association between etanercept exposure and adverse pregnancy outcomes, fetal death, or congenital malformations.

Certolizumab pegol is a Fab' antibody fragment conjugated to polyethylene glycol. Since there is no fragment crystallizable (Fc) region, there is minimal placental transfer and large scale studies have found no adverse pregnancy outcomes associated with certolizumab exposure. Certolizumab can be used safely throughout all phases of pregnancy and continued up to delivery without risk of fetal immunosuppression, and is recommended as an especially safe biologic medication to initiate during pregnancy.

Interleukin-17 A Inhibitors (Secukinumab, Ixekizumab, and Brodalumab)

Preclinical studies of these biologics have not found any adverse pregnancy outcomes or postnatal effects. A retrospective study of 292 cases of secukinumab exposure during pregnancies did not find any increased rates of spontaneous abortion, preterm deliveries, or congenital malformations to that of the general population.

Interleukin-23 Inhibitors (Guselkumab, Tildrakizumab, and Risankizumab)

Guselkumab preclinical studies did not identify any adverse pregnancy outcomes or postnatal immunologic effects to infants.

Interleukin-12/Interleukin-23 Inhibitors (Ustekinumab)

Prospective cohort studies examining ustekinumab use predominantly during the first and second trimester of pregnancy did not find any associated adverse pregnancy outcomes. Further it was not associated with increased risk of fetal death or congenital malformations following exposure.

Interleukin-4 Receptor Alpha Subunit Inhibitors (Dupilumab)

Dupilumab is a monoclonal IgG antibody directed against interleukin-4 (IL-4) receptor. Preclinical studies revealed that weekly dupilumab exposure during all trimesters of pregnancy did not result in any maternal-fetal complications, congenital malformations, or infantile immunosuppression.

Rituximab

Rituximab is not recommended during pregnancy and has been associated with an increased risk of neonatal hematologic abnormalities. Exposure to rituximab in utero can affect fetal B-cell development. Women should be counseled to avoid pregnancy for at least 12 months after rituximab exposure.

KEY POINTS

- *Prioritize safety*: Dermatological treatments during pregnancy and lactation should be carefully selected, focusing on medications with proven safety profiles for both mother and baby.
- *Topical first-line*: Mild corticosteroids, azelaic acid, and emollients are generally safe topical options, while retinoids and high-potency steroids should be avoided.
- Systemic-low dose corticosteroids or IVIg are the immunosuppressives which can be prescribed.
- Antibiotics (e.g., penicillins, cephalosporins, anti fungal like terbinafine and antihistaminics like loratadine and cetrizine) can be safely prescribed during pregnancy.

SUGGESTED READINGS

1. Patel MA, Aliporewala VM, Patel DA. Common Antifungal Drugs in Pregnancy: Risks and Precautions. J Obstet Gynaecol India. 2021;71(6):577-82.
2. Wolverton SE. Comprehensive Dermatologic Drug Therapy, 3rd edition. Philadelphia: Saunders; 2012.
3. Murase JE, Heller MM, Butler DC. Safety of dermatologic medications in pregnancy and lactation: Part I. Pregnancy. J Am Acad Dermatol. 2014;70(3):401.e1-14.
4. Puchner A, Gröchenig HP, Sautner J, Helmy-Bader Y, Juch H, Reinisch S, et al. Immunosuppressives and biologics during pregnancy and lactation: A consensus report issued by the Austrian Societies of Gastroenterology and Hepatology and Rheumatology and Rehabilitation. Wien Klin Wochenschr. 2019;131(1-2):29-44.
5. Liu D, Zhang C, Wu L, Zhang L, Zhang L. Fetal outcomes after maternal exposure to oral antifungal agents during pregnancy: A systematic review and meta-analysis. Int J Gynaecol Obstet. 2020;148(1):6-13.

Index

Page numbers followed by *b* refer to box, *f* refer to figure, *fc* refer to flowchart, and *t* refer to table.

A

B

C

D

E

I

J

K

L

N

O

P

Q

R

S

T

U

V